Newer Outpatient Therapies and Treatments

Editor

DOUGLAS PAAUW

MEDICAL CLINICS
OF NORTH AMERICA

www.medical.theclinics.com

Consulting Editor
DANIEL D. DRESSLER

September 2024 • Volume 108 • Number 5

ELSEVIER

1600 John F. Kennedy Boulevard • Suite 1800 • Philadelphia, Pennsylvania, 19103-2899

http://www.theclinics.com

MEDICAL CLINICS OF NORTH AMERICA Volume 108, Number 5
September 2024 ISSN 0025-7125, ISBN-13: 978-0-443-29696-3

Editor: Taylor Hayes
Developmental Editor: Malvika Shah

Medical Clinics of North America (ISSN 0025-7125) is published bimonthly by Elsevier Inc., 360 Park Avenue South, New York, NY 10010-1710. Months of publication are January, March, May, July, September, and November. Business and editorial offices: 1600 John F. Kennedy Boulevard, Suite 1800, Philadelphia, PA 19103-2899. Periodicals postage paid at New York, NY, and additional mailing offices. Subscription prices are USD $336.00 per year (US individuals), $100.00 per year (US Students), $433.00 per year (Canadian individuals), $200.00 per year for (foreign students), $100.00 per year for (Canadian students), $479.00 per year (foreign individuals). For institutional access pricing please contact Customer Service via the contact information below. To receive student/resident rate, orders must be accompanied by name of affiliated institution, date of term, and the signature of program/residency coordinator on institution letterhead. Orders will be billed at individual rate until proof of status is received. Foreign air speed delivery is included in all Clinics' subscription prices. All prices are subject to change without notice. Orders, claims, and journal inquiries: Please visit our Support Hub page https://service.elsevier.com for assistance.

Reprints. For copies of 100 or more of articles in this publication, please contact the Commercial Reprints Department, Elsevier Inc., 360 Park Avenue South, New York, NY 10010-1710. Tel.: 212-633-3874; Fax: 212-633-3820; E-mail: reprints@elsevier.com.

Medical Clinics of North America is also published in Spanish by McGraw-Hill Interamericana Editores S. A., P.O. Box 5-237, 06500 Mexico, D.F., Mexico.

Medical Clinics of North America is covered in *MEDLINE/PubMed (Index Medicus), Current Contents, ASCA, Excerpta Medica, Science Citation Index, and ISI/BIOMED.*

PROGRAM OBJECTIVE
The goal of the *Medical Clinics of North America* is to keep practicing physicians up to date with current clinical practice by providing timely articles reviewing the state of the art in patient care.

TARGET AUDIENCE
All practicing physicians and other healthcare professionals.

LEARNING OBJECTIVES
Upon completion of this activity, participants will be able to:
1. Review treatments for common dermatologic diagnoses addressed in primary care settings and new emerging treatments.
2. Explain emerging therapies and treatments for cardiovascular disease and mood and anxiety disorders.
3. Discuss new developments to help delay the onset of dementia, treat dementia in its earliest stages, and manage behavioral problems that occur in a person with dementia.

ACCREDITATION
The Elsevier Office of Continuing Medical Education (EOCME) is accredited by the Accreditation Council for Continuing Medical Education (ACCME) to provide continuing medical education for physicians.

The EOCME designates this journal-based CME activity for a maximum of 12 *AMA PRA Category 1 Credit*(s)™. Physicians should claim only the credit commensurate with the extent of their participation in the activity.

All other healthcare professionals requesting continuing education credit for this enduring material will be issued a certificate of participation.

DISCLOSURE OF CONFLICTS OF INTEREST
The EOCME assesses conflict of interest with its instructors, faculty, planners, and other individuals who are in a position to control the content of CME activities. All relevant conflicts of interest that are identified are thoroughly vetted by EOCME for fair balance, scientific objectivity, and patient care recommendations. EOCME is committed to providing its learners with CME activities that promote improvements or quality in healthcare and not a specific proprietary business or a commercial interest.

The planning committee, staff, authors, and editors listed below have identified no financial relationships or relationships to products or devices they or their spouse/life partner have with commercial interest related to the content of this CME activity:
Abdul Aziz A. Asbeutah, MD; Alison Bays, MD, MPH; Rachel S. Casas, MD, EdM; Sophie Clark, MD; Heidi Combs, MD, MS; Daniel D. Dressler, MD, MSc, MHM, FACP; Jeffrey D. Edelman, MD; Gregory C. Gardner, MD, MACP; Zachary D. Goldberger, MD, MS; Laura Granados, MD; Taylor Hayes; Talia A. Helman, MD; Mira John, MD; Thomas Johnson, MD; Nevin Kamal, MD; Kristen Lee, MD; Michelle Littlejohn; Jesse Markman, MD, MBA; Denise J. McCulloch, MD, MPH; Sarah Merriam, MD, MS; Garren Montgomery, MD; Kim M. O'Connor, MD; Douglas Paauw, MD, MACP; Merlin Packiam; Arsheya Patel, MD; Sheryl Pfeil, MD; Paul S. Pottinger, MD, FACP, FIDSA; Christine Prifti, MD; Katherine Runkel, MD; Malvika Shah; Nina Tan, MD; Jay C. Vary Jr, MD, PhD; Jeffrey Wallace, MD, MPH; Judith M.E. Walsh, MD, MPH; Jennifer Wright, MD; Emmanuelle Yecies, MD, MS

The planning committee, staff, authors, and editors listed below have identified financial relationships or relationships to products or devices they or their spouse/life partner have with commercial interest related to the content of this CME activity:
Grazia Aleppo, MD: *Consultant*: Dexcom, Insulet; *Research Support*: Fractyl Health, Insulet, MannKind, Tandem Diabetes Care, Welldoc

Brendan M. Browne, MD, MS: *Consultant*: Cook Medical

Savitha Subramanian, MD: *Advisor*: Abbott Diabetes Care

UNAPPROVED/OFF-LABEL USE DISCLOSURE
The EOCME requires CME faculty to disclose to the participants;
1. When products or procedures being discussed are off-label, unlabelled, experimental, and/or investigational (not US Food and Drug Administration [FDA] approved); and
2. Any limitations on the information presented, such as data that are preliminary or that represent ongoing research, interim analyses, and/or unsupported opinions. Faculty may discuss information about pharmaceutical agents that is outside of FDA-approved labelling. This information is intended solely for CME

and is not intended to promote off-label use of these medications. If you have any questions, contact the medical affairs department of the manufacturer for the most recent prescribing information.

TO ENROLL
To enroll in the *Medical Clinics of North America* Continuing Medical Education program, call customer service at 1-800-654-2452 or sign up online at http://www.theclinics.com/home/cme. The CME program is available to subscribers for an additional annual fee of USD 319.00.

METHOD OF PARTICIPATION
In order to claim credit, participants must complete the following;
1. Complete enrolment as indicated above.
2. Read the activity.
3. Complete the CME Test and Evaluation. Participants must achieve a score of 70% on the test. All CME Tests and Evaluations must be completed online.

CME INQUIRIES/SPECIAL NEEDS
For all CME inquiries or special needs, please contact elsevierCME@elsevier.com.

MEDICAL CLINICS OF NORTH AMERICA

FORTHCOMING ISSUES

November 2024
Perioperative and Consultative Medicine
Efren Manjarrez, *Editor*

January 2025
Point-of-Care Ultrasound in Clinical Care
Irene Ma, *Editor*

March 2025
**Approach to Urgent Neurologic Problems
for the Non-Neurologist**
James G. Greene, *Editor*

RECENT ISSUES

July 2024
Allergy and Immunology
Andrew Lutzkanin and
Kristen M. Lutzkanin, *Editors*

May 2024
**Patient Management with Stable
Ischemic Heart Disease**
Alexander Fanaroff and
John W. Hirshfeld Jr, *Editors*

March 2024
Sexually Transmitted Infections
Susan Tuddenham, *Editor*

Contributors

CONSULTING EDITOR

DANIEL D. DRESSLER, MD, MSc, MHM, FACP
Professor of Medicine, Emory University School of Medicine, Atlanta, Georgia

EDITOR

DOUGLAS PAAUW, MD, MACP
Professor of Medicine, Rathmann Family Foundation Endowed Chair for Patient-Centered Clinical Education, University of Washington School of Medicine, Seattle, Washington

AUTHORS

GRAZIA ALEPPO, MD
Professor of Medicine, Division of Endocrinology, Metabolism and Molecular Medicine, Feinberg School of Medicine, Northwestern University, Chicago, Illinois

ABDUL AZIZ A. ASBEUTAH, MD
Cardiology Fellow, Division of Cardiovascular Medicine, Department of Medicine, University of Wisconsin-Madison Hospitals and Clinics, Madison, Wisconsin

ALISON BAYS, MD, MPH
Assistant Professor, Division of Rheumatology, University of Washington, Seattle, Washington

BRENDAN M. BROWNE, MD, MS
Assistant Professor, Division of Urology, Department of Surgery, Emory University, Atlanta, Georgia

RACHEL S. CASAS, MD, EdM
Associate Professor, Division of General Internal Medicine, Department of Medicine, Penn State Milton S. Hershey Medical Center, Hershey, Pennsylvania

SOPHIE CLARK, MD
Assistant Professor, Division of Geriatric Medicine, University of Colorado School of Medicine, Aurora, Colorado

HEIDI COMBS, MD, MS
Professor, Department of Psychiatry and Behavioral Sciences, University of Washington School of Medicine, Seattle, Washington

JEFFREY D. EDELMAN, MD
Associate Professor, Department of Pulmonary, Critical Care and Sleep Medicine, University of Washington; Puget Sound Department of Veterans Affairs, Seattle, Washington

GREGORY C. GARDNER, MD, MACP
Emeritus Professor, Division of Rheumatology, University of Washington, Seattle, Washington

ZACHARY D. GOLDBERGER, MD, MS
Associate Professor, Division of Cardiovascular Medicine, Department of Medicine, University of Wisconsin-Madison Hospitals and Clinics, Madison, Wisconsin

LAURA GRANADOS, MD
Fellow, Department of Pulmonary, Critical Care and Sleep Medicine, University of Washington, Seattle, Washington

TALIA A. HELMAN, MD
Resident Physician, Division of Urology, Department of Surgery, Emory University, Atlanta, Georgia

MIRA JOHN, MD
Fellow, Department of Pulmonary, Critical Care and Sleep Medicine, University of Washington, Seattle, Washington

THOMAS JOHNSON, MD
Assistant Professor, Division of Geriatric Medicine, University of Colorado School of Medicine, Aurora, Colorado

NEVIN KAMAL, MD
Endocrinology Fellow, Division of Endocrinology, Metabolism and Molecular Medicine, Feinberg School of Medicine, Northwestern University, Chicago, Illinois

KRISTEN LEE, MD
Endocrinology Fellow, Division of Endocrinology, Metabolism and Molecular Medicine, Feinberg School of Medicine, Northwestern University, Chicago, Illinois

JESSE MARKMAN, MD, MBA
Associate Professor, Department of Psychiatry and Behavioral Sciences, University of Washington School of Medicine, Seattle, Washington

DENISE J. MCCULLOCH, MD, MPH
Assistant Professor, Vaccine and Infectious Disease Division, Fred Hutchinson Cancer Center, Seattle, Washington

SARAH MERRIAM, MD, MS
Assistant Professor of Medicine, Division of General Internal Medicine, University of Pittsburgh School of Medicine, VA Pittsburgh Healthcare System, Pittsburgh, Pennsylvania

GARREN MONTGOMERY, MD
Clinical Fellow, Division of Gastroenterology, Hepatology, and Nutrition, Ohio State University Wexner Medical Center, Columbus, Ohio

KIM M. O'CONNOR, MD
Associate Professor, Division of General Internal Medicine, Department of Internal Medicine, University of Washington, Seattle, Washington

ARSHEYA PATEL, MD
Clinical Fellow, Division of Gastroenterology, Hepatology, and Nutrition, Ohio State University Wexner Medical Center, Columbus, Ohio

SHERYL PFEIL, MD
Clinical Professor of Internal Medicine, Division of Gastroenterology, Hepatology, and Nutrition, Ohio State University Medical Center, Columbus, Ohio

PAUL S. POTTINGER, MD, FACP, FIDSA
Professor, Division of Allergy and Infectious Diseases, Department of Medicine, University of Washington School of Medicine, Seattle, Washington

CHRISTINE PRIFTI, MD
Assistant Professor, Department of General Internal Medicine, Chobanian and Avedisian School of Medicine, Boston University Medical Center, Boston, Massachusetts

KATHERINE RUNKEL, MD
Assistant Professor, Division of Geriatric Medicine, University of Colorado School of Medicine, Aurora, Colorado

SAVITHA SUBRAMANIAN, MD
Professor of Medicine, Division of Metabolism, Endocrinology and Nutrition, University of Washington, Seattle, Washington

NINA TAN, MD
Acting Instructor, Division of General Internal Medicine, Department of Internal Medicine, University of Washington, Seattle, Washington

JAY C. VARY Jr, MD, PhD
Associate Professor, Department of Dermatology, University of Washington, University of Washington Dermatology Center, Seattle, Washington

JEFFREY WALLACE, MD, MPH
Professor, Division of Geriatric Medicine, University of Colorado School of Medicine, Aurora, Colorado

JUDITH M.E. WALSH, MD, MPH
Professor, School of Medicine, University of California, San Francisco, San Francisco, California

JENNIFER WRIGHT, MD
Associate Professor, Division of General Internal Medicine, Department of Medicine, University of Washington, Seattle, Washington

EMMANUELLE YECIES, MD, MS
Clinical Assistant Professor (Affiliated), Department of Primary Care and Population Health, Stanford University School of Medicine (Affiliated), VA Palo Alto Healthcare System, Palo Alto, California

Contents

This article reviews the evaluation and management of several gastrointestinal disorders that are commonly encountered by gastroenterologists and primary care physicians. With a focus on newer therapies, we discuss the management of chronic constipation, irritable bowel syndrome, Clostridioides difficile infection, gastroparesis, steatotic liver disease, and diverticulitis.

Dermatologic concerns are discussed in about a third of all primary care visits. This review discusses treatments for common dermatologic diagnoses addressed in primary care settings, with an emphasis on new and emerging treatments. Topical, oral, and injectable treatment of common forms of alopecia, facial rashes, atopic dermatitis, psoriasis, seborrheic dermatitis, and stasis dermatitis will be discussed to help increase comfort in prescribing and alert providers to common side effects or complications of more intensive treatments used by dermatologists.

Seven of the 11 newer medications recently or soon to be approved to treat rheumatologic diseases discussed in this article are biologic agents and reflect the current ability of science to target specific components of the immune system. The other agents are molecules that are directed against specific immune pathway targets as well. All have shown superiority to placebo and in some cases have been compared to currently accepted therapies. Safety issues are generally centered around infections due to the immune-interrupting nature of these therapies.

Newer medications and devices, as well as greater understanding of the benefits and limitations of existing treatments, have led to expanded treatment options for patients with lung disease. Treatment advances have led to improved outcomes for patients with asthma, chronic obstructive pulmonary disease, interstitial lung disease, pulmonary hypertension, and cystic fibrosis. The risks and benefits of available treatments are substantially variable within these heterogeneous disease groups. Defining the role of newer therapies mandates both an understanding of these disorders and overall treatment approaches. This section will review general treatment approaches in addition to focusing on newer therapies for these conditions.

This article contains noninclusive language such as "females" and "women" when those terms were used in the research and historic context we are summarizing. New therapies have become available for vasomotor symptoms, postpartum depression, contraception, osteoporosis, recurrent yeast infections, acute and recurrent urinary tract infections, and female hypoactive sexual desire disorder. These therapies meet unique patient needs and change clinical practice for select groups. As is typical for new treatments, insurance coverage and access issues limit the adoption of some therapies.

Significant advances in atherosclerotic cardiovascular (ASCVD) risk stratification and treatment have occurred over the past 10 years. While the lipid panel continues to be the basis of risk estimation, imaging for coronary artery calcium is now widely used in estimating risk at the individual level. Statins remain first-line agents for ASCVD risk reduction but in high-risk patients, ezetimibe, proprotein convertase subtilisin kexin-9 inhibitors, and bempedoic acid can be added to further reduce individual cardiovascular risk based on results of cardiovascular outcomes trials. Results of randomized control trials do not support use of medications targeted at triglyceride lowering for ASCVD risk reduction, but icosapent ethyl can be considered.

Memory loss and dementia are among older adults' greatest health fears. This article provides insight into new developments to help delay the onset of dementia, to treat dementia in its earliest stages, and to manage behavioral problems that occur in persons with dementia. Urinary incontinence (UI) is another common problem in older adults that has a major impact on quality of life. This article evaluates newer medications for reducing urinary urge/UI and provides perspective in their role for managing UI.

For more than 20 years, the mainstay of pharmacologic treatment for depression and anxiety disorders has been serotonin reuptake inhibitors and selective serotonin and norepinephrine reuptake inhibitors. There are newer medications, many with novel mechanisms of action, that have come to market; however, first-line treatments remain the same. There are now more robust data on the use of various augmentation agents in the treatment of major depressive disorder providing better recommendations for use by the primary care provider. Data to support the use of psychedelic-assisted psychotherapy in the treatment of mood and anxiety disorders are not robust enough to recommend generalized use at this time.

New diabetes drugs such as glucagon-like peptide-1 receptor agonists (GLP-1 RAs) and glucose-dependent insulinotropic peptide/GLP-1 RAs have emerged to show hemoglobin A1c (HbA1c) reduction, weight loss, and cardiovascular benefits. Similarly, sodium-glucose cotransporter 2 inhibitors' benefits span from HbA1c decrease to cardiovascular and renoprotective effects. Diabetes technology has expanded to include type 2 diabetes mellitus, with literature supporting its use in T2DM on any insulin regimen. Connected insulin pens and insulin delivery devices have opened new solutions to insulin users and automated insulin delivery systems have become the standard of care therapy for type 1 diabetes mellitus.

Over the last decade, randomized clinical trials of several pharmacologic agents have demonstrated a reduction in cardiovascular mortality and other important secondary outcomes. Angiotensin-Neprilysin Inhibitors and Sodium-Glucose Co-transporter 2 inhibitors have now become pillars in the treatment of heart failure. Ivabradine is a negative chronotropic agent used as an adjunctive therapy in patients with heart failure. Two new hypertension therapies, zilebesiran and aprocitentan, are currently in investigational stages. Finally, mavacamten has emerged as a pharmacologic treatment for hypertrophic obstructive cardiomyopathy. Practitioners must be familiar with the indications and side effects of newer therapies as they are now frequently prescribed.

This article summarizes the situation with public health threats for primary care patients as of early 2024 and provides updates on strategies for the prevention, diagnosis, and treatment of common infections where new treatments and vaccines are available. For flu and COVID, an update on treatment is also provided—along with pearls useful for the busy primary care provider. The authors also discuss a new treatment option for drug-resistant vulvovaginal candidiasis and provide a balanced view of the increasingly popular technique of preventing bacterial sexually transmitted infections using doxycycline after condomless sex among men who have sex with men.

Benign prostate hyperplasia (BPH) affects a large number of men and can be treated with behavioral, medical, or surgical treatments. The newest addition to medical therapy is β3-agonists for overactive lower urinary tract symptoms. Multiple new surgical treatments have become available in the past decade, including several clinic-based minimally invasive surgical techniques (eg, UroLift, Rezum, Optilume BPH), OR treatments (eg, Aquablation, single port robotics), and prostate artery embolization. The growth of options allows providers to better tailor BPH treatment to the specific disease factors and patient preferences.

Foreword

Advances in Medical Therapies to Advance Patient Care

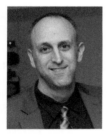

Daniel D. Dressler, MD, MSc, MHM, FACP
Consulting Editor

New medications and new medical interventions often lead to evolution and improvement in clinical care and patient outcomes over time. At times, new therapeutics can transform care in major ways, for example, as seen with medications like sodium–glucose cotransporter-2 inhibitors, which have had dramatic impacts on diabetes care and even heart failure care,[1] and with possible impacts to reduce kidney stones,[2] gout exacerbations,[3] and other adverse conditions. And occasionally new therapies can revolutionize care, as we have witnessed with various immunologic and biologic medications that treat—and in some situations cure—a variety of autoimmune and oncologic conditions, in addition to some rare genetic disorders.

Each year, on average, a few dozen new medications are approved by the US Food and Drug Administration for therapeutic applications to patients. The current issue of *Medical Clinics of North America*, eloquently synthesized by Guest Editor Dr Douglas Paauw, delineates some of the most recent advances in outpatient clinical care, explaining some of the newest therapies and interventions in the fields of cardiology, dermatology, endocrinology (diabetes), gastroenterology, pulmonology, rheumatology, and infectious diseases. Included are detailed discussions of a new therapy for managing hypertrophic cardiomyopathy and new therapeutic interventions for managing constipation and gastroparesis as well as prevention of recurrent *Clostridium difficile* infection. New interventions to manage respiratory syncytial virus, influenza, and COVID-19 are detailed within the infectious diseases article. In addition, various new biologic agents for the treatment of pulmonary diseases, skin diseases, and rheumatologic conditions are explained.

Furthermore, this issue of *Medical Clinics of North America* delves into some of the newest therapeutics and interventions related to women's health—including treatment of vasomotor symptoms of menopause, osteoporosis care, and advances in the

Med Clin N Am 108 (2024) xv–xvi
https://doi.org/10.1016/j.mcna.2024.04.009
0025-7125/24/© 2024 Published by Elsevier Inc.

medical.theclinics.com

management of postpartum depression, contraception, osteoporosis, and more—as well as one of the most common conditions affecting men's health—benign prostatic hypertrophy—detailing the novel medications available as well as the newest innovative procedural interventions to manage the condition.

As clinicians, one of our primary goals—and often one of our greatest challenges—rests with staying abreast of the newest modalities that can contribute to the care of our patients, including considerations of when and how to apply those new therapeutics and how they compare with predecessor treatments. This issue of *Medical Clinics of North America* assists readers in achieving that goal, focusing on the most recent advances related to clinical conditions that patients and their physicians encounter on a regular basis.

Daniel D. Dressler, MD, MSc, MHM, FACP
Emory University Hospital
1364 Clifton Road Northeast
Atlanta, GA 30322, USA

E-mail address:
ddressl@emory.edu

REFERENCES

1. Vaduganathan M, Docherty KF, Claggett BL, et al. SGLT-2 inhibitors in patients with heart failure: a comprehensive meta-analysis of five randomised controlled trials. Lancet 2022;400:757–67. https://doi.org/10.1016/S0140-6736(22)01429-5.
2. Paik JM, Tesfaye H, Curhan GC, et al. Sodium-glucose cotransporter 2 inhibitors and nephrolithiasis risk in patients with type 2 diabetes. JAMA Intern Med 2024;184(3): 265–74. https://doi.org/10.1001/jamainternmed.2023.7660. PMID: 38285598; PMCID: PMC10825784.
3. McCormick N, Yokose C, Wei J, et al. Comparative effectiveness of sodium-glucose cotransporter-2 inhibitors for recurrent gout flares and gout-primary emergency department visits and hospitalizations: a general population cohort study. Ann Intern Med 2023;176(8):1067–80. https://doi.org/10.7326/M23-0724. Epub 2023 Jul 25. PMID: 37487215.

Preface

What Are the New Therapeutic Options in the Outpatient World?

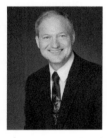

Douglas Paauw, MD, MACP
Editor

In 2023, the FDA approved 55 new drugs. The average number of new drug approvals over the last decade has been about 45 per year. This is a remarkable number of medications for physicians to keep track of, and it is easy to miss important therapies that become available. Beyond knowing all the new available therapies, understanding the role of these therapies and when they are actually worth the very high prices of newly released drugs is a very important part of being a good health care professional in 2024. Further complicating our roles with our patients are that many of the new medications that are released are heavily advertised, and our patients may have much more familiarity with them before we do. Many newer surgical procedures and medical devices are developed each year, and the ambulatory medical professional is expected to be familiar with these as well to help answer patient questions and weigh in on benefit.

This issue of *Medical Clinics of North America* is devoted to updating newer therapies used in the outpatient arena. Several of the articles heavily cover newer, biologic agents that are the cornerstone of new drug development in the specialties (rheumatology and pulmonary medicine). Other articles cover quite a bit of technology and surgical procedures, as these have become a focus of practice in these areas (diabetes and men's health). The article on therapy of viral respiratory infections does an excellent job covering two of the hot topics in infectious disease in the last several years (therapy for COVID-19 and the new RSV vaccine). Several of the authors have singled out challenging topics and integrated the new therapies that have been released, and

Med Clin N Am 108 (2024) xvii–xviii
https://doi.org/10.1016/j.mcna.2024.03.008
0025-7125/24/© 2024 Elsevier Inc. All rights reserved.

how and when they should be used. I hope you find this issue helpful in keeping up with the rapid changes and developments in therapies in the outpatient setting.

Douglas Paauw, MD, MACP
University of Washington School of Medicine
Seattle, WA, USA

E-mail address:
dpaauw@uw.edu

Treatment and Management of Gastrointestinal Disorders

Garren Montgomery, MD[a],*, Arsheya Patel, MD[a], Sheryl Pfeil, MD[b]

KEYWORDS

- Constipation • IBS • *Clostridioides difficile* • Diverticulosis • Steatotic liver disease

KEY POINTS

- Several newer pharmacologic therapies effective for constipation include lubiprostone, linaclotide, plecanatide, and prucalopride.
- Gut-directed psychotherapies are an often underutilized treatment option in irritable bowel syndrome (IBS); a new US Food and Drug Administration (FDA)-approved smartphone app (Mahana IBS) is a self-directed cognitive behavioral therapy that can be an effective part of your IBS management plan.
- Fecal microbiota encapsulated spores (Vowst) and the rectal microbiota suspension (Rebyota) are new promising FDA-approved therapies to prevent recurrent *Clostridioides difficile* infection.
- While not yet FDA-approved for this indication, prucalopride has been shown to improve gastric motility and may be an effective medication for gastroparesis with fewer side effects than metoclopramide.
- Steatotic liver disease has recently seen a change in nomenclature from nonalcoholic fatty liver disease/nonalcoholic steatohepatitis to metabolic dysfunction-associated steatotic liver disease/metabolic dysfunction-associated steatohepatitis. Cornerstones of therapy remain weight loss and control of underlying diabetes mellitus and hyperlipidemia, though a recently approved medication resmetirom appears promising.

CHRONIC CONSTIPATION
Introduction

Constipation can be described as infrequent bowel movements (typically fewer than 3 bowel movements per week), straining during defecation or sensation of incomplete evacuation, hard stools, or the need for manual maneuvers to facilitate defecation.[1] Constipation can be a primary disorder of the function of the colon or rectum (functional constipation) or a secondary to other underlying processes. Functional

[a] Division of Gastroenterology, Hepatology, and Nutrition, Ohio State University Wexner Medical Center, Columbus, OH, USA; [b] Division of Gastroenterology, Hepatology, and Nutrition, Ohio State University Medical Center, Columbus, OH, USA
* Corresponding author. 395 West 12th Avenue, Columbus, OH 43210.
E-mail address: garren.montgomery@osumc.edu

Med Clin N Am 108 (2024) 777–794
https://doi.org/10.1016/j.mcna.2024.03.010
0025-7125/24/© 2024 Elsevier Inc. All rights reserved.

constipation can be further classified into slow transit constipation (due to delayed fecal passage) or rectal outlet dysfunction, which is secondary to insufficient rectal propulsive forces or increased resistance to evacuation.[2]

Evaluation

A detailed history and physical examination are necessary to identify secondary causes of constipation including mechanical obstruction, medications (opioids, calcium channel blockers), systemic illness (hypothyroidism, diabetes mellitus), and neurologic disorders (Parkinson's disease).[2] It is important to identify individuals with alarm symptoms such as weight loss, unexplained anemia, rectal bleeding, or age greater than 45 years without a history of prior colorectal cancer screening, as these individuals should be referred for colonoscopy to exclude an underlying neoplastic process.[3]

The initial evaluation for constipation is the digital rectal examination (DRE), which is best completed in the left lateral decubitus or jackknife positions. A DRE can help identify structural abnormalities that contribute to or result from constipation (hemorrhoids, masses, anal fissures, rectocele) and also those patients with underlying pelvic floor dysfunction or dyssynergic defecation.[4]

When evaluating for pelvic floor dysfunction, attention should be paid to the patient's resting sphincter tone, ability to tighten their anal sphincter, and abdominal wall, pelvic floor, and anal sphincter movement when pushing for simulated defecation. When the DRE is nondiagnostic but there remains concern for pelvic floor dysfunction or dyssynergic defecation, anorectal manometry or balloon expulsion testing can be obtained to clarify whether these disorders are present. In patients without evidence of dyssynergic defecation who are not responding to therapy, the next step in evaluation typically involves obtaining a colon transit study or a "sitz marker study," which can identify those with slow intestinal transit as the cause of constipation.[5]

Management

The initial management includes lifestyle interventions such as increasing dietary fiber intake toward a goal of 20 to 35 g of fiber per day, increasing physical activity, and encouraging adequate hydration.[3] The soluble fiber psyllium is often recommended as an initial supplement, though its use is sometimes poorly tolerated due to side effects of bloating and flatulence. Several studies have shown that fiber supplementation in the form of kiwifruit is as effective as psyllium in the management of constipation, but with fewer side effects.[6–8]

If lifestyle measures fail to adequately improve constipation, a trial of laxatives is warranted. Initial management should include the osmotic laxatives such as polyethylene glycol (PEG) or magnesium oxide. The stimulant laxative, senna, can also be considered. Short term (4 weeks or less) or occasional use of bisacodyl can be considered as rescue therapy. Additionally, the use of the osmotic laxative, lactulose, is another option for patients who have had inadequate response to these other over-the-counter agents.[9] Of note, while the stool softener docusate is still often prescribed for constipation, multiple studies have shown it to be an ineffective treatment, and its use for this indication is not recommended.[10–12]

Other pharmacologic options that have emerged for treatment of chronic constipation include the secretagogues such as lubiprostone, linaclotide, and plecanatide and the 5-hydroxytryptamine receptor 4 (5-HT4) agonist prucalopride (**Table 1**). Lubiprostone, a chloride channel activator, increases the number of spontaneous bowel movements per week, improves stool consistency, and improves abdominal

Table 1
Medications for chronic idiopathic constipation

Drug[a]	Mechanism of Action	Dosing	Side Effects	Cost (Monthly)[b]	Comments
Linaclotide	Guanylate cyclase-C agonist	Initial: 72–145 mcg daily Maximum: 290 mcg daily	Diarrhea (though often improves after 1–2 wk on therapy)	$523–$649	Should be taken without food, at least 30 min before the first meal of the day.
Plecanatide	Guanylate cyclase-C agonist	3 mg daily	Diarrhea	$569–$670	Contraindicated in patients under 6 y of age and should be avoided in those under 18 y of age.
Prucalopride	5-HT4 agonist	Initial: 1 mg daily Maximum: 2 mg daily	Diarrhea, abdominal pain, headache, nausea	$568–$637	Suicide attempts reported in clinical trials but there has been no causal association between use of prucalopride and suicide.
Lubiprostone	Chloride channel activator	24 mcg twice daily	Nausea, diarrhea	$374–$423	Nausea is dose-dependent and may be improved by taking with meals.

[a] Note that all of these medications are contraindicated in the setting of known or suspected mechanical bowel obstruction.

[b] Approximate cost without insurance. Costs are estimated based on recent ACG/AGA guidelines (Chang et al,[9] 2023) and pricing data available on the online database Lexi-Drug (UpToDate Lexidrug, Lexi-Drugs Online. Waltham, MA: UpToDate, Inc, https://online.lexi.com). The listed prices are not exact and are likely to vary.

discomfort and bloating compared to placebo.[13–15] Linaclotide is a guanylate cyclase-C agonist that improves the number of spontaneous bowel movements per week, stool consistency, and rates of global relief compared to placebo.[16,17] Additionally, it reduces symptoms of abdominal bloating and discomfort in individuals with chronic constipation.[18] Plecanatide, another guanylate cyclase-C agonist, is similar in efficacy as well as tolerability to linaclotide in adults,[19] though of note is contraindicated in children under 6 years and should be avoided in patients under 18 years due to the lack of safety data in this population. Prucalopride, a 5-HT4 agonist, improves the number of spontaneous bowel movements per day compared to placebo.[20–22] Suicide attempts and suicidal ideation, however, have been reported in clinical trials and the label does caution patients and providers to be alert to any sudden changes in thoughts, behaviors, or mood.[23]

For those patients identified as having an underlying defecatory disorder or pelvic floor dyssynergia, pelvic floor retraining in the form of biofeedback therapy has been shown to be effective. Randomized controlled trials have demonstrated symptomatic improvements in 50% to 80% of patients with an underlying defecatory disorder.[24,25] Furthermore, these symptomatic improvements have been shown to be long-lasting in several trials with follow-up periods lasting greater than 6 months.[26,27]

IRRITABLE BOWEL SYNDROME
Introduction

Irritable bowel syndrome (IBS) is a functional bowel disorder that is characterized by chronic abdominal pain and changes in stool frequency and/or character.[28] While there are multiple hypotheses regarding the underlying etiology, it is felt to be chiefly a disorder of the brain–gut interaction, with many patients with IBS displaying lower sensory thresholds to pain, a phenomenon known as visceral hypersensitivity.[29,30]

IBS is a common disorder with an estimated prevalence of 6.1% in the United States.[31] It is one of the most common reasons for outpatient primary care and gastroenterology visits and is associated with significant health care expenditures, with the yearly cost of managing IBS in the United States estimated at over $1 billion.[32]

Evaluation

IBS is a clinical diagnosis based on Rome IV criteria. Patients must have had abdominal pain occurring at least once per week over the last 3 months with 2 or more of the following: a change in stool frequency, a change in stool form, or pain related to defecation.[28] Prior to diagnosing IBS, it is important to evaluate for alarm symptoms that require further evaluation including symptom onset after age 50 years, weight loss, gastrointestinal bleeding, unexplained anemia, or family history of gastrointestinal (GI) malignancies or inflammatory bowel disease.[28] Based on history and examination, limited testing may be necessary to exclude conditions that can mimic IBS such as inflammatory bowel disease, microscopic colitis, or celiac disease. However, extensive testing is not warranted when diagnostic criteria are met and alarm features are excluded.[1]

Once the diagnosis of IBS is made, accurate categorization by subtype is necessary to determine the most appropriate therapies. The 4 subtypes of IBS are delineated later and are distinguished by the predominant stool consistency. Stool consistency is best assessed using the Bristol Stool Form Scale (BSFS), which assigns stools based on form a number from 1 to 7, with lower numbers indicating harder stools and higher number indicating softer to more liquid stools.[33]

- IBS-C: greater than 25% of stools associated with BSFS 1 or 2, with less than 25% of stools with BSFS 6 or 7
- IBS-D: greater than 25% of stools associated with BSFS 6 or 7, with less than 25% of stools with BSFS 1 or 2
- IBS-M: greater than 25% of stools with BSFS 1 or 2 and greater than 25% of stools with BSFS 6 or 7
- IBS-U: unclassified, no predominant stool consistency able to be identified.[33]

Management

Numerous lifestyle and over-the-counter (OTC) therapies exist for the management of IBS. Soluble fiber, such as psyllium, remains a first-line therapy for the management of global symptoms of IBS.[34] The low FODMAP (fermentable oligosaccharides, disaccharides, monosaccharides, and polyols) diet has been shown to improve abdominal pain, bloating, and distension in patients with IBS compared to alternative treatment.[35] Notably, the diet should be implemented under the supervision of a GI dietician in order to avoid nutritional deficiencies.[33] Probiotics are currently not recommended for the management of IBS as they have shown no benefit.[33,36] Peppermint is a popular natural therapy that acts as an antispasmodic, with trials suggesting some benefit for treatment of both abdominal pain and overall symptoms in IBS. It is generally well tolerated with minimal side effects, though may cause heartburn in some patients.[37] While other antispasmodics such as hyoscyamine and dicyclomine are commonly used to treat abdominal pain, limited data support their role in IBS treatment and their use is not universally endorsed by societal guidelines.[33,38,39]

Owing to dysregulation of the gut–brain axis in IBS, gut-directed psychotherapies have garnered increasing support as a treatment option. These psychotherapies include cognitive behavioral therapy (CBT) as well as gut-directed hypnotherapy, with CBT currently having more evidence to support its efficacy.[33] While CBT is an effective treatment of IBS, its implementation is limited by factors including cost and therapist availability. Consequently, a new prescription digital therapeutic known as Mahana IBS was developed and recently approved by the US Food and Drug Administration (FDA) in 2021 for patients aged 22 years and older. Mahana IBS is an app-based, self-directed CBT program and can be completed in sessions that take less than 10 minutes per day.[40]

In addition to gut-directed psychotherapies, neuromodulators such as tricyclic antidepressants are commonly prescribed for the management of abdominal pain in IBS. These medications reduce central and visceral pain by modulating ascending visceral sensory afferents and central transmission.[41] Tricyclic antidepressants (TCAs) have been evaluated in numerous randomized controlled trial (RCTs), with a recent systematic review and meta-analysis showing significant improvement in global symptoms of patients with IBS treated with TCA compared to placebo.[42]

For the treatment of IBS-C, while PEG is frequently used due to its availability and favorable side effect profile, current studies have not shown a significant improvement in abdominal pain symptoms in this patient population.[43] Newer therapies for IBS-C including lubiprostone, linaclotide, plecanatide, and tenapanor have been shown to be effective in treating both constipation and the global symptoms of IBS[33,38] **(Table 2)**.

For the treatment of IBS-D, loperamide is commonly used first line to reduce diarrhea frequency, although data regarding its ability to improve symptoms of abdominal discomfort are sparse.[44,45] Bile acid sequestrants including cholestyramine can be used in IBS-D if bile acid malabsorption is suspected.[33] More recent therapies for the treatment of IBS-D include rifaximin, alosetron, and eluxadoline

Table 2
Irritable bowel syndrome-C medications

Drugs	Mechanism of Action	Dosing	Side Effects	Cost (Monthly)[a]	Comments
Linaclotide	Guanylate cyclase-C agonist	290 mcg daily	Diarrhea (though often improves after 1–2 wk on therapy)	$523–$649	Should be taken without food, at least 30 min before the first meal of the day.
Plecanatide	Guanylate cyclase-C agonist	3 mg daily	Diarrhea	$569–$670	Contraindicated in patients under 6 y of age and should be avoided in those under 18 y of age.
Lubiprostone	Chloride channel activator	8 mcg twice daily	Nausea, diarrhea	$374–$423	Nausea is dose-dependent and may be improved by taking with meals. Only FDA-approved for treatment of IBS-C in women.[b]
Tenapanor	Inhibitor of the gastrointestinal sodium/hydrogen (Na/H) exchanger	50 mg twice daily	Diarrhea	$2143	

[a] Approximate cost without insurance. Costs are estimated based on recent ACG/AGA guidelines (Chang et al,[9] 2023) and pricing data available on the online database Lexi-Drug (UpToDate Lexidrug, Lexi-Drugs Online. Waltham, MA: UpToDate, Inc, https://online.lexi.com). The listed prices are not exact and are likely to vary.

[b] The clinical efficacy of lubiprostone was not conclusively demonstrated in trials for men with IBS-C.

Table 3
Irritable bowel syndrome-D medications

Drug	Mechanism of Action	Dosing	Side Effects	Cost[a]	Comments
Rifaximin	Nonabsorbable antibiotic	550 mg 3 times daily for 14 d course.	Minimal, though nausea, URI, and UTI have been reported	$2744 (for 14 d course)	If symptoms recur after initial 14 d treatment course, up to 2 additional retreatments can be considered
Alosetron	5-HT3 antagonist	0.5 mg twice daily, can be titrated at 4 wk intervals to maximum dose of 1 mg twice daily	Constipation (can be severe), ischemic colitis	$1767–$2067 (monthly)	Patients must be monitored closely for constipation and drug discontinued or dose lowered if this develops. Should only be used in women with severe IBS-D failing other traditional therapies.
Eluxadoline	Mixed mu- and kappa-opioid receptor agonist/partial delta-opioid receptor antagonist	100 mg twice daily, though 75 mg twice daily recommended for those unable to tolerate higher dose, those with mild–moderate hepatic impairment, or those taking other OATP1B1 inhibitors	Constipation, nausea, abdominal pain	$1921 (monthly)	Contraindicated in those without a gallbladder, a history of pancreatitis, and in those who consume >3 alcoholic beverages daily.

[a] Approximate cost without insurance. Costs are estimated based on pricing data available on the online database Lexi-Drug (UpToDate Lexidrug, Lexi-Drugs Online. Waltham, MA: UpToDate, Inc, https://online.lexi.com). The listed prices are not exact and are likely to vary.
Abbreviations: URI, upper respiratory infection; UTI, urinary tract infection.

(**Table 3**). Rifaximin, a nonabsorbable antibiotic, both improves diarrhea frequency and reduces global symptoms of IBS including abdominal discomfort and bloating.[46] Those who experience recurrent symptoms after the initial treatment course can be retreated with up to 2 additional courses.[39] Alosetron, a 5-HT3 antagonist, improves the global IBS symptoms, abdominal discomfort, stool consistency, and urgency but is only approved in women with severe, chronic (>6 months) IBS-D who have failed traditional therapies.[39] Eluxadoline is a mixed opioid agonist/antagonist shown to be effective at reducing abdominal pain, stool consistency, and urgency.[47] While effective in treating IBS-D, it is contraindicated in individuals without a gallbladder, any personal history of pancreatitis, history of alcohol use disorder, or current consumption of greater than 3 alcoholic beverages per day.[33]

CLOSTRIDIOIDES DIFFICILE INFECTION
Introduction

Clostridioides difficile infection (CDI) is a toxin-mediated disease resulting in diarrheal illness, though in more severe cases can lead to ileus, toxic megacolon, and pseudo-membranous colitis. The most significant risk factors for CDI are antibiotic use, age 65 years or older, and prior hospitalization.[48] While there are effective treatments for CDI, the rate of recurrent infection approaches 20%,[49] and as such therapies including fecal microbiota transplantation (FMT) and newer live biotherapeutic products have emerged as effective options for those with recurrent CDI.

Management

For an initial episode of CDI, treatment options include oral vancomycin and fidaxomicin. While both options have comparable initial cure rates, fidaxomicin results in greater rates of sustained clinical response (lower likelihood of recurrent infection) compared to vancomycin.[50,51] It is important to note that while metronidazole has previously been used for CDI, its use is no longer recommended as the cure rate is inferior to oral vancomycin.[52]

For those experiencing recurrent CDI, treatment varies depending on the number of recurrences (**Fig. 1**). In addition to standard-of-care antibiotics, for patients who are at

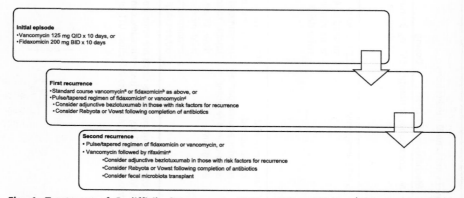

Fig. 1. Treatment of *C. difficile*. [a]Vancomycin 125 mg QID × 10 days. [b]Fidaxomicin 200 mg BID × 10 days. [c]Fidaxomicin 200 mg BID × 5 days, then 200 mg every other day × 20 days. [d]Vancomycin 125 mg QID × 10–14 days, then 125 mg BID × 7 days, then 125 mg daily × 7 days, then 125 mg every other day for 2-8 weeks. [e]Vancomycin 125 mg QID × 10 days, then Rifaximin 400 mg TID × 20 days.

high risk for subsequent recurrences (age > 65 years, immunocompromised, severe CDI on presentation), bezlotoxumab, a monoclonal antibody against *C. difficile* toxin B, should be considered as an adjunctive therapy. Bezlotoxumab (when used in conjunction with standard-of-care antibiotics) results in higher rates of sustained cure at 12 weeks compared to antibiotics alone.[53]

Patients experiencing multiple recurrent CDI (second or further recurrences) should be considered for FMT. Since 2013, multiple studies[54,55] have shown FMT via endoscopy to be an efficacious therapy for the treatment and prevention of recurrent CDI.[56] However, despite its efficacy, traditional FMT is not yet approved by the FDA and is associated with a risk of transmission of infectious agents. Some agents that have been reported include Shiga toxin-producing *Escherichia coli*, extended-spectrum beta-lactamase-producing *E coli*, and norovirus infection.[57–59]

Fecal microbiota encapsulated spores (Vowst) and the rectal microbiota suspension (Rebyota) are alternative forms of FMT that do not require endoscopic administration and have recently been FDA-approved for the prevention of recurrent infection in patients with at least one episode of recurrent CDI. Both therapies have been shown to reduce CDI recurrence compared to placebo and are administered around 48 to 72 hours after completion of standard-of-care antibiotics.[60–62] While further studies are needed comparing Vowst and Rebyota to traditional methods of FMT, these therapies are promising.

GASTROPARESIS
Introduction

Gastroparesis is a disorder characterized by delayed emptying of contents from the stomach after eating in the absence of mechanical obstruction. The syndrome is caused by neuromuscular dysfunction resulting in reduced gastric body/fundus accommodation, gastric antral hypomotility, and impaired pyloric relaxation.[63] Cardinal symptoms include early satiety, postprandial fullness, nausea, vomiting, belching, bloating, and epigastric abdominal pain.[64]

Limited data exist regarding the epidemiology of gastroparesis given its substantial symptom overlap with functional dyspepsia. Recent population-based studies, however, suggest a prevalence of definite gastroparesis of 9.6 per 100,000 persons for men and 37.9 per 100,000 for women in the United States.[65] Greater than 90% of patients with gastroparesis have either diabetic (DGP), postsurgical, or idiopathic gastroparesis (IGP), with IGP being the most common etiology.

Evaluation

The current gold standard for the diagnosis of gastroparesis is the 4 hour gastric emptying scintigraphy (GES). Gastric emptying is not static and patients with gastroparesis can have normal, delayed, or even rapid gastric emptying on GES.[66] Notably, certain medications can affect gastric emptying including opiates and antispasmodics (atropine, dicyclomine, loperamide), and these should be discontinued 48 hours prior to a GES. Alternative methods of diagnosis include the gastric emptying breath test (GEBT) and wireless motility capsule (WMC). The GEBT measures the amount of 13-carbon isotope exhaled at specific intervals after a meal and correlates well with GES.[67] Unlike GES, however, GEBT does not use radiation and is more cost-effective.[68] WMC utilizes a wireless capsule to measure regional and whole gut transit times. WMC also correlates well with GES but provides the added benefit of measuring small bowel and colonic transit times which can be abnormal in two-thirds of patients with gastroparesis.[69]

Management

Traditionally, management of gastroparesis includes initiation of a low residue diet with frequent, small meals. For those patients with DGP, improved glycemic control is recommended. Currently, the only FDA-approved medication for the treatment of gastroparesis is the dopamine receptor antagonist (DRA), metoclopramide. Metoclopramide and domperidone (another DRA not available in the United States) have both been shown to improve gastric emptying as well as curtail symptoms of gastroparesis. While generally considered safe, metoclopramide can rarely lead to tardive dyskinesia (risk of 0.1% per 1000 patient-years) which typically occurs only after long-term use in patients who are elderly, female, diabetic, or concomitant antipsychotic medications.[70] Over time, however, patients can develop tachyphylaxis to metoclopramide which has led physicians to seek alternative treatment options.

More recently, serotonergic agonists have gained traction for the treatment of gastroparesis. Prucalopride, currently only FDA-approved to treat chronic idiopathic constipation, improves gastric emptying and gastroparesis symptoms[71] and is frequently used by gastroenterologists to treat patients with gastroparesis and constipation. Similarly, granisetron, a serotonergic antiemetic, also improves gastroparesis symptoms in the majority of those who take the medication.[72] Aprepitant, a neurokinin neurokinin-1 (NK1) receptor antagonist used to treat chemotherapy-induced or postoperative nausea, can improve postprandial gastric volumes and compliance and in randomized controlled trials has improved gastroparesis symptoms.[73]

For carefully selected patients with refractory symptoms, nonpharmacologic treatment options are available and may be considered in consultation with a gastroenterologist and gastrointestinal surgeon. Neuromodulation in the form of gastric electric stimulators operate by treating the visceral hypersensitivity associated with gastroparesis thereby improving gastroparesis symptoms. Few randomized controlled trials have shown any benefit, however, and device implantation carries significant risk.[74] Pylorus-directed therapies such as botulinum injection have been shown to improve gastric emptying, but not symptom severity.[75,76] Similarly, transpyloric stenting can improve gastric emptying but confers a substantial risk of stent migration. More recently, several initial case studies and series have demonstrated gastric peroral endoscopic myotomy to improve gastric emptying and gastroparesis symptoms with minimal side effects.[77] Further prospective, randomized control trials will be needed, however, to verify its efficacy.

STEATOTIC LIVER DISEASE
Introduction

Steatotic liver disease (SLD) is the most common chronic liver disease worldwide. Historically, SLD encompassed nonalcoholic fatty liver disease (NAFLD), nonalcoholic steatohepatitis (NASH), and alcoholic liver disease (ALD). While ALD was diagnosed based on alcohol consumption, NAFLD and NASH were typically diagnoses of exclusion. In recent years, due to a better understanding of pathogenesis and the potential stigmatizing nature of the existing terminology, efforts were made to create new nomenclature that did not rely on exclusionary criteria and more accurately reflected the root cause of these diseases.

Under the new terminology, SLD remains the overarching diagnosis; however, NAFLD is replaced with metabolic dysfunction-associated SLD (MASLD), and NASH is replaced with metabolic dysfunction-associated steatohepatitis (MASH). MASLD is diagnosed in patients with hepatic steatosis, one or more cardiometabolic risk factors, and no other clear cause of hepatic steatosis. Patients who have MASLD and elevated transaminases or biopsy-proven steatohepatitis meet criteria for MASH. A new category, metabolic dysfunction associated steatotic liver disease and alcohol-associated liver disease (MetALD), was created for those patients who meet criteria for MASLD but also consume more than a mild amount of alcohol (30–60 g of alcohol daily for men, 20–50 g daily for women). If patients consume greater amounts of alcohol on a regular basis, they meet criteria for ALD. Since the introduction of this new nomenclature, numerous studies report a near-complete overlap between the MASLD-defined and the NAFLD-defined population.[78,79] Consequently, there have been no changes to the management of these patients.

Management

Weight loss remains the cornerstone of therapy. The loss of at least 10% total body weight has been shown to lead to resolution of hepatic steatosis, reversal of fibrosis, and reduction in cardiovascular disease, the principal cause of death among patients with MASLD.[80] While no specific diet is superior to another, the Mediterranean diet is often recommended due to its sustainability and cardiovascular benefits. Additionally, coffee consumption (caffeinated or not) of at least 3 cups per day has been associated with a decreased risk for MASLD and hepatic fibrosis.[81]

Unfortunately, the majority of the patients with MASLD cannot sustain meaningful weight loss through lifestyle changes. Bariatric surgery, recommended in patients with a body mass index (BMI) $\geq$40 or $\geq$35 kg/m^2 with weight-related comorbidities, should be considered for those patients without cirrhosis who fail conservative treatments for weight loss. Bariatric surgery can resolve MASH and improve hepatic fibrosis while simultaneously decreasing all-cause morbidity and mortality.[82–84] Expectedly, these results are dependent on patients maintaining sustained postsurgical weight loss.

Pharmacologic therapy for the management of MASLD is a growing field. Historically, vitamin E was used in patients without diabetes as it was shown to improve MASH histology (not fibrosis), but did carry numerous risks including hemorrhagic strokes and prostate cancer.[85] For patients with diabetes or obesity, newer agents such as glucagon-like peptide-1 (GLP-1) agonists and sodium/glucose cotransporter 2 (SGLT-2) inhibitors have been shown to improve hepatic steatosis, resolve MASH, and potentially delay the progression of hepatic fibrosis in addition to their established cardiorenal protective effects.[86,87] Statins, generally underutilized in patients with MASLD due to concern for drug-induced liver injury, are recommended for patients with MASLD and dyslipidemia as they have been shown to reduce all-cause mortality and potentially prevent or delay hepatocellular carcinoma.[88,89] Most recently, resmetirom, a thyroid hormone receptor agonist, gained approval by the FDA in March 2024 for treatment of MASH associated with moderate-to-severe fibrosis. While studies are still ongoing, initial results of a phase 3 clinical trial showed resmetirom to be superior to standard of care (diet and exercise) in regard to MASH resolution or improvement in fibrosis by at least one stage.[90]

COLONIC DIVERTICULITIS
Introduction

Colonic diverticulitis is a common gastrointestinal disease in the US population. Acute uncomplicated diverticulitis refers to the acute onset of diverticular inflammation, without associated complication. Acute complicated diverticulitis refers to acute diverticular inflammation with abscess or perforation. Although colonic diverticula are common, and more prevalent with increasing age, the risk of progression to diverticulitis is low.[91] Risk factors for diverticulitis include age, tobacco use, nonsteroidal anti-inflammatory drug (NSAID) use, and obesity.[92]

Evaluation

The majority of the patients with diverticulitis have acute uncomplicated diverticulitis and are managed in the outpatient setting.[93] Patients present with acute, usually lower left-sided, abdominal pain. They may have associated fever or leukocytosis. The diagnosis of diverticulitis is determined by abdominal–pelvic computed tomography (CT) scan, which demonstrates diverticula and characteristic pericolonic inflammatory changes. CT scans also help determine the severity and exclude any complications such as abscess formation or perforation.

Management

Patients who have acute uncomplicated diverticulitis who are immunocompetent and without significant comorbidities may be managed in the outpatient setting. A clear liquid diet is generally advised during an episode of acute uncomplicated diverticulitis. Antibiotics should be used selectively, rather than routinely, in immunocompetent patients with mild uncomplicated diverticulitis.[92,94,95] Antibiotic treatment is advised in patients who are immunocompromised, have comorbidities, frailty, or evidence of severe disease or complicated diverticulitis.[91,92] When antibiotics are indicated, outpatient treatment of mild uncomplicated diverticulitis most commonly includes either a combination of an oral fluoroquinolone and metronidazole or monotherapy with oral amoxicillin–clavulanate. Following resolution of a first episode of diverticulitis, a colonoscopy should be performed approximately 6 to 8 weeks later, in order to exclude a colonic malignancy if not done within the past 1 year.[95]

To reduce the risk of recurrence, patients should consume a diet rich in fruits, vegetables, and whole grains and low in red meat. Evidence does not support the traditional recommendation of avoiding specific dietary elements such as fruits with small seeds (strawberries), corn, popcorn, and nuts.[96] Additionally, patients should be counseled to avoid tobacco and NSAID use (except aspirin for secondary cardiovascular prophylaxis). An elective segmental resection should not be advised based solely on the number of episodes of diverticulitis. Instead, surgical resection should be an individualized recommendation, after consideration of risks, consultation among the care providers, and discussion with the patient.

CLINICS CARE POINTS

- Pelvic floor dysfunction, or dyssynergic defecation, should be considered in individuals with chronic constipation, particularly in those who fail to respond to lifestyle measures and a trial of laxatives. This can be diagnosed with a digital rectal examination or anorectal manometry and can be managed with pelvic floor physical therapy.

- Management of irritable bowel syndrome can require a multimodal approach including dietary modification, pharmacologic therapy, and gut-directed psychotherapies.

- While both fidaxomicin and oral vancomycin have similar initial cure rates when treating Clostridioides difficile infection, fidaxomicin is associated with a lower risk of recurrent infection. However, fidaxomicin's high cost can limit its utilization.

- Weight loss remains the cornerstone of therapy for metabolic dysfunction-associated liver disease (MASLD). However, resmetirom, the first FDA-approved medication for MASLD/MASH is a promising new therapy.

- For immunocompetent patients with uncomplicated mild diverticulitis, antibiotics are not always necessary.
- Patients with diverticulitis should be counseled on NSAID avoidance, smoking cessation, and weight loss (if overweight) to reduce the risk of recurrence.

DISCLOSURES

The authors have no disclosures.

REFERENCES

1. Mearin F, Lacy BE, Chang L, et al. Bowel disorders. Gastroenterology 2016. https://doi.org/10.1053/j.gastro.2016.02.031.
2. Camilleri M, Brandler J. Refractory constipation: how to evaluate and treat. Gastroenterol Clin North Am 2020;49(3):623–42.
3. Cho YS, Lee YJ, Shin JE, et al. 2022 seoul consensus on clinical practice guidelines for functional constipation. J Neurogastroenterol Motil 2023;29(3):271–305.
4. Tantiphlachiva K, Rao P, Attaluri A, et al. Digital rectal examination is a useful tool for identifying patients with dyssynergia. Clin Gastroenterol Hepatol 2010;8(11):955–60.
5. Bharucha AE, Dorn SD, Lembo A, et al. American Gastroenterological Association medical position statement on constipation. Gastroenterology 2013;144(1):211–7.
6. Bayer SB, Heenan P, Frampton C, et al. Two gold kiwifruit daily for effective treatment of constipation in adults-a randomized clinical trial. Nutrients 2022;(19):14.
7. Chey SW, Chey WD, Jackson K, et al. Exploratory comparative effectiveness trial of green kiwifruit, psyllium, or prunes in us patients with chronic constipation. Am J Gastroenterol 2021;116(6):1304–12.
8. Van Der Schoot A, Katsirma Z, Whelan K, et al. Systematic review and meta-analysis: Foods, drinks and diets and their effect on chronic constipation in adults. Aliment Pharmacol Ther 2023. https://doi.org/10.1111/apt.17782.
9. Chang L, Chey WD, Imdad A, et al. American Gastroenterological Association-American College of Gastroenterology clinical practice guideline: pharmacological management of chronic idiopathic constipation. Gastroenterology 2023; 164(7):1086–106.
10. Fakheri RJ, Volpicelli FM. Things we do for no reason: prescribing docusate for constipation in hospitalized adults. J Hosp Med 2019;14(2):110–3.
11. Fleming V, Wade WE. A review of laxative therapies for treatment of chronic constipation in older adults. Am J Geriatr Pharmacother 2010;8(6):514–50.
12. Tarumi Y, Wilson MP, Szafran O, et al. Randomized, double-blind, placebo-controlled trial of oral docusate in the management of constipation in hospice patients. J Pain Symptom Manage 2013;45(1):2–13.
13. Barish CF, Drossman D, Johanson JF, et al. Efficacy and safety of lubiprostone in patients with chronic constipation. Dig Dis Sci 2010;55(4):1090–7.
14. Fukudo S, Hongo M, Kaneko H, et al. Lubiprostone increases spontaneous bowel movement frequency and quality of life in patients with chronic idiopathic constipation. Clin Gastroenterol Hepatol 2015;13(2):294–301.e5.
15. Johanson JF, Morton D, Geenen J, et al. Multicenter, 4-week, double-blind, randomized, placebo-controlled trial of lubiprostone, a locally-acting type-2 chloride channel activator, in patients with chronic constipation. Official journal of the American College of Gastroenterology | ACG 2008;103(1):170–7.

16. Lembo AJ, Schneier HA, Shiff SJ, et al. Two randomized trials of linaclotide for chronic constipation. N Engl J Med 2011;365(6):527–36.

17. Fukudo S, Miwa H, Nakajima A, et al. High-dose linaclotide is effective and safe in patients with chronic constipation: A phase III randomized, double-blind, placebo-controlled study with a long-term open-label extension study in Japan. Neuro Gastroenterol Motil 2019;31(1):e13487.

18. Lacy BE, Schey R, Shiff SJ, et al. Linaclotide in chronic idiopathic constipation patients with moderate to severe abdominal bloating: a randomized, controlled trial. PLoS One 2015;10(7):e0134349.

19. Shah ED, Kim HM, Schoenfeld P. Efficacy and tolerability of guanylate cyclase-c agonists for irritable bowel syndrome with constipation and chronic idiopathic constipation: a systematic review and meta-analysis. Official journal of the American College of Gastroenterology | ACG 2018;113(3):329–38.

20. Tack J, van Outryve M, Beyens G, et al. Prucalopride (Resolor) in the treatment of severe chronic constipation in patients dissatisfied with laxatives. Gut 2009;58(3): 357–65.

21. Camilleri M, Kerstens R, Rykx A, et al. A placebo-controlled trial of prucalopride for severe chronic constipation. N Engl J Med 2008;358(22):2344–54.

22. Quigley EM, Vandeplassche L, Kerstens R, et al. Clinical trial: the efficacy, impact on quality of life, and safety and tolerability of prucalopride in severe chronic constipation–a 12-week, randomized, double-blind, placebo-controlled study. Aliment Pharmacol Ther 2009;29(3):315–28.

23. Administration USFaD. Prucalopride - full prescribing information. Available at: https://www.accessdata.fda.gov/drugsatfda_docs/label/2018/210166s000lbl. pdf. [Accessed 10 December 2023].

24. Simón MA, Bueno AM, Otero P, et al. A randomized controlled trial on the effects of electromyographic biofeedback on quality of life and bowel symptoms in elderly women with dyssynergic defecation. Int J Environ Res Public Health 2019;16(18).

25. Özkütük N, Eşer İ, Bor S. Effectiveness of biofeedback therapy on quality of life in patients with dyssynergic defecation disorder. Turk J Gastroenterol 2021; 32(1):22–9.

26. Ba-Bai-Ke-Re MM, Wen NR, Hu YL, et al. Biofeedback-guided pelvic floor exercise therapy for obstructive defecation: an effective alternative. World J Gastroenterol 2014;20(27):9162–9.

27. Van Outryve M, Pelckmans P. Biofeedback is superior to laxatives for normal transit constipation due to pelvic floor dyssynergia. Gastroenterology 2006; 131(1):333–4 [author reply 334].

28. Hung TH, Wang CY, Lee HF. Update in diagnosis and management of irritable bowel syndrome. Tzu Chi Med J Oct-Dec 2023;35(4):306–11.

29. Naliboff BD, Munakata J, Fullerton S, et al. Evidence for two distinct perceptual alterations in irritable bowel syndrome. Gut 1997;41(4):505–12.

30. Accarino AM, Azpiroz F, Malagelada JR. Selective dysfunction of mechanosensitive intestinal afferents in irritable bowel syndrome. Gastroenterology 1995; 108(3):636–43.

31. Almario CV, Sharabi E, Chey WD, et al. Prevalence and burden of illness of rome iv irritable bowel syndrome in the united states: results from a nationwide cross-sectional study. Gastroenterology 2023;165(6):1475–87.

32. Inadomi JM, Fennerty MB, Bjorkman D. Systematic review: the economic impact of irritable bowel syndrome. Aliment Pharmacol Ther 2003;18(7):671–82.

33. Lacy BE, Pimentel M, Brenner DM, et al. ACG clinical guideline: management of irritable bowel syndrome. Am J Gastroenterol 2021;116(1):17–44.

34. Moayyedi P, Quigley EM, Lacy BE, et al. The effect of fiber supplementation on irritable bowel syndrome: a systematic review and meta-analysis. Am J Gastroenterol 2014;109(9):1367–74.

35. Dionne J, Ford AC, Yuan Y, et al. A systematic review and meta-analysis evaluating the efficacy of a gluten-free diet and a low FODMAPs diet in treating symptoms of irritable bowel syndrome. Am J Gastroenterol 2018;113(9):1290–300.

36. Su GL, Ko CW, Bercik P, et al. AGA clinical practice guidelines on the role of probiotics in the management of gastrointestinal disorders. Gastroenterology 2020; 159(2):697–705.

37. Alammar N, Wang L, Saberi B, et al. The impact of peppermint oil on the irritable bowel syndrome: a meta-analysis of the pooled clinical data. BMC Complement Altern Med 2019;19(1):21.

38. Chang L, Sultan S, Lembo A, et al. AGA clinical practice guideline on the pharmacological management of irritable bowel syndrome with constipation. Gastroenterology 2022;163(1):118–36.

39. Lembo A, Sultan S, Chang L, et al. AGA clinical practice guideline on the pharmacological management of irritable bowel syndrome with diarrhea. Gastroenterology 2022;163(1):137–51.

40. Brenner DM, Ladewski AM, Kinsinger SW. Development and current state of digital therapeutics for irritable bowel syndrome. Clin Gastroenterol Hepatol 2023. https://doi.org/10.1016/j.cgh.2023.09.013.

41. Fadgyas Stanculete M, Dumitrascu DL, Drossman D. Neuromodulators in the brain-gut axis: their role in the therapy of the irritable bowel syndrome. J Gastrointestin Liver Dis 2021;30(4):517–25.

42. Ford AC, Lacy BE, Harris LA, et al. Effect of antidepressants and psychological therapies in irritable bowel syndrome: an updated systematic review and meta-analysis. Am J Gastroenterol 2019;114(1):21–39.

43. Chapman RW, Stanghellini V, Geraint M, et al. Randomized clinical trial: macrogol/PEG 3350 plus electrolytes for treatment of patients with constipation associated with irritable bowel syndrome. Am J Gastroenterol 2013;108(9):1508–15.

44. Lavö B, Stenstam M, Nielsen AL. Loperamide in treatment of irritable bowel syndrome–a double-blind placebo controlled study. Scand J Gastroenterol Suppl 1987;130:77–80.

45. Hovdenak N. Loperamide treatment of the irritable bowel syndrome. Scand J Gastroenterol Suppl 1987;130:81–4.

46. Chang L, Lembo A, Sultan S. American gastroenterological association institute technical review on the pharmacological management of irritable bowel syndrome. Gastroenterology 2014;147(5):1149–72.e2.

47. Lembo AJ, Lacy BE, Zuckerman MJ, et al. Eluxadoline for irritable bowel syndrome with diarrhea. N Engl J Med 2016;374(3):242–53.

48. Davies K, Lawrence J, Berry C, et al. Risk factors for primary clostridium difficile infection; results from the observational study of risk factors for clostridium difficile infection in hospitalized patients with infective diarrhea (ORCHID). Front Public Health 2020;8:293.

49. Finn E, Andersson FL, Madin-Warburton M. Burden of clostridioides difficile infection (CDI) - a systematic review of the epidemiology of primary and recurrent CDI. BMC Infect Dis 2021;21(1):456.

50. Beinortas T, Burr NE, Wilcox MH, et al. Comparative efficacy of treatments for Clostridium difficile infection: a systematic review and network meta-analysis. Lancet Infect Dis 2018;18(9):1035–44.

51. Al Momani LA, Abughanimeh O, Boonpheng B, et al. Fidaxomicin vs vancomycin for the treatment of a first episode of clostridium difficile infection: a meta-analysis and systematic review. Cureus 2018;10(6):e2778.

52. Johnson S, Louie TJ, Gerding DN, et al. Vancomycin, metronidazole, or tolevamer for Clostridium difficile infection: results from two multinational, randomized, controlled trials. Clin Infect Dis 2014;59(3):345–54.

53. Wilcox MH, Gerding DN, Poxton IR, et al. Bezlotoxumab for prevention of recurrent clostridium difficile infection. N Engl J Med 2017;376(4):305–17.

54. van Nood E, Vrieze A, Nieuwdorp M, et al. Duodenal infusion of donor feces for recurrent Clostridium difficile. N Engl J Med 2013;368(5):407–15.

55. Kelly CR, Khoruts A, Staley C, et al. Effect of fecal microbiota transplantation on recurrence in multiply recurrent clostridium difficile infection: a randomized trial. Ann Intern Med 2016;165(9):609–16.

56. Moayyedi P, Yuan Y, Baharith H, et al. Faecal microbiota transplantation for Clostridium difficile-associated diarrhoea: a systematic review of randomised controlled trials. Med J Aust 2017;207(4):166–72.

57. Zellmer C, Sater MRA, Huntley MH, et al. Shiga toxin-producing escherichia coli transmission via fecal microbiota transplant. Clin Infect Dis 2021;72(11):e876–80.

58. DeFilipp Z, Bloom PP, Torres Soto M, et al. Drug-resistant e. coli bacteremia transmitted by fecal microbiota transplant. N Engl J Med 2019;381(21):2043–50.

59. Schwartz M, Gluck M, Koon S. Norovirus gastroenteritis after fecal microbiota transplantation for treatment of Clostridium difficile infection despite asymptomatic donors and lack of sick contacts. Am J Gastroenterol 2013;108(8):1367.

60. Gonzales-Luna AJ, Carlson TJ, Garey KW. Review article: safety of live biotherapeutic products used for the prevention of clostridioides difficile infection recurrence. Clin Infect Dis 2023;77(Supplement_6):S487–96.

61. Bancke L, Su X. 167. Efficacy of Investigational Microbiota-Based Live Biotherapeutic RBX2660 in Individuals with Recurrent Clostridioides difficile Infection: Data from Five Prospective Clinical Studies. Open Forum Infect Dis 2021; 8:S100–1.

62. Feuerstadt P, Louie TJ, Lashner B, et al. SER-109, an oral microbiome therapy for recurrent clostridioides difficile infection. N Engl J Med 2022;386(3):220–9.

63. Grover M, Farrugia G, Stanghellini V. Gastroparesis: a turning point in understanding and treatment. Gut 2019;68(12):2238–50.

64. Camilleri M, Chedid V, Ford AC, et al. Gastroparesis. Nat Rev Dis Primers 2018; 4(1):41.

65. Grant BF, Chou SP, Saha TD, et al. Prevalence of 12-Month Alcohol Use, High-Risk Drinking, and DSM-IV Alcohol Use Disorder in the United States, 2001-2002 to 2012-2013: Results From the National Epidemiologic Survey on Alcohol and Related Conditions. JAMA Psychiatr 2017;74(9):911–23.

66. Bharucha AE, Camilleri M, Forstrom LA, et al. Relationship between clinical features and gastric emptying disturbances in diabetes mellitus. Clin Endocrinol 2009;70(3):415–20.

67. Szarka LA, Camilleri M, Vella A, et al. A stable isotope breath test with a standard meal for abnormal gastric emptying of solids in the clinic and in research. Clin Gastroenterol Hepatol 2008;6(6):635–643 e1.

68. Sharma A, Coles M, Parkman HP. Gastroparesis in the 2020s: New Treatments, New Paradigms. Curr Gastroenterol Rep 2020;22(5):23.

69. Siegfried WY, Rattanakovit K, Mack A, et al. Su1454 Is gastroparesis a pan-enteric neuropathic disorder: investigation with wireless motility capsule. Gastroenterology 2015;148(4). S-516-S-517.

70. Al-Saffar A, Lennernas H, Hellstrom PM. Gastroparesis, metoclopramide, and tardive dyskinesia: Risk revisited. Neuro Gastroenterol Motil 2019;31(11):e13617.

71. Carbone F, Van den Houte K, Clevers E, et al. Prucalopride in gastroparesis: a randomized placebo-controlled crossover study. Am J Gastroenterol 2019; 114(8):1265-74.

72. Midani D, Parkman HP. Granisetron transdermal system for treatment of symptoms of gastroparesis: a prescription registry study. J Neurogastroenterol Motil 2016;22(4):650-5.

73. Pasricha PJ, Yates KP, Sarosiek I, et al. Aprepitant has mixed effects on nausea and reduces other symptoms in patients with gastroparesis and related disorders. Gastroenterology 2018;154(1):65-76 e11.

74. Levinthal DJ, Bielefeldt K. Systematic review and meta-analysis: Gastric electrical stimulation for gastroparesis. Auton Neurosci 2017;202:45-55.

75. Arts J, Holvoet L, Caenepeel P, et al. Clinical trial: a randomized-controlled crossover study of intrapyloric injection of botulinum toxin in gastroparesis. Aliment Pharmacol Ther 2007;26(9):1251-8.

76. Friedenberg FK, Palit A, Parkman HP, et al. Botulinum toxin A for the treatment of delayed gastric emptying. Am J Gastroenterol 2008;103(2):416-23.

77. Mekaroonkamol P, Li LY, Dacha S, et al. Gastric peroral endoscopic pyloromyotomy (G-POEM) as a salvage therapy for refractory gastroparesis: a case series of different subtypes. Neuro Gastroenterol Motil 2016;28(8):1272-7.

78. Song SJ, Lai JC, Wong GL, et al. Can we use old NAFLD data under the new MASLD definition? J Hepatol 2023. https://doi.org/10.1016/j.jhep.2023.07.021.

79. Ratziu V, Boursier J. Fibrosis AGftSoL. Confirmatory biomarker diagnostic studies are not needed when transitioning from NAFLD to MASLD. J Hepatol 2023. https://doi.org/10.1016/j.jhep.2023.07.017.

80. Long MT, Noureddin M, Lim JK. AGA clinical practice update: diagnosis and management of nonalcoholic fatty liver disease in lean individuals: expert review. Gastroenterology 2022;163(3):764-774 e1.

81. Chen YP, Lu FB, Hu YB, et al. A systematic review and a dose-response meta-analysis of coffee dose and nonalcoholic fatty liver disease. Clin Nutr 2019; 38(6):2552-7.

82. Fakhry TK, Mhaskar R, Schwitalla T, et al. Bariatric surgery improves nonalcoholic fatty liver disease: a contemporary systematic review and meta-analysis. Surg Obes Relat Dis 2019;15(3):502-11.

83. Lee Y, Doumouras AG, Yu J, et al. Complete resolution of nonalcoholic fatty liver disease after bariatric surgery: a systematic review and meta-analysis. Clin Gastroenterol Hepatol 2019;17(6):1040-1060 e11.

84. Lassailly G, Caiazzo R, Ntandja-Wandji LC, et al. Bariatric surgery provides long-term resolution of nonalcoholic steatohepatitis and regression of fibrosis. Gastroenterology 2020;159(4):1290-1301 e5.

85. Violi F, Cangemi R. Pioglitazone, vitamin E, or placebo for nonalcoholic steatohepatitis. N Engl J Med 2010;363(12):1185-6 [author reply 1186].

86. Armstrong MJ, Gaunt P, Aithal GP, et al. Liraglutide safety and efficacy in patients with non-alcoholic steatohepatitis (LEAN): a multicentre, double-blind, randomised, placebo-controlled phase 2 study. Lancet 2016;387(10019):679-90.

87. Newsome PN, Buchholtz K, Cusi K, et al. A placebo-controlled trial of subcutaneous semaglutide in nonalcoholic steatohepatitis. N Engl J Med 2021;384(12): 1113–24.
88. Bril F, Portillo Sanchez P, Lomonaco R, et al. Liver safety of statins in prediabetes or t2dm and nonalcoholic steatohepatitis: post hoc analysis of a randomized trial. J Clin Endocrinol Metab 2017;102(8):2950–61.
89. Kaplan DE, Serper MA, Mehta R, et al. Effects of hypercholesterolemia and statin exposure on survival in a large national cohort of patients with cirrhosis. Gastroenterology 2019;156(6):1693–1706 e12.
90. Harrison SA, Bedossa P, Guy CD, et al. A phase 3, randomized, controlled trial of resmetirom in nash with liver fibrosis. N Engl J Med 2024;390(6):497–509.
91. Peery AF. Management of colonic diverticulitis. BMJ 2021;372:n72.
92. Peery AF, Shaukat A, Strate LL. AGA clinical practice update on medical management of colonic diverticulitis: expert review. Gastroenterology 2021;160(3): 906–911 e1.
93. Bharucha AE, Parthasarathy G, Ditah I, et al. Temporal trends in the incidence and natural history of diverticulitis: a population-based study. Am J Gastroenterol 2015;110(11):1589–96.
94. Au S, Aly EH. Treatment of uncomplicated acute diverticulitis without antibiotics: a systematic review and meta-analysis. Dis Colon Rectum 2019;62(12):1533–47.
95. Hall J, Hardiman K, Lee S, et al. The American Society of Colon and Rectal Surgeons clinical practice guidelines for the treatment of left-sided colonic diverticulitis. Dis Colon Rectum 2020;63(6):728–47.
96. Young-Fadok TM. Diverticulitis. N Engl J Med 2018;379(17):1635–42.

Treatment of Common Dermatologic Conditions

Nina Tan, MD[a],*, Jay C. Vary Jr, MD, PhD[b], Kim M. O'Connor, MD[a]

KEYWORDS

- Dermatology treatment updates • Primary care • Topical steroids • Atopic dermatitis
- Psoriasis • Alopecia • Acne rosacea • Acne vulgaris • Periorificial dermatitis
- Seborrheic dermatitis • Stasis dermatitis

KEY POINTS

- Safely and appropriately prescribe topical steroids and steroid-sparing agents such as calcineurin inhibitors, retinoids, topical, and oral antimicrobials to manage common dermatologic conditions seen in primary care.
- Provide counseling about common side effects or complications of advanced dermatologic therapies such as biologics or JAK inhibitors.
- Recognize the clinical presentation of common dermatologic conditions in skin of varying degrees of pigmentation.

INTRODUCTION

Comfort in diagnosing common skin conditions is important for primary care providers and was addressed in a previous article in this journal.[1,2] Conveniently, many skin conditions will respond to similar therapies so learning how to prescribe topical and systemic medications such as steroids, steroid-sparing agents like calcineurin inhibitors, retinoids, antibiotics, and antifungals is the foundation to treating many conditions. Many newer agents such as biologics or JAK inhibitors may be prescribed by dermatologists so familiarity with the common side effects or complications of these treatments is also important in primary care. In this review, we will discuss the treatment of common forms of alopecia, facial rashes, atopic dermatitis, psoriasis, seborrheic dermatitis, and stasis dermatitis. Additionally, studies have shown that almost half of dermatologists feel they didn't have adequate training to treat skin disease in African-Americans, likely because general medicine and dermatology educational materials contain few images of darker skin tones.[3,4] In line with the recommendations

[a] Department of Internal Medicine, Division of General Internal Medicine, University of Washington, Box 354760, 4245 Roosevelt Way Northeast, 3rd Floor, Seattle, WA 98105, USA;
[b] Department of Dermatology, University of Washington, University of Washington Dermatology Center, Box 354697, 4225 Roosevelt Way NE, 4th Floor, Seattle, WA 98105, USA
* Corresponding author.
E-mail address: ninat@uw.edu

Med Clin N Am 108 (2024) 795–827
https://doi.org/10.1016/j.mcna.2024.02.002
0025-7125/24/© 2024 Elsevier Inc. All rights reserved.

from researchers studying these disparities, in this chapter we provide information and images that may be helpful when managing these common skin conditions in all skin types. The authors also encourage referencing the various patient-led and academic resources that focus on dermatology in skin of color which can be found with a simple internet search or in this reference.[5]

DISCUSSION
Topical Vehicles

Topical therapies are the mainstay of dermatologic treatment. Whether using cortico-steroids, antimicrobials, or comedolytics, topical therapies allow a high concentration of localized medication while minimizing systemic side effects.

Providers can take advantage of the different characteristics of topical vehicles to prescribe therapies that may be more effective and safer to use on different sites of the body (**Table 1**). The choice of vehicle affects medication efficacy, which is inversely related to ease of use and can influence patient adherence (**Fig. 1**). All med-ications containing water require the use of preservatives, which can cause allergic contact dermatitis, so nonaqueous ointments are preferable when this is a concern. The alcohol content in gels and lotions provides drying benefits but may also cause stinging and burning if applied to open skin. Greasier medications such as ointments penetrate the hydrophobic epidermis more readily, so they are more potent but may be less cosmetically pleasing in some areas.[6]

Topical therapies are more easily applied to moist skin. Advise patients to apply a thin layer to all affected areas as over-application is not more efficacious. Daily to twice daily dosing is adequate.[7] The concept of the "fingertip unit" (FTU) can be useful in advising how much to apply based on location (**Fig. 2**).

Topical Steroids

Topical corticosteroids are the most prescribed class of topical medications. In the U.S., these are grouped by varying efficacy from class 1 (very high potency) to class 7 (low potency). Potency is based on both the class of medication and its absorption,

Table 1
Use of topical vehicles

Vehicles	Uses
Gels	Drying (high alcohol content). May cause burning sensation. Use on scalp and hairy areas.
Lotions	Cooling and sometimes drying depending upon alcohol content. Use on oozing lesions, areas with hair.
Creams	Mix of water in oil with preservatives, fragrances, emulsifiers More moisturizing than lotions Occlusion increases potency. Absorbs into skin. Use in cosmetically important and intertriginous areas.
Ointments	Lubricating and occlusive (little or no alcohol). No burning or stinging. Typically contain petrolatum and the active ingredient without added preservatives or fragrances. Most potent (self-occlusive) Use on dry, thick, hyperkeratotic lesions. Avoid use in hairy areas, intertriginous (maceration, folliculitis)
Foams/shampoos/oil	Scalp and ear canals

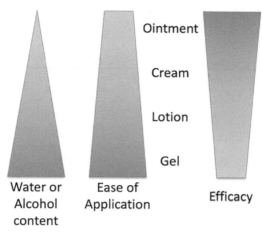

Fig. 1. Characteristics of topical vehicles. Gels contain more alcohol so have a drying effect and may be easier to use, though not as potent as ointments which have little water or alcohol and may be more difficult to use.

which is why a steroid can fall into several classes depending on the vehicle it is carried in. For example, fluocinonide 0.05% cream is class 3, while fluocinonide 0.05% ointment is class 2 due to the occlusive effect of ointments. Potency is important when considering the location of the application and the type of skin lesion (**Table 2**). More potent steroids are necessary for severe skin conditions, though in general, high-potency steroids should be avoided on the face, dorsum of hands, and intertriginous areas.

Side effects of topical corticosteroids include striae distensae (stretch marks), bruising, telangiectasias, skin fragility, and hypopigmentation. If used over extensive areas for long periods of time, there can be suppression of the hypothalamic-pituitary-adrenal axis.[6] Hypopigmentation is more likely to occur in more darkly pigmented skin; however, repigmentation typically occurs weeks to months after discontinuation. Steroid rosacea is more common with fluorinated steroids such as dexamethasone, triamcinolone, betamethasone, and beclomethasone. Ointments have little to no preservatives, fragrances, or emulsifiers, so they are the best choice if contact dermatitis is suspected.

Fingertip Unit (FTU)	Location	FTU
	Face	2.5
	Trunk-Front	7
	Trunk-Back	7
	One arm	3
	One hand	1
	One leg	6
	One foot	2

Fig. 2. One FTU is a line of topical medication from a standard tube that extends along the distal phalanx of the index finger. This is equivalent to about 0.5 g of medication, which should cover one hand.

Table 2
Potency and use of topical steroids

Class	Use (Examples)	Avoid	Length of Use and Maximum Use
1* (very high potency) Clobetasol propionate 0.05% ointment or cream Betamethasone dipropionate 0.05% augmented ointment Halobetasol 0.05% ointment or cream	Thick, hyperkeratotic lesions Psoriasis Severe atopic dermatitis Lichen simplex chronicus Options for scalp treatments include foams, shampoos, sprays, solutions.	Face, dorsum of the hands, genitals, intertriginous areas	1–2 wk Not to exceed 1 mo of continuous use Not to exceed 100 g/week to reduce risk of hypothalamic pituitary axis suppression
2 (high potency) Betamethasone dipropionate 0.05% augmented cream Mometasone furoate 0.1% ointment FluocinoNIDE 0.05% ointment 3 (high potency) FluocinoNIDE 0.05% cream Triamcinolone 0.5% ointment or cream Betamethasone valerate 0.1% ointment	Same as 1	Same as 1	1–2 wk Not to exceed 1 mo of continuous use
4 (medium potency) Triamcinolone 0.1% ointment or cream Mometasone furoate 0.1% cream FluocinoLONE 0.025% ointment 5 (medium potency) Betamethasone valerate 0.1% cream Desonide 0.05% ointment FluocinoLONE 0.025% cream	Rashes Moderate atopic dermatitis Large surface areas (nonfacial)		4–5 wk Not to exceed 3 mo of continuous use
6 (low potency) Desonide 0.05% cream FluocinoLONE 0.01% cream	Facial dermatitis Intertrigo		6–7 wk Not to exceed 3 mo of continuous use
7 (low potency) Hydrocortisone 0.1% to 2.5% cream Hydrocortisone 2.5% ointment or cream Hydrocortisone 1% or lower (OTC)	Same as 6	Palms/soles (too weak to be effective on thicker skin)	6–7 wk Not to exceed 3 mo of continuous use

If topical steroids are required for maintenance therapy, consider "pulse dose" therapy to decrease side effects. For example, once a condition is under better control, topical steroids can be applied on weekends or weekdays only. In many conditions, topical calcineurin inhibitors can be used on the off days if needed. A conservative rule of thumb is that a steroid can be used for as many weeks as its class number without concern for side effects. Use of very high-potency steroids for longer than 4 weeks should be avoided both to decrease the risk of side effects and to prevent rebound symptoms upon discontinuation. If needed, gradually taper very high-potency steroids by reducing both the potency and dosing frequency at 2-week intervals until discontinuation. Only resume topical steroids after a steroid-free period of at least 1 week.

Cost can be a concern with many topical steroids. Choosing generic formulations can increase adherence but generics are not always inexpensive either. Steroid potency can be increased several-fold through occlusion, for example, by wrapping the area with plastic wrap overnight. Avoid occlusion of very high-potency steroids and when using steroids on the face, dorsal hands, or intertriginous areas.

Treatment of Itching

Pruritus (itch) is described as the desire to scratch and can vary from a minor annoyance to a debilitating condition. Chronic itch in the US has been estimated to cost society about 88 billion USD/year and disproportionately affects ethnic minorities.[8,9] There are many causes of itch from the direct release of histamine with hives to less understood pathways in inflammatory skin conditions such as eczema or psoriasis, systemic causes such as liver failure, an internal malignancy such as lymphoma, or psychogenic causes. The etiology and workup for pruritus are beyond the scope of this article and have been well reviewed elsewhere.[10]

Treatment of itch will bring your patient great relief while also elevating your status in their eyes as a master clinician. While histamine is responsible for acute itch and produces a hive when injected into the skin, chronic pruritus is associated with a variety of nonhistamine mediators that are less well characterized, and treatments are numerous.

Chronic itch can be treated with many topical and systemic options. The traditional treatments, such as antihistamines, topical steroids, and topical anesthetics are still first line and are cost effective. Recent additions to this list are denoted with a "c" in **Table 3** and are universally much more expensive. Topical options include the PDE4 inhibitor, crisabarole, or the JAK inhibitor, ruxolitinib. These are generally considered very safe, although the list of side effects with oral JAK inhibitors is quite long and there is not enough data on the topical formulation to be well informed on the potential hazards. Ruxolitinib is limited to 20% BSA for atopic dermatitis and 10% BSA for vitiligo, which should reduce the risk of systemic side effects.

Many opiates cause pruritus due to action on the mu-opiate receptor, so it is not a surprise that in people who are not taking opiates, yet experience itch for other reasons, they may find that naltrexone in standard or even very low doses can be helpful. Unlike the mu-opiate receptor, the kappa-opiate receptor actually suppresses itch and its agonist, difelikefalin, is approved for renal pruritus. In 2023, Kim, and colleagues showed difelikefalin can also be helpful for the very common scapular itch diagnosis, notalgia paresthetica and though likely cost prohibitive in many instances, may provide a path to future novel treatments as well.[11] Fortunately, newer biologic drugs targeting IL-4, IL-13, and IL-31 of the Th2 pathway as well as PDE4 and JAK inhibitors can help tremendously by interfering with many of the signals of the chronic pruritus pathway. Their use is limited by cost, however, and there is no

Table 3
Medications for Pruritus and/or Atopic Dermatitis

References[67,68] and FDA Prescribing Information	Mechanism of Action	Half Life	Side Effects	Monitoring
Topicals				
Corticosteroids	Multiple		Atrophy, striae, purpura, pigment changes	
Pimecrolimus Tacrolimus	Calcineurin inhibitor		Stinging with application Malignancy risk from these topicals has been called into question[69,70]	
Crisaborole[17,c]	Phosphodiesterase-4 (PDE4) inhibitor		Mild stinging with application	
Ruxolitinib[16,c]	Janus Kinase (JAK)1/2 inhibitor		Acne. Oral JAK inhibitors carry other risks of uncertain relevance for topical. 10%–20% max Body Surface Area (BSA)	Consider pretreatment tuberculosis (TB) testing to screen for latent tuberculosis infection (LTBI)
Lidocaine	Sodium channel blockade		Safe when used on limited BSA	
Pramoxine	Sodium channel blockade		Safe when used on limited BSA	
Camphor/Menthol	Activates temperature sensitive receptors			
N-palmitoylethanolamine (N-PEA)	Endocannabinoid			
Ketamine-Lidocaine-Amitriptyline	Multiple			
Capsaicin	Desensitization of temperature sensitive receptors		Burning with application.	
Narrow Band Ultraviolet B exposure (NB-UVB)	Cutaneous immunosuppression		Skin burn, hyperpigmentation, photoaging, skin cancer	Annual skin examination for skin cancer
Systemics				
Diphenhydramine	First generation H1 blocker	4 h	Sedation, caution in older adults	
Hydroxyzine		20 h		

Drug	Class/Mechanism	Half-life	Adverse effects	Screening/Monitoring
Fexofenadine Loratadine Cetirizine	Second generation H1 blocker	14.4 h 8–11 h 8.3 h	Sedation	
Selective serotinin reuptake inhibitor (SSRI)	Serotonin reuptake inhibitor	Varied	Varied	
Tricyclic Antidepressant (TCA)	Serotonin and/or norepinephrine reuptake inhibitor	Varied	Varied	
Gabapentin	Uncertain	5–7 h	Sedation	
Pregabalin	Uncertain	6.3 h	Sedation	
Naltrexone	Mu-opioid receptor competitive antagonist	4 h	Sedation	
Difelikefalin[c]	Kappa-opioid receptor agonist	23–31 h	Sedation, vomiting, diarrhea	
Dupilumab[15,c]	Anti-IL-4 receptor	10–12 wk	Conjunctivitis, facial rash	Avoid live vaccines
Tralokinumab[14,c] Lebrikizumab[a,c]	Anti-IL-13	3 wk 3 wk	Conjunctivitis	Avoid live vaccines
Nemolizumab[a,c]	Anti-IL-31 receptor	17 d		
Abrocitinib[13,c] Upadacitinib[27,c]	JAK1 inhibitor	5 h 9–14 h	Acne LTBI reactivation Lymphoma Solid tumor malignancies Nonmelanoma skin cancer (NMSC) Leukopenias Thrombosis Stroke Intestinal perforation Major Adverse Cardiovascular Event (MACE)	Pretreatment screening: TB, Human Immunodeficiency Virus (HIV), Hepatis B Virus (HBV) Hepatitis C Virus (HCV) Complete Blood Count (CBC), Liver Function Tests (LFTs) and Lipids Monitoring: CBC, LFTs (upadacitinib), lipids q3m
Baricitinib[12 b,c] Gusacitinib[a,b,c]	JAK1/2 inhibitor Pan-JAK/SYK inhibitor	12 h 7 h	Presumably similar to JAK1 inhibitors	Presumably similar to JAK1 inhibitors

A nonexhaustive list of topical and systemic approaches to treatment of pruritus and/or atopic dermatitis. Green shaded boxes are more likely to be prescribed only by dermatologists as their high costs often require extensive authorization with insurance.

[a] Not approved in US currently.
[b] Off label for atopic dermatitis.
[c] More likely to be prescribed by dermatologists as their high costs often require extensive authorization with insurance.

FDA-approved IL-31 inhibitor at the time of this publication. Many of these newer medicines may not be prescribed by generalists but their widespread use necessitates awareness of potential side effects and monitoring requirements as some carry significant risk.[12–17]

As mentioned above, the JAK inhibitors carry a long list of potential serious side effects, though the most common side effect patients describe is worsening acne, the so called "JAKne," which can be treated like typical acne.[18] Severe complications like thrombosis, stroke, major adverse coronary events (MACE), intestinal perforation, skin cancer, and solid tumor malignancies are concerns especially when treating older patients. Please see the psoriasis discussion below for a discussion about perioperative use, with live vaccinations, and use in pregnancy.

Atopic Dermatitis

Atopic dermatitis (AD) is a common condition usually starting in infancy that often improves with age but persists in many adults as well. Often described as the "itch that rashes," it is usually distributed on the cheeks in infants, progresses to the neck and flexural folds in the toddler years and persists in these areas but is often less predictably localized (ie, *atopic*) in adults (**Fig. 3**). In addition to the intense pruritus and scaly erythematous involved skin, postinflammatory hyperpigmentation (PIH) can occur in areas of intense inflammation. These changes occur in all skin types but are most pronounced in more richly melanized baseline skin and can lead to unwanted pigmentary changes even long after the rash is controlled. AD is felt to be due to a defective barrier in the stratum corneum early in life that allows irritants and microbes to penetrate the superficial skin and trigger an immune response that leads to the rash and pruritus characteristic of the disease.

Treatment of AD is usually based on 4 pillars that must all be addressed for a successful outcome: addressing dry skin, inflammation, pruritus, and infection. These are critically important to manage this chronic condition and have been well reviewed elsewhere, so we will focus on relatively recent additions to our armamentarium for the treatment of inflammation and pruritus, all of which were discussed in the pruritus section above.[19]

Topical treatments for AD have expanded from the still effective mainstays of treatments such as topical steroids and calcineurin inhibitors to include FDA approvals for a PDE4 inhibitor and a topical JAK inhibitor (see **Table 3**). As is the case for many new

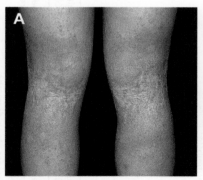
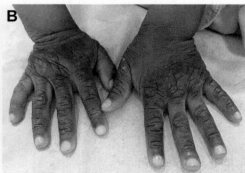

Fig. 3. (*A, B*) Ill-defined erythematous plaques with scale and varying degrees of hyperpigmentation in atopic dermatitis. ([*A*] *From* James WD et al: Andrews' diseases of the skin, ed 12, Philadelphia, 2016, Elsevier, Figure E2 [*B*] Robert G. Micheletti et al., Andrews' Diseases of the Skin Clinical Atlas, 2nd edition, 2023, Elsevier.)

medicines, cost is the biggest side effect of treatment for both creams. Systemic treatments for AD have exploded in number since the approval of the anti-IL4 antibody, dupilumab, in 2017 which is the first drug to shut down the inflammatory pathways that make atopic dermatitis miserable without broad immunosuppression. Subsequently, biologic agents targeting the similar IL13 are approved or in the pipeline and a novel anti-IL31 inhibitor is likely to be approved soon that may target the pruritus of AD more directly. A number of small molecules targeting the JAK pathway are also approved or in the pipeline for AD and some are also used for psoriasis. These oral medicines may be more appealing than the injected biologics, but they come with a longer list of potentially serious side effects as previously discussed. Please see the psoriasis discussion below for a discussion about use perioperatively, with live vaccinations, and use in pregnancy.

Psoriasis

Plaque psoriasis is the most common variant of psoriasis and typically develops in young adulthood (**Figs. 4** and **5**). Treatment of cutaneous plaque psoriasis with phototherapy, topical steroids, calcineurin inhibitors, calcipotriene, coal tar, and salicylic acid, as well as systemics like methotrexate and cyclosporine are all mainstays of treatment of mild to moderate psoriasis that are best-reviewed elsewhere.[20–22] They should remain first-line options for treatment as they are effective both for psoriasis and for cost control.

Two topicals have been approved more recently for plaque psoriasis. Roflumilast cream is a PDE4 inhibitor that is associated with a risk of diarrhea that is far better than its systemic cousin, apremilast, yet may limit treatment in those affected.[23] Tapinarof cream is the first approved aryl hydrocarbon receptor agonist and is well tolerated, with folliculitis and contact dermatitis being its primary side effects.[24] In addition, tapinarof is also produced by some bacteria which may make this "natural" attribute more appealing to some patients.[25]

An array of systemic agents has also been developed for psoriasis recently, from the biologic agents to the similarly expensive PDE4, JAK, and TYK inhibitors (**Table 4**). All of these are usually prescribed by dermatology but often have side effects of which generalists should be aware when comanaging these patients.

The first biologics approved for psoriasis were the TNF inhibitors in 1998. TNF inhibition poses a significant risk of reactivation and dissemination for those with LTBI so testing prior to initiation and then annually is recommended for TNF inhibitors. Pretreatment tests for HIV, HBV, and HCV are also important so that treatment can be initiated prior to starting long term immunosuppression. Newer biologics such as inhibitors of IL-17A, IL12/23, and IL23 carry similar, though likely lower risks, and all carry similar recommendations for pretreatment testing and ongoing TB monitoring.

The small molecule inhibitors to PDE4, JAK1, JAK3, and TYK2 may carry similar infectious and malignancy risks while also posing unique additional risks. JAK inhibitors may raise the risk of solid tumors and nonmelanoma skin cancers.[26,27] The JAK and TYK inhibitors carry a risk of intestinal perforation and may raise lipids, though it's unclear if this is clinically relevant.[26–28] The TYK2 inhibitor may be associated with rhabdomyolysis as well.[28]

Given that all biologics are at least narrowly immunosuppressive, patients needing to schedule surgery are often advised to stop their biologic in advance. The guidelines of the joint American Academy of Dermatology and National Psoriasis Foundation (AAD-NPF) recommend continuing biologic medications for any surgery that will not breach contaminated tissues such as known infections or the respiratory,

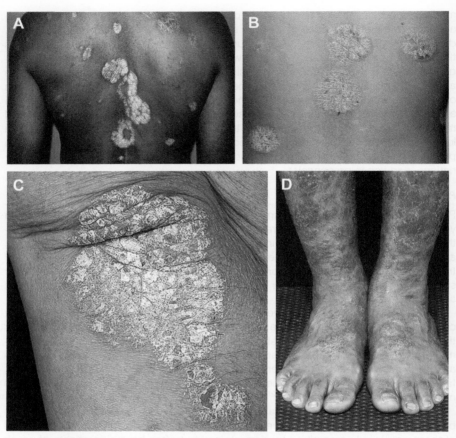

Fig. 4. (*A-D*) Note the well-defined erythematous plaques with adherent scale seen on the back and extensor surfaces predominantly. ([*A*] Robert G. Micheletti et al., Andrews' Diseases of the Skin Clinical Atlas, 2nd edition, 2023, Elsevier. [*B*] With permission from Julie V. Schaffer, MD. [*C*] *From* Ball, J.W., Dains, J.E., Flynn, J.A., Solomon, B.S., & Stewart, R.W. (2023). Seidel's guide to physical examination, (10th ed.). St. Louis: Elsevier. [*D*] Farrar, J., Garcia, P. J., Hotez, P. J., Junghanss, T., Kang, G., Lalloo, D., & White, N. J. Manson's Tropical Diseases, 24th edition, 2023 Elsevier.)

genitourinary, or intestinal tracts in which contamination with flora would be expected. Orthopedic, ophthalmic, and breast surgeries are examples of typically low risk surgeries. For higher risk surgeries, it is recommended to stop the biologic for 3 to 4 half-lives prior to surgery and restart 2 weeks postoperatively if no complications have arisen.[29] There are no clear guidelines for the small molecule inhibitors to PDE4, JAK1/3, and TYK2, yet their shorter half-lives make cessation perioperatively easier.

Live vaccines are not recommended while on any of these biologics or small molecule inhibitors. AAD-NPF recommends stopping for 2 to 3 half-lives of a biologic prior to a live vaccine and restarting 2 weeks after vaccination.[29]

TNF inhibitors are considered generally safe in pregnancy while a lack of data for the remaining IL12/23, IL17 A, IL23 inhibitor biologics and the PDE4, JAK1/3, and TYK2 inhibitors prevents recommendations for pregnancy risk.[29]

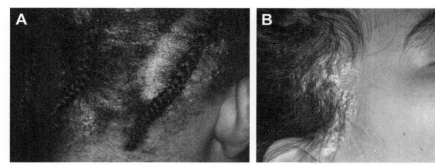

Fig. 5. (*A*, *B*) Scalp psoriasis with well-defined erythematous plaques and adherent, powdery, white, thickened scale. ([A] Amy S Paller, Anthony J. Mancini, Paller and Mancini - Hurwitz Clinical Pediatric Dermatology, 6th edition, 2021, Elsevier. [B] Lemmi F, Lemmi C: Physical assessment findings CD-ROM, Philadelphia, 2013, Saunders.)

Alopecia

One of the more common dermatologic complaints seen by dermatologists and primary care physicians is alopecia or hair loss. For a discussion of the numerous inflammatory, genetic, infectious, and other causes of alopecia, please see our previous article.[2] Here we will update treatments for pattern hair loss as well as pathogenesis and treatment updates for Central Centrifugal Cicatricial Alopecia (CCCA).

Pattern Hair Loss

Historically, androgenetic alopecia (AGA) or male pattern hair loss (MPHL) were used to describe the pattern of bitemporal and/or vertex recession more common in cisgender men while female pattern hair loss (FPHL) described a pattern of crown thinning without hairline recession more common in cisgender women (**Fig. 6**). As either pattern can be seen in either gender, the term pattern hair loss (PHL) has become accepted.[30]

Any discussion of treatment should include acceptance, as PHL is common. Coverup techniques can be effective and there are many nonmedical treatments for PHL such as platelet-rich plasma injection, hair transplantation, or laser/light treatment we will not discuss here as they are unlikely to be performed by a primary care clinician. Topical minoxidil and oral finasteride are both approved for PHL, and spironolactone is commonly used as an off-label treatment due to its effect on androgen levels. The only recent new addition to our treatments of PHL is low dose minoxidil (LDM) (**Table 5**).

Minoxidil is an antihypertensive that results in generalized hypertrichosis by an unknown mechanism and is commonly used as a topical preparation to encourage the growth of hairs with thicker diameter and length. LDM has the potential benefit of also lowering blood pressure. Side effects tend to be dose dependent, with hypertrichosis being by far the most common side effect, and less commonly, pedal edema and hypotension. Doses used in males are all off label, but usually 2.5-5 mg daily and in females 1.25 to 2.5 mg daily. The sex-based dosing difference is likely due to its effect on hypertrichosis, which is more often unwanted in people assigned female at birth, but it's important to work with each individual to find what dose is most appropriate for their goals.

It is worth noting that topical minoxidil, LDM, and spironolactone are classes of medicines used in primary care, and generalists should feel comfortable offering these

Table 4
Medications for psoriasis

Drug	Mechanism of Action	Half Life	Side Effects	Testing Required
Topicals				
Corticosteroids	Multiple		Atrophy, striae, purpura, pigment changes	
Pimecrolimus Tacrolimus	Calcineurin inhibitor		Stinging with application Malignancy risk from these topicals has been called into question[69,70]	
Calcipotriene	Vitamin D analog			
Salicylic acid	Comedolytic			
Coal Tar	Multiple		Staining of skin	
Roflumilast[23]	PDE4 inhibitor		Diarrhea, nausea, headache	
Tapinarof[26]	Aryl hydrocarbon receptor agonist		Folliculitis, Contact Dermatitis	
Narrow Band Ultraviolet B exposure (NB-UVB)	Cutaneous immunosuppression		Skin burn, hyperpigmentation, photoaging, skin cancer	Annual skin examination for skin cancer
Systemics				
Methotrexate	Dihydrofolate reductase inhibitor prevents T lymphocyte proliferation		Hepatotoxicity, pulmonary fibrosis, teratogenic, nausea, fatigue, hair loss	Pretreatment screening: HIV, HBV, HCV, CBC, CMP, HCG (if applicable) Monitoring: CBC, CMP, HCG (if applicable)
Cyclosporine	Calcineurin inhibitor		Hypertension, renal failure, hypomagnesemia, immunosuppression, hypertrichosis	Monitoring: Weekly blood pressure checks, CBC, Creatinine, Magnesium

Drug	Class	Half-life	Adverse effects	Screening/Monitoring
Acitretin	Vitamin A analog		Hepatotoxicity, teratogenic, hypertriglyceridemia, dry skin	Monitoring: CBC, CMP, Triglycerides, HCG (if applicable)
Etanercept[a]	Tumor Necrosis Factor (TNF) inhibitor	3.5 d	LTBI reactivation	Pretreatment screening: TB (skin test or interferon gamma release assay), HIV, HBV, HCV; Monitoring: Annual TB screening recommended. There are no other specific monitoring recommendations.
Adalimumab[a]		14 d	Hepatitis B reactivation	
Infliximab[a]		10 d	Invasive Fungal Infections	
Ustekinumab[a]	IL12/23 inhibitor	21 d	Lymphoma	
Guselkumab[a]	IL23 inhibitor	18 d	Demyelinating disease	
Risankizumab[a]		11 d	CHF exacerbation	
Tildrakizumab[a]		23 d		
Ixekizumab[a]	IL17 A inhibitor	13 d	Same as above and also:	
Secukinumab[a]		27 d	Inflammatory bowel disease	
Brodalumab[a]		11 d	Oral or esophageal candidiasis. Brodalumab specifically also carries an additional risk of suicide	
Apremilast[a]	PDE4 inhibitor	6–9 h	Diarrhea; Risk of suicide	Pretreatment screening: none; Monitoring: Annual TB screening recommended. There are no other specific monitoring recommendations.
Upadacitinib[27,a]	JAK1 inhibitor	9–14 h	Acne; LTBI reactivation; Lymphoma; Solid tumor malignancies; NMSC; Leukopenias; Intestinal perforation; Thrombosis; Stroke; Major adverse coronary events	Pretreatment screening: TB, HIV, HBV, HCV, CBC, LFTs, and Lipids; Monitoring: CBC, LFTs, Lipids q3m
Tofacitinib[26,a]	JAK1/3 inhibitor	3 h		

(continued on next page)

Table 4
(continued)

Drug	Mechanism of Action	Half Life	Side Effects	Testing Required
Deucravacitinib[a]	Tyrosine Kinase 2 (TYK2) inhibitor	10 h	LTBI reactivation Lymphoma Rhabdomyolysis	Pretreatment screening: TB, HIV, HBV, HCV, Creatinine, LFTs, and Triglycerides Monitoring: Triglycerides q3m, and additionally LFTs if concern for liver disease

[a] More likely to be prescribed by dermatologists as their high costs often require extensive authorization with insurance.
A nonexhaustive list of topical and systemic approaches to treatment of psoriasis.

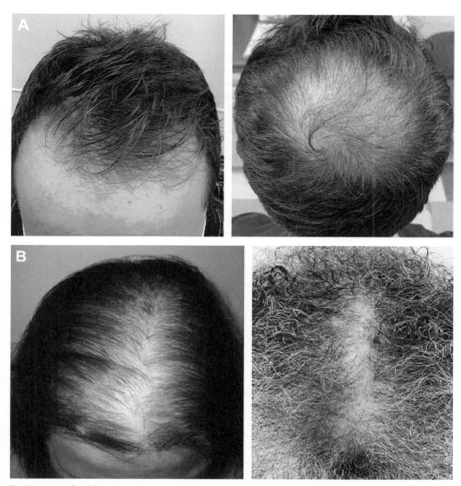

Fig. 6. Note the bitemporal recession seen in pattern hair loss (PHL) most common in cisgender and transgender men (*Upper*) or the widened partline or generalized thinning of the crown seen in PHL commonly in cisgender women (*Lower*). ([*Upper*] Murad Alam, Jeffrey S. Dover, Procedures in Cosmetic Dermatology: Hair Restoration, 1st Edition, 2022, Elsevier. [*Lower*] Murad Alam, Jeffrey S. Dover, Procedures in Cosmetic Dermatology: Hair Restoration, 1st Edition, 2022, Elsevier.)

to their patients without consultation with a dermatologist as the ratio of people with PHL to board-certified dermatologists in the US is approximately 6000:1.

Central centrifugal cicatricial alopecia

CCCA is a pattern of permanent scarring hair loss most common in women of African ancestry living in the United States and is often misdiagnosed as PHL. As its name suggests, it starts centrally near the vertex of the scalp and expands outward leaving behind scarring hair loss in its wake. It sometimes results in obvious scar lacking any hairs, but more commonly spares many hairs giving the clinical appearance of a thinned crown similar to PHL (**Fig. 7**). Originally termed "hot comb alopecia" for its

Table 5
Medications for alopecia

Drug	Dosing	Side Effects	Mechanism of Action
Minoxidil topical	2% solution for women—BID 5% solution for men—BID 5% foam for either men BID or women once daily	Local irritation is more common in the solution formulas due to propylene glycol[71] Tachycardia and presyncopal symptoms are similar to placebo[71] Hypertrichosis from accidental application to other areas.	Unknown
Minoxidil oral, low dose	1.25-5 mg daily	Hypertrichosis of facial and body hair Pedal edema Tachycardia and hypotension at higher doses	Unknown
Finasteride oral	1 mg daily	Contraindicated in pregnancy and donating blood is not recommended within 1 mo of taking finasteride. Erectile dysfunction, loss of libido in 1%–10% of males[72] Reduction in PSA may interfere with prostate cancer screening	Type II 5-alpha-reductase inhibitor
Dutasteride oral	0.5 mg daily	Similar to finasteride	Type I & II 5-alpha-reductase inhibitor
Spironolactone oral	50–200 mg daily	Gynecomastia, breast tenderness, irregular menses at higher doses Contraindicated in pregnancy Hypotension Hyperkalemia May be a banned substance for competitive athletes	Inhibits testosterone production. Competitively inhibits the androgen receptor

A nonexhaustive list of topical and systemic nonsurgical approaches to treatment of pattern hair loss.

correlation with the use of heated metal combs for hair straightening, it has been attributed to various hair care practices for decades though the actual evidence for this has been called into question as these practices are common and may result from confirmation bias.[31,32] Recently, a potentially causative mutation in PADI3 was identified in about a third of patients with CCCA that may result in hair shaft rupture and subsequent scarring inflammation.[33] CCCA differs from traction alopecia in which

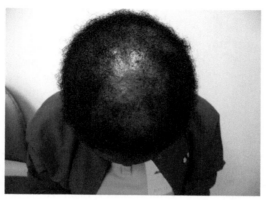

Fig. 7. Thinning of hair on the crown seen in CCCA, which can mimic Pattern Hair Loss as the inflammation and scarring present can be subtle on clinical examination. (*From* Tosti A. Diseases of Hair and Nails. In: Goldman L and Cooney KA, eds. Goldman-Cecil Medicine. Volume 1. 27th Edition. Elsevier; 2024 : 2747–2755, Figure 409.8.)

scarring occurs from tight hairstyles, often along the frontal or temporal hairlines, however, tension may play a role in CCCA as well. There are no standard recommendations for hair styling for CCCA, and specific recommendations require cultural humility and familiarity with a variety of hair care practices. Avoiding traction hairstyles and manipulation at the vertex as well as avoiding chemical treatments such as relaxers or hair dyes may be helpful as general recommendations. Initial treatment is with topical or intralesionally injected corticosteroids, systemic antibiotics such as tetracyclines, and early referral to a dermatologist to help slow progression.[32]

Facial Rashes

In this section we will discuss the treatment of acne vulgaris, acne rosacea, periorificial dermatitis, and seborrheic dermatitis.

Acne vulgaris

Acne vulgaris is the most common skin condition affecting young adults. Although most cases of acne vulgaris start in adolescence and resolve by the mid-20s, up to 50% of patients will have symptoms into later adulthood.[34] Acne vulgaris is a chronic, inflammatory condition that significantly impacts quality of life and mental health. Acute treatment followed by maintenance therapy can improve dermatologic and quality of life outcomes.

Understanding the pathogenesis of acne vulgaris helps to clarify the treatment approach. Androgen-induced increased sebum production in the pilosebaceous unit followed by abnormal keratinization leads to occlusion of the follicle, creating a microcomedone. Bacterial colonization of the hair follicle with *Cutibacterium* (formally *Propionibacterium) acnes* triggers a host immune response leading to the development of inflammatory lesions.[34,35] Areas with the highest sebaceous gland activity are most affected including the face, back, chest, shoulders, and torso.

Acne vulgaris can range in severity from mild comedonal (**Fig. 8**A) to inflammatory to severe nodulocystic (**Fig. 8**B). Regardless of the type of acne vulgaris, a topical comedolytic is necessary to address the abnormal keratinization and microcomedone formation that is a hallmark of this condition. Setting appropriate expectations for management is also important. Treatments for acne vulgaris do not address lesions

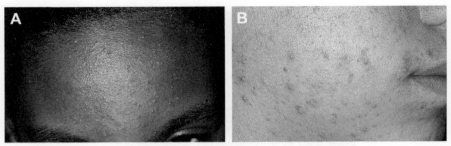

Fig. 8. (*A*) Acne vulgaris presenting predominantly as comedones (*B*) Acne vulgaris presenting as inflammatory and nodulocystic acne. ([*A*] *From* Paller AS, Mancini AJ: Hurwitz clinical pediatric dermatology, a textbook of skin disorders of childhood and adolescence, ed 5, Philadelphia, 2016, Elsevier, Figure E2. [*B*] Thomas P. Habif (2018), Skin Disease-Diagnosis & Treatment:First South Asia Edition, 1st edition, Elsevier India.)

that are already present but do prevent the development of new lesions. It takes approximately 8 weeks for a microcomedone to mature so patients should be counseled that they may not see improvement in their skin for several months. It is also important to counsel patients to apply medications to the entire location affected by acne rather than spot treatments for active lesions. For acne involving the shoulders, chest, and torso, benzoyl peroxide (BP) washes will be easiest to apply and provide both comedolytic and antiinflammatory activity.

Topical comedolytics are available over the counter or by prescription (**Table 6**.) The Global Alliance to Improve Outcomes in Acne Group recommends topical retinoids as first-line agents when possible since they are more efficacious than other comedolytics and improve penetration of other topical agents such as antibiotics.

Traditionally, topical retinoids were applied at night because tretinoin can be deactivated by light and increase the risk of photosensitivity. However, many newer formulations are more stable in light but can still cause photosensitivity. Side effects include

Table 6
Treatment of primarily comedonal acne

Comedolytic	Options	Considerations
Topical retinoids	• Tretinoin (Rx) • Tazarotene (Rx) • Adapalene (OTC and Rx) • Trifarotene (Rx)	• Tretinoin: Least expensive • Tazarotene: Most potent • Adapalene: Least irritating to skin • All may decrease post inflammatory hyperpigmentation • Avoid use during pregnancy
Benzoyl peroxide (BP)-OTC and Rx		• May bleach clothes, towels, etc
Azelaic acid-Rx		• Good for sensitive skin • May cause hypopigmentation
Salicylic acid-OTC		• Good for sensitive skin
Tea Tree oil-OTC		• May cause contact dermatitis

Abbreviations: OTC, over the counter; Rx, by prescription.
Topical comedolytic medications to be used for both initial and maintenance therapy for acne. Consider adding combined oral contraceptive and/or spironolactone in females to any treatment above.

redness, dry skin, peeling, and burning. Starting at a lower potency every few nights and titrating to the highest potency up to nightly as tolerated will improve efficacy and decrease side effects. To improve adherence, it is important to counsel patients that treatment will often trigger a pustular flare and their skin may worsen before it improves.

Retinoid formulations vary based on cost and side effects. Tretinoin is the least expensive option, tazarotene is the most potent, and adapalene is the least likely to irritate the skin and the only over-the-counter option. If cost or tolerance of retinoid side effects is a barrier, then tea tree oil, salicylic acid, and benzoyl peroxide can be used and are similarly efficacious for the treatment of comedonal acne, though also carry their own side effects (see **Table 6**). Patients with more pigmented skin are at higher risk of developing PIH and scarring, such as keloids, from acne vulgaris lesions and from skin irritation due to the products used to treat acne. Prevention is key. Slow titration of topical agents can lessen the risk of skin irritation. Since some PIH is caused by visible light, the use of iron oxide containing sunscreens can help block both UV light and visible light and prevent the progression of hyperpigmentation.[36] Different shades of iron oxide are used in many tinted sunscreens which patients may find appealing if their goal is to decrease the cosmetic appearance of PIH. To accelerate the resolution of hyperpigmentation, topical retinoids or azelaic acid can be added to acne treatment regimens.[37]

For primarily inflammatory acne, an antibiotic can be used in addition to the comedolytic (**Tables 7** and **8**). Antibiotics should not be used as monotherapy because even with primarily inflammatory acne, the base lesion is still the microcomedone which is treated with comedolytic maintenance therapy. To decrease the

Table 7
Treatment of Primarily Inflammatory Acne (mild to moderate)

Treatment	Topical Options	Considerations
Topical retinoid alone	See **Table 6**	
Benzoyl peroxide alone	Gel, lotion, cream, foam, wash	• May bleach clothes, towels, etc
Topical retinoid + benzoyl peroxide		• May bleach clothes, towels, etc
Topical antibiotic + benzoyl peroxide	• Clindamycin • Minocycline • Dapsone • Sulfur/sulfacetamide • Erythromycin	• Clindamycin: Least costly • Minocycline: More expensive • Dapsone: expensive. Okay with G6PD deficiency and sulfur allergy. Avoid use with BP as can cause temporary yellow-orange skin/hair discoloration. • Erythromycin: Refrigerate. Increasing rates of resistance. Not first line.
Topical retinoid + topical antibiotic + benzoyl peroxide		Most effective

Regimens to treat inflammatory acne may include monotherapy or a combination of medications with different mechanisms of action. Continue comedolytic (retinoid, BP or azelaic acid) for maintenance therapy. Add BP to decrease antibiotic resistance if antibiotics to be used longer than 2 mo. Try to discontinue antimicrobials at 3 months. Consider adding combined oral contraceptive and/or spironolactone in females to any treatment above.

Table 8
Treatment of primarily Inflammatory Acne (moderate to severe)

Treatment	Options	Side Effects	Dosing
Topical retinoid + oral antibiotic + benzoyl peroxide	• Doxycycline • Minocycline • Sarecycline • Azithromycin (if allergic to tetracyclines)	• Doxycycline: pill esophagitis, GI upset, photosensitivity, contraindicated in pregnancy • Minocycline: vestibular symptoms, irreversible bluish-grey discoloration to skin, drug-induced lupus, contraindicated in pregnancy • Azithromycin: GI upset, QT prolongation in high-risk patients	• Doxycycline 100 mg po qd or bid • Minocycline 100 mg po qd or bid • Sarecycline dosing is weight based • Azithromycin 500 mg po 3 x per week x 1 mo, then 500 mg 2 x per week x 1 mo, then 500 mg weekly x 1 mo OR 500 mg on day 1 followed by 250 mg daily for 4, repeated on 1st and 15th of every month for 3 mo
Topical benzoyl peroxide + topical antibiotic + oral antibiotic			
Topical retinoid + topical antibiotic + oral antibiotic + benzoyl peroxide			

Regimens to treat inflammatory acne may include monotherapy or a combination of medications with different mechanisms of action. Continue comedolytic (retinoid, BP or azelaic acid). Add BP if antibiotics to be used longer than 2 mo. Try to discontinue antimicrobials at 3 months, continue comedolytic long term. Refer to dermatology for oral isotretinoin if severe or refractory acne. Consider adding combined oral contraceptive and/or spironolactone in females to any treatment above.

development of *C. acnes* antibiotic resistance, use of topical and oral antibiotics should be limited to patients who really need them and for the least amount of time possible, ideally no more than 3 months of therapy.[34,38,39] If topical or oral antibiotics are needed for longer than 2 months, evidence suggests that topical benzoyl peroxide should also be started because its nonspecific antimicrobial activity can prevent selective resistance at sites of application.[34,40] It is best to apply topical antibiotics and benzoyl peroxide in the morning and retinoid in the evening as benzoyl peroxide can decrease the stability of topical tretinoin. Once acne has improved, antibiotics should be discontinued and comedolytic medication should be continued for maintenance therapy.[33,38]

The anti-inflammatory rather than antibacterial properties of antibiotics are likely the most helpful effect in the treatment of acne vulgaris and acne rosacea.[40] Consequently, treatment has shifted to using topical antibiotics and/or sub-antimicrobial dose oral antibiotics. Data demonstrate that sub-antimicrobial doses are effective in treating acne with potentially less risk for antibiotic resistance.[38] Topical antibiotic options include clindamycin, minocycline, dapsone, sulfur/sulfacetamide or erythromycin, some of which are combined with a retinoid or benzoyl peroxide. Studies have demonstrated that combination antibiotic-comedolytic medications are more effective in treating inflammatory acne than monotherapy.[40] Topical dapsone 5% is also used in the treatment of acne and is safe in patients with G6PD deficiency or sulfonamide allergies.[40,41] There have been no direct comparisons of topical dapsone to topical clindamycin or erythromycin. Some early data in India suggests that topical minocycline may be more effective than topical clindamycin.[42] The cost of topical dapsone and minocycline compared to these other agents likely outweighs any benefits of these products at this time. Due to increasing evidence of antibacterial resistance to C acnes with erythromycin, the other topical antibiotics are preferred. In 2020, the FDAapproved clascoterone, a topical androgen receptor inhibitor. Data from two phase 3 randomized trials demonstrated improved efficacy compared to placebo in patients with moderate to severe acne. Side effects include local skin irritation and some reports of hypothalamic-pituitary axis suppression.[43]

Oral antibiotics may be necessary to treat moderate to severe inflammatory acne (see **Table 8**). Tetracyclines such as doxycycline, minocycline, or sarecycline are mainstays of therapy. There is no difference in efficacy between doxycycline and minocycline, however because of the side effect profiles of both, doxycycline is generally recommended as the first-line agent.[40] Doxycycline side effects include gastrointestinal upset, pill esophagitis, and photosensitivity. Minocycline may cause vestibular symptoms, irreversible bluish-grey skin discoloration, and drug-induced lupus. Sarecycline has a narrower spectrum of antibiotic activity, lower propensity to promote C acnes resistance, and potentially less disruption of the gut microbiome. Side effects are otherwise similar to other tetracyclines.[44] Traditional dosing for doxycycline and minocycline is 100 mg once or twice daily however studies demonstrate equal or improved efficacy with sub-antimicrobial dosing regimens such as doxycycline 40 mg ER daily or 20 mg twice a day with less side effects.[45] Sarecycline dosing is weight based. For those who are allergic to tetracyclines, the macrolide azithromycin is an option. Randomized controlled trials comparing azithromycin to doxycycline, minocycline, and tetracycline demonstrate that it is at least equally effective and, in some cases, even more effective. In these studies, azithromycin was pulse-dosed; however, a recommended dosing regimen has yet to be determined.[40] Due to concerns about rising antibiotic resistance to azithromycin, tetracyclines should be used if possible, however, azithromycin is a safe option during pregnancy and breastfeeding, whereas all tetracyclines are contraindicated due to the risk of permanent teeth discoloration. Not enough data exists to determine if cephalosporins, trimethoprim-sulfamethoxazole, or fluoroquinolones are effective in the treatment of acne.[40]

Postmenarchal females with moderate to severe acne may benefit from the use of combined oral contraceptives and/or spironolactone. Spironolactone is typically dosed at 50 to 100 mg daily, where side effects are rare and evaluation of potassium levels is generally unnecessary in otherwise healthy females under the age of 45. There may be additional benefit when hormonal agents are combined with other topical therapies. Finally, patients with severe nodulocystic acne or acne that is refractory to treatment can be referred to dermatology to discuss oral isotretinoin.

Clinics Care Points: Acne Vulgaris

- A topical comedolytic such as retinoids or benzoyl peroxide should be used throughout treatment.
- Topical or oral antibiotics should be used in conjunction with a comedolytic medication, not as monotherapy.

- Patients with darkly pigmented skin are at higher risk of developing postinflammatory hyperpigmentation (PIH). The use of iron oxide sunscreen blocks visible light in addition to UV light and can help prevent the progression of PIH, while topical retinoids or azelaic acid can be used to lighten PIH.

- For acne that doesn't respond to first-line treatment, consider adding combined oral contraceptive and/or spironolactone in females

Acne rosacea

Like acne vulgaris, acne rosacea is a chronic inflammatory disorder with periods of exacerbation and remission. It typically presents in the 30-60s and affects the central face, nose, cheeks, eyelids, forehead and chin in all skin colors. Symptoms include flushing, nontransient erythema, telangiectasias, papules, pustules, nodules, cysts or sebaceous gland hypertrophy (eg, rhinophyma) (**Fig. 9**). Ocular involvement with blepharitis or conjunctivitis is present in more than 50% of patients and may be found in the absence of other skin manifestations of rosacea.[46] Rosacea appears to be due to a combination of factors including abnormalities in innate immunity, inflammatory reactions to cutaneous microorganisms, ultraviolet damage, and vascular dysfunction, although the pathogenesis is not well understood. Topical and oral therapies work well for papules and pustules but less so or not at all for flushing, redness, or telangiectasias. Patients should be counseled to avoid excessive sun exposure, that it may take 2 to 3 months of treatment before improvement is seen, and that since this is a chronic condition maintenance therapy is recommended.[47]

The topical agents ivermectin, metronidazole, and azelaic acid are first-line treatments for rosacea (**Table 9**). Randomized controlled trials demonstrate improved efficacy of topical ivermectin compared to topical metronidazole and azelaic acid, however the cost is significantly higher.[48,49] Data demonstrate that azelaic acid is at least equally and possibly more efficacious to topical metronidazole, although topical metronidazole is better tolerated and less expensive.[50] Topical minocycline 1.5% foam is effective but costly and no studies are available comparing it to other topical options.[51] Topical sulfacetamide 10%/sulfur 5% or combination benzoyl peroxide/clindamycin is also an option, however the data for efficacy is less robust. Data supporting monotherapy with topical clindamycin or erythromycin is limited and due to the potential risk of antibiotic resistance should be avoided.[40] Data is limited on whether

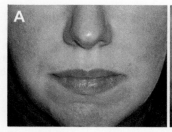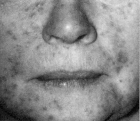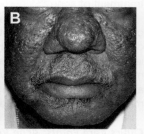

Fig. 9. (*A*) Flushing, papules and pustules seen with acne rosacea (*B*) Sebaceous gland hypertrophy of the nose, also known as rhinophyma, seen with severe acne rosacea. ((a) Richard L. Gallo, et al., Standard classification and pathophysiology of rosacea: The 2017 update by the National Rosacea Society Expert Committee, Journal of the American Academy of Dermatology, 78 (1), 2018, 148-155, https://doi.org/10.1016/j.jaad.2017.08.037. (b) *With permission from* James W, Elston D, McMahon PJ. Andrews' diseases of the skin clinical atlas. Elsevier; 2018, Figure 27.31.)

Table 9
Treatment of papulopustular lesions of rosacea

Treatment[a,b]	Considerations
Topical ivermectin	Most effective. Expensive
Topical metronidazole	Well tolerated
Topical azelaic acid	May cause hypopigmentation
Topical minocycline foam	Expensive
Oral antibiotics • Doxycycline • Minocycline	• See side effect profiles in **Table 8** • Use sub-antimicrobial dosing for mild-moderate disease and full dose for moderate to severe • Full dose 100 mg po QD or BID • Doxycycline DR 40 mg PO QD. Expensive • Doxycycline 20 mg PO BID • Doxycycline 25 mg/5 mL suspension 25 mg PO BID
Oral isotretinoin	Refer to dermatology if severe or refractory rosacea or development of sebaceous gland hyperplasia

[a] Combine topical and oral options for increased effectiveness. Once symptoms improve, discontinue oral antibiotics.
[b] Continue topical treatments long term for maintenance.

topical retinoids are effective in the treatment of the papulopustular lesions of rosacea.[52]

Oral antibiotics should be considered for moderate to severe rosacea not responding to topical therapies, and for ocular rosacea. The only systemic FDA-approved therapy for rosacea is once daily extended-release sub-antimicrobial dose (40 mg) doxycycline, which has been shown to have similar efficacy to doxycycline 100 mg dose regimens but with substantially fewer adverse effects, such as gastrointestinal symptoms.[52] Maintenance therapy with a topical agent should be continued long term. For severe cases, a few studies demonstrate added benefit when combining oral antibiotics with topical metronidazole and topical ivermectin.[53,54] Oral isotretinoin also may be effective. Referral to dermatology should be considered for patients with moderate to severe disease or development of focal enlargement due to sebaceous gland hypertrophy (eg, rhinophyma) to help reduce the risk of poor cosmetic outcomes.

Flushing can be a particularly bothersome symptom of rosacea. A variety of agents have been tried including clonidine, beta-blockers, antidepressants, and gabapentin but data is limited and side effects can be significant. Avoidance of triggers such as extremes of temperature, sunlight, spicy foods, and alcohol may be effective but difficult to adhere to. For patients with papulopustular rosacea, topical antibiotics may reduce facial erythema but no high-quality studies have evaluated efficacy in patients without papulopustular lesions. The topical alpha-agonists, brimonidine 0.33% gel and oxymetazoline 1% cream, can reduce fixed facial erythema and telangiectasias through transient vasoconstriction of superficial blood vessels but are costly, infrequently covered by insurance, have mixed outcomes, and do not improve papulopustular lesions.[55] Both agents are recommended for daily use and will reduce facial erythema within 30 minutes of application and peak around 3 to 6 hours after application, after which effects progressively diminish. Both agents can cause burning and contact dermatitis. Brimonidine may be more effective than oxymetazoline; however, the risk of worsening redness and rebound erythema with prolonged use is greater with brimonidine. Oxymetazoline may worsen papulopustular lesions.[52] Some patients may consider using either of these agents on an as needed basis for special occasions.

To help reduce cost, over-the-counter oxymetazoline nasal spray can be mixed with a moisturizer and used preventatively or as needed after symptom onset. Referral to dermatology for pulsed light therapy and laser therapy can be considered for the treatment of telangiectasias and nontransient erythema.

Clinics Care Points: Acne Rosacea

- Topical metronidazole, azelaic acid, or ivermectin are first-line therapies. If suboptimal response to topical therapies, oral antibiotics such as doxycycline can be added to topical maintenance therapy. Oral isotretinoin may also be effective.

- Treatment of flushing can be challenging. Counsel patients on avoidance of triggers. Trials of topical alpha-agonists such as brimonidine and oxymetazoline may be helpful, though they may also be costly.

- Refer to dermatology early if severe presentation and/or sebaceous gland hypertrophy (eg, rhinophyma) to help reduce the risk of poor cosmetic outcomes. Dermatologists can also use pulsed light therapy and/or laser therapy to treat flushing.

Periorificial dermatitis

Periorificial dermatitis, or perioral dermatitis, typically presents with multiple small inflammatory papules around the mouth, nose or eyes often sparing the vermillion border, though can also present as scaly, hypopigmented macules and patches in darkly pigmented skin (**Fig. 10**). Although the name suggests an eczematous appearance, it most closely resembles an acneiform or rosacea-like eruption with or without eczematous features. Exposure to external elements likely triggers these lesions with the strongest association with topical or inhaled corticosteroids and the use of masks. Other triggers may include fluorinated toothpastes, heavy face creams, and moisturizers, especially those with a petrolatum or paraffin base, and certain cosmetics like lipsticks.[56]

The most important intervention is to discontinue the inciting agent which is called "zero therapy." Periorificial dermatitis may self-resolve within a few months if triggers can be eliminated. However, stopping the inciting agent can cause an initial flare of the rash, leading many patients to request therapy. When caused by topical steroids, tapering from a higher potency to a lower potency steroid such as hydrocortisone

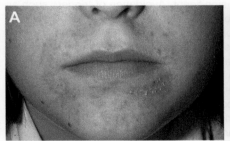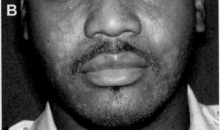

Fig. 10. (*A*) Perioral papules sparing the vermillion border in periorificial dermatitis, (*B*) Hypopigmentation due to seborrheic dermatitis. ([*A*] Habif, T. P. (2015). Clinical Dermatology: A Color Guide to Diagnosis and Therapy. Saunders. [*B*] With permission from Scott Norton, MD.)

1% over a few months and then discontinuing entirely may reduce the likelihood of a significant flare but this approach has not been well studied.[57] For mild to moderate cases, consider using topical calcineurin inhibitors. Most of the placebo controlled randomized trial data supports the use of pimecrolimus 1% cream twice a day with most benefit shown in the first few weeks of therapy.[58,59] Therapy should continue for about 4 to 8 weeks and then either be discontinued if effective or changed to a different therapy if ineffective. A less costly option would be the use of topical metronidazole or erythromycin, both of which have shown better efficacy when compared to placebo.

The use of oral tetracycline has also demonstrated efficacy in small, randomized controlled trials when compared to topical therapy.[60,61] Both groups showed improvement in lesion counts however the oral antibiotic group improved faster. There are no studies examining the efficacy of doxycycline or minocycline; however, these regimens are often tried for 8 weeks because of their advantage of fewer restrictions on timing of administration. Dosing is similar to the treatment of acne vulgaris and acne rosacea. If patients are allergic to tetracyclines, azithromycin can be used but dosing is unclear. Small, uncontrolled studies or case reports have shown some benefit with azelaic acid 20% cream, topical tetracycline, topical adapalene 0.1% gel, topical clindamycin with or without hydrocortisone 1%, and topical sulfacetamide-sulfur plus oral tetracyclines.

Clinics Care Points: Periorificial Dermatitis

- Assess for possible triggers (eg: topical or oral steroids, masks, fluorinated toothpaste) and recommend discontinuation if appropriate. If topical steroid use is a trigger, recommend tapering from higher potency to low-potency steroid use for weeks to months and counsel patients that the condition may flare before improving after discontinuing topical steroid use.

- Topical calcineurin inhibitors such as pimecrolimus may be used for 4 to 8 weeks for treatment though if cost is a concern, trial topical metronidazole or erythromycin instead.

- Oral tetracycline has been shown to be more effective than topical metronidazole. Other oral antibiotics that may be helpful include doxycycline and minocycline. Topical therapy should be continued.

Seborrheic dermatitis

Erythema accompanied by greasy looking, yellowish scale in the eyebrows, glabella, lateral nasal areas, and melolabial folds is characteristic of seborrheic dermatitis (**Fig. 11**). The mustache and beard areas, scalp, external auditory canals, chest, axilla, and groin may also be affected. Seborrheic dermatitis is a chronic, relapsing condition that flares with psychological stress, changes in weather, or lack of regular shampooing; therefore, acute treatment followed by maintenance therapy is needed.

The only new therapy for the treatment of seborrheic dermatitis, is the addition of roflumilast foam, a PDE4 inhibitor described for psoriasis, previously (**Table 10**). For acute treatment, either topical low-potency corticosteroids or topical calcineurin inhibitors may be used once or twice a day until symptoms resolve. These will rapidly improve the inflammation but are not appropriate for maintenance use. Two doses of oral fluconazole separated by a week can temporarily clear the skin quickly but is not appropriate as maintenance therapy due to the risk of liver dysfunction and drug interactions. For maintenance therapy of facial symptoms, intermittent use of topical antifungal creams or antifungal/antiseborrheal shampoos to wash the face can be effective though are slower to show initial benefit. In more heavily pigmented skin,

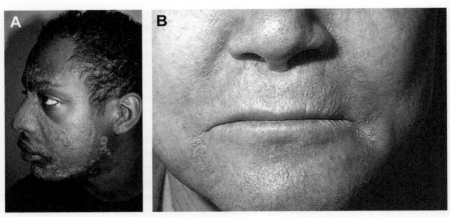

Fig. 11. (*A*) Discolored, scaly plaques with or without erythema can be seen in seborrheic dermatitis, (*B*) Discolored, scaly plaques with or without erythema can be seen in seborrheic dermatitis. (*From*: (A) James WD et al: Andrews' diseases of the skin, ed 12, Philadelphia, 2016, Elsevier, figure E3(B) Morse SA, Holmes KK, Ballard RC, Moreland AA: Atlas of Sexually Transmitted Diseases and AIDS, 4th ed, Philadelphia, Saunders Elsevier, 2010, p 9, see Fig. 1.24.).

SD may cause hypopigmentation that typically resolves with treatment, though pimecrolimus can treat both SD and hypopigmentation.[62] For scalp symptoms, antifungal shampoos are effective and rotating between different active ingredients with each shampooing is usually even more effective. For those who wash their hair less often, ketoconazole foam or roflumilast foam can be applied to the scalp and left in, though patients should also be counseled that infrequent hair washing can lead to product build-up that leads to scalp irritation which exacerbates SD symptoms.[63] Compared to natural hairstyles, use of hair extensions may also contribute to scalp irritation and inflammation that leads to SD.[63] Over-the-counter antidandruff shampoos can be used but these often contain sodium lauryl sulfate which can be irritating and cause hair breakage, further damaging hair that has undergone heat or chemical relaxer treatments.[63,64]

CLINICS CARE POINTS: SEBORRHEIC DERMATITIS

- For treatment of acute episodes, topical low-potency corticosteroids or calcineurin inhibitors can be used until symptoms resolve. Alternatively, 2 doses of oral fluconazole can also clear acute symptoms.
- Maintenance therapy options include antifungal creams or shampoos and antidandruff shampoos.
- Pimecrolimus can treat both SD and associated hypopigmentation.
- For those who wash their hair less often, ketoconazole foam or roflumilast foam can be applied and left on the scalp though patients should also be counseled that product build-up may irritate the scalp and exacerbate SD symptoms.

Stasis Dermatitis

Stasis dermatitis is a common complication of chronic lower extremity edema. When this chronic edema acutely worsens, the skin can become red and scaly with serous

Table 10
Treatment of seborrheic dermatitis

Medication	Formulation	Side Effects
Hydrocortisone, topical	2.5% cream BID PRN flares	Steroid atrophy, pigment changes, telangiectasias, purpura, acne, rosacea, perioral dermatitis
Desonide, topical	0.05% cream BID PRN flares	Same as above
Triamcinolone, topical	0.1% cream for 1 week PRN flares	Same as above
Pimecrolimus, topical	1% cream BID PRN flares	Stinging or burning with application May help treat hypopigmentation associated with SD
Roflumilast, topical	0.3% foam daily	Nasopharyngitis, nausea, and headache. Foam is flammable. High cost
Ciclopirox, topical	0.77% cream BID or 1% shampoo with each hair washing or alternating with another similar shampoo	
Fluconazole, Oral	400 mg PO weekly for 2 wk	Drug interactions
Zinc Pyrithione, topical	1% shampoo with each hair washing or alternating with another similar shampoo	
Selenium Sulfide, topical	1%–2.5% shampoo with each hair washing or alternating with another similar shampoo	
Ketoconazole, topical	2% cream or foam BID or 1%–2% shampoo with each hair washing or alternating with another similar shampoo	
Salicylic acid, topical	3% shampoo with each hair washing or alternating with another similar shampoo	

drainage and crust (dried serum) and can mimic cellulitis or erysipelas. In stasis dermatitis, erythema involves only the leg, respecting the anatomic boundaries of the ankle and knee, typically only on the lower half of the shin and calf (**Fig. 12**). The bilateral nature of the skin changes coupled with the slow development of symptoms over weeks rather than hours or days suggests dermatitis rather than cellulitis. Pruritis is usually the predominant complaint in dermatitis.

The prevention of dermatitis is important and can be achieved by gentle cleansing, treatment of xerosis with emollients, leg elevation, and the use of compression stockings (at least 20–30 mm Hg or use two 15–20 mm Hg worn on top of each other). A 2012 Cochrane review demonstrated that horse chestnut extract dosed at 300 mg twice a day (50 mg escin-active component) may decrease leg volume and circumference at ankle and calf through venoconstriction. Side effects are rare but may cause an increase in bleeding, gastrointestinal symptoms and worsen kidney disease.[65] Micronized purified flavonoid fraction (MPFF-diosmiplex) dosed at 450 mg micronized purified Diosmin twice a day in conjunction with compression demonstrated improved healing of venous ulcers (<10 mm in size), edema and pain compared to placebo with minimal side effects.[66]

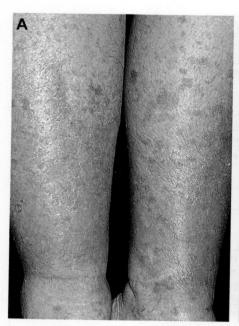 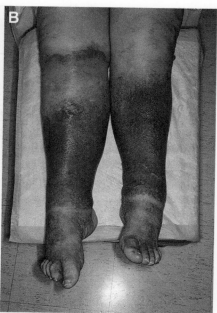

Fig. 12. (*A*) Erythema and scaling of the skin over the lower legs seen with stasis dermatitis, (*B*) Erythema and scaling of the skin over the lower legs seen with stasis dermatitis. ([*A*] *From Swartz MH. Textbook of Physical Diagnosis. 4th ed. Philadelphia: Elsevier; 2001, Figure 3.27 [B] Thomas P. Habif et al., Skin Disease: Diagnosis and Treatment, 4th Edition, 2018, Elsevier.*)

Once statis dermatitis develops, acute inflammation can be treated using a moderate potency topical corticosteroid such as triamcinolone 0.1% ointment applied twice a day to the affected areas. Systemic treatment with a short course of prednisone can be helpful in severe cases. Exudative eczematous changes can be addressed by applying wet dressings saturated with tap water or saline and covered with light, air permeable, dry cotton to the legs for 2 to 3 hours up to three times per day followed by the application of emollients. Wet dressings may be used in conjunction with topical corticosteroids to increase penetration and absorption.

SUMMARY

Patients often present to primary care providers with dermatologic complaints. When considering topical therapies, it is important to remember that the vehicle also carries therapeutic benefits and potential side effects. Many common dermatologic conditions will respond to similar medications including topical steroids, steroid-sparing agents such as topical calcineurin inhibitors, retinoids, antifungal medications, and antibiotics. Although most of the newer biologic agents and JAK inhibitors are typically prescribed by dermatologists, familiarity with the common side effects or complications of these treatments is important for primary care clinicians caring for these patients long term. Recognizing when conditions are chronic and require maintenance therapy provides better long-term outcomes, and discontinuing therapies when no longer indicated reduces adverse events. We hope to have provided useful approaches for treatment of conditions commonly encountered in the primary care setting.

DISCLOSURE

The authors have no conflicts of interest to report including no financial conflicts of interest.

REFERENCES

1. Lowell BA, Froelich CW, Federman DG, et al. Dermatology in primary care: Prevalence and patient disposition. J Am Acad Dermatol 2001;45(2):250–5.
2. Vary JC, O'Connor KM. Common dermatologic conditions. Med Clin North Am 2014;98(3):445–85.
3. K. B, L. Y, C. E. Confidence and skill in managing skin disorders in African-Americans. J Invest Dermatol 2011;131.
4. Adelekun A, Onyekaba G, Lipoff JB. Skin color in dermatology textbooks: An updated evaluation and analysis. J Am Acad Dermatol 2021;84(1):194–6.
5. Chang MJ, Lipner SR. Resources for skin of color images. J Am Acad Dermatol 2021;84(6):e275–7.
6. Vincent CY, Li MMUC, Chowdhury MM. Dermatological pharmacology: topical agents, Medicine. Medicine 2021;49(6):350–4.
7. Samarasekera EJ, Sawyer L, Wonderling D, et al. Topical therapies for the treatment of plaque psoriasis: systematic review and network meta-analyses. Br J Dermatol 2013;168(5):954–67.
8. Shive M, Linos E, Berger T, et al. Itch as a patient-reported symptom in ambulatory care visits in the United States. J Am Acad Dermatol 2013;69(4):550–6.
9. Whang KA, Khanna R, Williams KA, et al. Health-Related QOL and Economic Burden of Chronic Pruritus. J Invest Dermatol 2021;141(4):754–60.e1.
10. Roh YS, Choi J, Sutaria N, et al. Itch: Epidemiology, clinical presentation, and diagnostic workup. J Am Acad Dermatol 2022;86(1):1–14.
11. Kim BS, Bissonnette R, Nograles K, et al. Phase 2 Trial of Difelikefalin in Notalgia Paresthetica. N Engl J Med 2023;388(6):511–7.
12. OLUMIANT Lilly. (baricitinib) [package insert]. U.S. Food and Drug Administration website. Available at: https://www.accessdata.fda.gov/drugsatfda_docs/label/2022/207924s006lbl.pdf.RevisedMay2022. [Accessed 7 January 2024].
13. Pfizer. CIBINQOTM (abrocitinib). [package insert]. U.S. Food and Drug Administration website. Available at: https://www.accessdata.fda.gov/drugsatfda_docs/label/2022/213871s000lbl.pdf. [Accessed 7 January 2024].
14. LEO Pharma Inc. ADBRY (tralokinumab-ldrm) [package insert]. U.S. Food and Drug Administration website. https://www.accessdata.fda.gov/drugsatfda_docs/nda/2022/761180Orig1s000lbl.pdf. [Accessed 7 January 2024].
15. Sanofi, Regeneron Pharmaceuticals, Inc. DUPIXENT (dupilumab) [package insert]. U.S. Food and Drug Administration website. Available at: https://www.accessdata.fda.gov/drugsatfda_docs/label/2017/761055lbl.pdf. [Accessed 7 January 2024].
16. Incyte. OPZELURA (ruxolitinib) [package insert]. U.S. Food and Drug Administration website. Available at: https://www.accessdata.fda.gov/drugsatfda_docs/label/2022/215309s001lbl.pdf. [Accessed 7 January 2024].
17. Pfizer. EUCRISA (crisaborole) [package insert]. U.S. Food and Drug Administration website. Available at: https://www.accessdata.fda.gov/drugsatfda_docs/label/2020/207695s007s009s010lbl.pdf. [Accessed 7 January 2024].
18. Correia C, Antunes J, Filipe P. Management of acne induced by JAK inhibitors. Dermatol Ther 2022;35(9). https://doi.org/10.1111/DTH.15688.

19. Sidbury R, Alikhan A, Bercovitch L, et al. Guidelines of care for the management of atopic dermatitis in adults with topical therapies. J Am Acad Dermatol 2023; 89(1):e1–20.

20. Elmets CA, Korman NJ, Prater EF, et al. Joint AAD-NPF Guidelines of care for the management and treatment of psoriasis with topical therapy and alternative medicine modalities for psoriasis severity measures. J Am Acad Dermatol 2021;84(2): 432–70.

21. Menter A, Gelfand JM, Connor C, et al. Joint American Academy of Dermatology-National Psoriasis Foundation guidelines of care for the management of psoriasis with systemic nonbiologic therapies. J Am Acad Dermatol 2020;82(6):1445–86.

22. Elmets CA, Lim HW, Stoff B, et al. Joint American Academy of Dermatology-National Psoriasis Foundation guidelines of care for the management and treatment of psoriasis with phototherapy. J Am Acad Dermatol 2019;81(3):775–804.

23. Arcutis Biotherapeutics, Inc. ZORYVE (roflumilast) [package insert]. U.S. Food and Drug Administration website. Available at: https://www.accessdata.fda.gov/drugsatfda_docs/label/2022/215985s000lbl.pdf. [Accessed 7 January 2024].

24. Dermavant. VTAMA (tapinarof). [package insert]. U.S. Food and Drug Administration website. https://www.accessdata.fda.gov/drugsatfda_docs/label/2022/215272s000lbl.pdf. [Accessed 7 January 2024].

25. Smith SH, Jayawickreme C, Rickard DJ, et al. Tapinarof Is a Natural AhR Agonist that Resolves Skin Inflammation in Mice and Humans. J Invest Dermatol 2017; 137(10):2110–9.

26. Pfizer. XELJANZ (tofacitinib) [package insert]. U.S. Food and Drug Administration website. Available at: https://www.accessdata.fda.gov/drugsatfda_docs/label/2018/203214s018lbl.pdf. [Accessed 7 January 2024].

27. AbbVie Inc. RINVOQ (upadacitinib) [package insert]. U.S. Food and Drug Administration website. Available at: https://www.accessdata.fda.gov/drugsatfda_docs/label/2022/211675s003lbl.pdf. [Accessed 7 January 2024].

28. Bristol-Myers Squibb Company. SOTYKTU™ (deucravacitinib) [package insert]. U.S. Food and Drug Administration website. Available at: https://www.accessdata.fda.gov/drugsatfda_docs/label/2022/214958s000lbl.pdf. [Accessed 7 January 2024].

29. Menter A, Strober BE, Kaplan DH, et al. FROM THE ACADEMY Joint AAD-NPF guidelines of care for the management and treatment of psoriasis with biologics. J Am Acad Dermatol 2019;80(4):1029–72.

30. Gao JL, Sanz J, Tan N, et al. Androgenetic alopecia incidence in transgender and gender diverse populations: A retrospective comparative cohort study. J Am Acad Dermatol 2023;89(3):504–10.

31. Dlova NC, Jordaan FH, Sarig O, et al. Autosomal dominant inheritance of central centrifugal cicatricial alopecia in black South Africans. J Am Acad Dermatol 2014;70(4):679–82.e1.

32. George EA, Matthews C, Roche FC, et al. Beyond the hot comb: updates in epidemiology, pathogenesis, and treatment of central centrifugal cicatricial alopecia from 2011 to 2021. Am J Clin Dermatol 2023;24(1):81–8.

33. Malki L, Sarig O, Romano MT, et al. Variant PADI3 in central centrifugal cicatricial alopecia. N Engl J Med 2019;380(9):833–41.

34. Thiboutot D, Gollnick H, Bettoli V, et al. New insights into the management of acne: an update from the Global Alliance to Improve Outcomes in Acne group. J Am Acad Dermatol 2009;60(5 Suppl). https://doi.org/10.1016/J.JAAD.2009.01.019.

35. Williams HC, Dellavalle RP, Garner S. Acne vulgaris. Lancet 2012;379(9813): 361–72.
36. Iron oxides in novel skin care formulations attenuate blue light for enhanced protection against skin damage. J Cosmet Dermatol 2020. https://doi.org/10.1111/jocd.13803.
37. Elbuluk N, Grimes P, Chien A, et al. The pathogenesis and management of acne-induced post-inflammatory hyperpigmentation. Am J Clin Dermatol 2021;22(6): 829–36.
38. Simonart T. Newer approaches to the treatment of acne vulgaris. Am J Clin Dermatol 2012;13(6):357–64.
39. Gamble R, Dunn J, Dawson A, et al. Topical antimicrobial treatment of acne vulgaris: an evidence-based review. Am J Clin Dermatol 2012;13(3):141–52.
40. Mays RM, Gordon RA, Wilson JM, et al. New antibiotic therapies for acne and rosacea. Dermatol Ther 2012;25(1):23–37.
41. Stotland M, Shalita AR, Kissling RF. Dapsone 5 gel: A review of its efficacy and safety in the treatment of acne vulgaris. Am J Clin Dermatol 2009;10(4):221–7.
42. Shah B, Mistry D, Gonsalves N, et al. A Prospective, randomized, comparative study of topical minocycline gel 4% with topical clindamycin phosphate gel 1% in indian patients with acne vulgaris. Antibiotics 2023;12(9). https://doi.org/10.3390/ANTIBIOTICS12091455.
43. Hebert A, Thiboutot D, Stein Gold L, et al. Efficacy and safety of topical clascoterone cream, 1%, for treatment in patients with facial acne: two phase 3 randomized clinical trials. JAMA Dermatol 2020;156(6):621–30.
44. Zhanel G, Critchley I, Lin LY, et al. Microbiological profile of sarecycline, a novel targeted spectrum tetracycline for the treatment of acne vulgaris. Antimicrob Agents Chemother 2018;63(1). https://doi.org/10.1128/AAC.01297-18.
45. Moore A, Ling M, Bucko A, et al. Efficacy and safety of subantimicrobial dose, modified-release doxycycline 40 mg versus doxycycline 100 mg versus placebo for the treatment of inflammatory lesions in Moderate and Severe Acne: A Randomized, Double-Blinded, Controlled Study. J Drugs Dermatol JDD 2015;14(6): 581–6.
46. Gallo R, Drago F, Paolino S, et al. Rosacea treatments: What's new and what's on the horizon? Am J Clin Dermatol 2010;11(5):299–303.
47. van Zuuren EJ, Fedorowicz Z, Tan J, et al. Interventions for rosacea based on the phenotype approach: an updated systematic review including GRADE assessments. Br J Dermatol 2019;181(1):65–79.
48. Taieb A, Ortonne JP, Ruzicka T, et al. Superiority of ivermectin 1% cream over metronidazole 0·75% cream in treating inflammatory lesions of rosacea: a randomized, investigator-blinded trial. Br J Dermatol 2015;172(4):1103–10.
49. Taieb A, Khemis A, Ruzicka T, et al. Maintenance of remission following successful treatment of papulopustular rosacea with ivermectin 1% cream vs. metronidazole 0.75% cream: 36-week extension of the ATTRACT randomized study. J Eur Acad Dermatol Venereol 2016;30(5):829–36.
50. May D, Kelsberg G, Safranek S. What is the most effective treatment for acne rosacea? J Fam Pract 2011;60(2):100c–8a.
51. Gold LS, Rosso JQ Del, Kircik L, et al. Open-label extension study evaluating long-term safety and efficacy of FMX103 1.5% minocycline topical foam for the treatment of moderate-to-severe papulopustular rosacea. J Clin Aesthet Dermatol 2020;13(11):44. Available at: http://pmc/articles/PMC7716737/. [Accessed 2 January 2024].

52. van Zuuren EJ. Rosacea. In: Solomon CG, editor. N Engl J Med 2017;377(18): 1754–64. https://doi.org/10.1056/NEJMCP1506630.

53. Schaller M, Kemény L, Havlickova B, et al. A randomized phase 3b/4 study to evaluate concomitant use of topical ivermectin 1% cream and doxycycline 40-mg modified-release capsules, versus topical ivermectin 1% cream and placebo in the treatment of severe rosacea. J Am Acad Dermatol 2020;82(2):336–43.

54. Sanchez J, Somolinos AL, Almodóvar PI, et al. A randomized, double-blind, placebo-controlled trial of the combined effect of doxycycline hyclate 20-mg tablets and metronidazole 0.75% topical lotion in the treatment of rosacea. J Am Acad Dermatol 2005;53(5):791–7.

55. Okwundu N, Cline A, Feldman SR. Difference in vasoconstrictors: oxymetazoline vs. brimonidine. J Dermatolog Treat 2021;32(2):137–43.

56. Lipozenčić J, Hadžavdić SL. Perioral dermatitis. Clin Dermatol 2014;32(1): 125–30.

57. Hasan Hafeez Z. Perioral dermatitis: an update. Int J Dermatol 2003;42(7):514–7.

58. Oppel T, Pavicic T, Kamann S, et al. Pimecrolimus cream (1%) efficacy in perioral dermatitis - results of a randomized, double-blind, vehicle-controlled study in 40 patients. J Eur Acad Dermatol Venereol 2007;21(9):1175–80.

59. Schwarz T, Kreiselmaier I, Bieber T, et al. A randomized, double-blind, vehicle-controlled study of 1% pimecrolimus cream in adult patients with perioral dermatitis. J Am Acad Dermatol 2008;59(1):34–40.

60. Weber K, Thurmayr R, Meisinger A, et al. Journal of Dermatological Treatment A topical erythromycin preparation and oral tetracycline for the treatment of perioral dermatitis: a placebo-controlled trial A topical erythromycin preparation and oral tetracycline for the treatment of perioral dermatitis: a placebo-controlled trial. Journal of Dermatological Trearmenr 1993;4:57–9.

61. Veien NK, Munkvad JM, Otkjaer Nielsen A, et al. Topical metronidazole in the treatment of perioral dermatitis. J Am Acad Dermatol 1991;24(2 Pt 1):258–60.

62. High WA, Pandya AG. Pilot trial of 1% pimecrolimus cream in the treatment of seborrheic dermatitis in African American adults with associated hypopigmentation. J Am Acad Dermatol 2006;54(6):1083–8.

63. Elgash M, Dlova N, Ogunleye T, et al. Seborrheic dermatitis in skin of color: clinical considerations. J Drugs Dermatol 2019;18(1):24–7.

64. Chatrath S, Bradley L, Kentosh J. Dermatologic conditions in skin of color compared to white patients: similarities, differences, and special considerations. Arch Dermatol Res 2023;315(5):1089–97.

65. Underland V, Sæterdal I, Nilsen ES. Cochrane summary of findings: horse chestnut seed extract for chronic venous insufficiency. Glob Adv Health Med 2012; 1(1):122.

66. Guilhou JJ, Dereure O, Marzin L, et al. Efficacy of Daflon 500 mg in venous leg ulcer healing: a double-blind, randomized, controlled versus placebo trial in 107 patients. Angiology 1997;48(1):77–85.

67. Wolverton SE. Comprehensive dermatologic drug therapy. Published online 2007:1099.

68. Sutaria N, Adawi W, Goldberg R, et al. Itch: Pathogenesis and treatment. J Am Acad Dermatol 2022;86(1):17–34.

69. Devasenapathy N, Chu A, Wong M, et al. Cancer risk with topical calcineurin inhibitors, pimecrolimus and tacrolimus, for atopic dermatitis: a systematic review and meta-analysis. Lancet Child Adolesc Health 2023;7(1):13–25.

70. Asgari MM, Tsai AL, Avalos L, et al. Association between topical calcineurin inhibitor use and keratinocyte carcinoma risk among adults with atopic dermatitis. JAMA Dermatol 2020;156(10):1066–73.
71. Olsen EA, Whiting D, Bergfeld W, et al. A multicenter, randomized, placebo-controlled, double-blind clinical trial of a novel formulation of 5% minoxidil topical foam versus placebo in the treatment of androgenetic alopecia in men. J Am Acad Dermatol 2007;57(5):767–74.
72. Kaufman KD, Olsen EA, Whiting D, et al. Finasteride in the treatment of men with androgenetic alopecia. Finasteride Male Pattern Hair Loss Study Group. J Am Acad Dermatol 1998;39(4 Pt 1):578–89.

Newer Therapies in Rheumatology

Alison Bays, MD, MPH, Gregory C. Gardner, MD, MACP*

KEYWORDS

- Treatment • Spondyloarthropathy • Gout • Polymyalgia rheumatica
- Systemic lupus • Scleroderma • Rheumatoid arthritis • Psoriatic arthritis

KEY POINTS

- A variety of new medications have recently been approved to treat rheumatologic diseases.
- These therapies harness the increasing knowledge of the immune system.
- Most of the newer therapies are biologic agents that affect specific components of the immune system.
- Side effects of concern are primarily infection related due to the impact of these therapies on immune function.

INTRODUCTION

1998 was a landmark year in rheumatology with the introduction of etanercept as the first biologic medication available to treat a rheumatologic illness namely rheumatoid arthritis (RA). Since then, a multitude of new agents, principally biologics, have been introduced to treat inflammatory rheumatologic illnesses. Even the nonbiologic agents have become more specific in their immune activity. This article will discuss newer agents to treat rheumatologic illnesses and the disease for which they have been approved to provide context and structure.

AXIAL SPONDYLOARTHRITIS AND NON-RADIOGRAPHIC SPONDYLOARTHRITIS

Axial spondylitis (AS) is an inflammatory form of arthritis that affects the axial skeleton especially in men with peak onset in the 20s and 30s. Some patients with AS signs and symptoms but no radiographic changes are referred to as having non-radiographic spondyloarthritis (NrSpA).

Division of Rheumatology, University of Washington, 1959 Pacific Street, Box 356428, Seattle, WA 98195, USA
* Corresponding author. 1959 Pacific Street, Box 356428, Seattle, WA 98195.
E-mail address: rheumdoc@uw.edu

Med Clin N Am 108 (2024) 829–842
https://doi.org/10.1016/j.mcna.2024.02.004
0025-7125/24/© 2024 Elsevier Inc. All rights reserved.
medical.theclinics.com

UPADACITINIB (RINVOQ)

Upadacitinib, a Janus kinase (JAK) inhibitor, was approved for AS in April 2022 for patients with AS who have had an inadequate response to 1 or more tumor necrosis factor (TNF) inhibitors. The approval of upadacitinib was based on data from 2 studies that demonstrated its efficacy compared to placebo for both AS and NrSpA.[1,2] The primary endpoint of the studies was the ASAS 40. ASAS stands for assessment in ankylosing spondylitis and is a patient-reported instrument that has 4 components. ASAS 40 is at least a 40% response in 3 of the 4 categories and no worsening in the fourth.

EFFICACY

1. The approved dose is 15 mg of upadacitinib once a day.
2. 52% of the upadacitinib group with AS achieved an ASAS 40 response compared to 26% in the placebo group. The NrSpA group data were similar (45% vs 23%). Both results were statistically significant.
3. Patients taking upadacitinib for AS and NrSpA also demonstrated significant reduction of inflammation of the spine and sacroiliac joints on MRI scan compared to placebo.

SAFETY

Upadacitinib has been approved for several other inflammatory diseases and there is a wealth of safety data available.[3] No new safety signals were seen in the studies for AS/NrSpA. Patients taking upadacitinib can develop an asymptomatic elevation in total creatinine kinase, especially in those who are physically active. The package insert–indicated serious side effects (SEs) can include infection, cancer, thromboembolic disease, and cardiovascular events in those over 50 years old with at least 1 cardiovascular risk factor.

CONCLUSION

Upadacitinib is a welcome addition to the growing armamentarium for treating AS and NrSpA. Its ability to influence MRI changes is an indication of its ability to influence the underlying inflammatory process in these diseases.

GOUT

Gout is one of the most common forms of inflammatory arthritis affecting over 9.2 million people in the United States, representing 3.9% of the population.

CANAKINUMAB (ILARIS)

Canakinumab is a recently approved medication (August 2023) for the treatment of gouty flares in people in whom nonsteroidal anti-inflammatory drugs (NSAIDs) or colchicine is contraindicated, not tolerated, or provides inadequate response. It is also indicated for people in whom repeated courses of corticosteroids may not be appropriate.

Canakinumab is a monoclonal antibody that neutralizes interleukin (IL)-1β an important cytokine that is produced during a gouty attack. It has been approved for other conditions where IL-1 is a key cytokine such as periodic fever syndromes, systemic juvenile inflammatory arthritis, and adult-onset Still's disease. It has a long half-life of 27.2 days and makes it useful for specific aspects of gout therapy.[4]

EFFICACY

Data were presented to the Food and Drug Administration (FDA) in 2011 for approval in gout treatment but the application was rejected at that time due to insufficient data on safety. Three randomized controlled trials serve as the foundation for the recent FDA approval.[5-7] Two were done in patients who were not candidates for therapy with NSAIDs or colchicine. The third was done to compare canakinumab with colchicine prophylaxis while initiating urate-lowering therapy (ULT). Findings from the 3 trials indicate the following:

1. The optimum dose of canakinumab is 150 mg by subcutaneous injection.
2. A single dose of canakinumab was superior to the comparator medication, triamcinolone (TA) 40 mg intramuscularly with regards to pain reduction and swelling but not redness beginning at 6 hours after dosing and at 72 hours which was the primary objective time point.
3. Canakinumab is also superior to TA at preventing recurrent flares of gout up to 60 days after dosing.
4. Canakinumab even at doses lower than 150 mg can prevent flares of gouty arthritis with the initiation of ULT and is superior to colchicine prophylaxis. Flare after starting ULT is a common problem and results when serum uric acid is lowered and leads to resorption of urate from tissue deposition sites.

SAFETY ISSUES

Overall canakinumab is well tolerated with SEs being mild to moderate in severity.[8] In the 3 trials, canakinumab has slightly more infections than the comparator agents (7.0%–20.4% vs 7.0%–12.2%) and headache (5.7%–11.3% vs 5.7%). Less than 1.2% of patients stopped the medication due to SEs.

CONCLUSION

Canakinumab can be a useful addition to the treatment options for patients with gout. Quality of life benefits are also positive. The major roadblock to use is the price tag of $16,000 dollars for a single injection.

POLYMYALGIA RHEUMATICA

Polymyalgia rheumatica (PMR) is an inflammatory disorder affecting people over the age of 50.[9] The American College of Rheumatology (ACR) endorsed guidelines in 2015 regarding the treatment of PMR, including initial steroid dosing, tapering, and initiation of methotrexate for patients at higher risk of relapse.[10] More than half of patients with PMR relapse with steroid taper. However, there were no FDA-approved medications prior to sarilumab.

SARILUMAB (KEVZARA)

Sarilumab was approved by the FDA for the treatment of PMR in 2023. It is a human monoclonal antibody that binds the IL-6α receptor, blocking the IL-6 pathway, which is important in PMR.

EFFICACY

Efficacy and safety of IL-6 blockade were shown in trials with tocilizumab, PMR-SPARE (Tocilizumab in Patients with New Onset Polymyalgia Rheumatica) and

SEMAPHORE (Safety and Efficacy of Tocilizumab vs Placebo in Polymyalgia Rheumatica with Glucocorticoid Dependence).[11,12] The FDA approval for sarilumab was based on the phase 3 SAPHYR (Evaluation of the Efficacy and Safety of Sarilumab in Patients With Polymyalgia Rheumatica) trial of 118 participants who were diagnosed with PMR, had at least 1 disease flare, and were on prednisone at a dose of 7.5 mg daily or higher.[13] Participants had a mean disease duration of 300 days and median prednisone dose of 10 mg. Participants were assigned to a 52-week steroid taper or sarilumab with a 14-week prednisone taper, and sarilumab 200 mg twice monthly. The trial was ended early due to recruitment during the coronavirus disease 19 pandemic but showed efficacy with sustained remission, improved quality of life, and reduction in the cumulative glucocorticoid dose.

SAFETY ISSUES

Neutropenia is a common SE (15%) and the most common reason for medication discontinuation. Diarrhea (12%) was also a common SE. Sarilumab has a black box warning for serious infections. Gastric perforation has been seen with sarilumab in those with and without diverticulitis, but it does not carry the black box warning for gastrointestinal perforation as with tocilizumab.

CONCLUSION

Sarilumab for patients with PMR and difficulty tapering prednisone leads to an improved quality of life, less relapses, and lower cumulative glucocorticoid doses.

PSORIATIC ARTHRITIS

Psoriatic arthritis is an inflammatory arthritis that can be erosive and deforming. It has many presentations and may co-occur with psoriasis or present prior to or after psoriasis. Classes of medications previously approved include the anti-TNFα therapies, anti-IL17 therapies, and combined IL-12/23 therapies, as well as JAK inhibitors. Though highly effective, there are various contraindications to medication groups, making this an important new approval.

GUSELKUMAB (TREMFYA)

Guselkumab was approved in 2020 by the FDA as the first IL-23 inhibitor for psoriatic arthritis. IL-23 has 2 subunits and guselkumab targets the P19 subunit of IL-23.[14] It was approved in 2017 to treat moderate to severe plaque psoriasis based on 3 phase 3 trials.[15–17]

EFFICACY

Approval was based on the DISCOVER-1 (Guselkumab in Patients with Active Psoriatic Arthritis who were Biologic-Naive Or Had Previously Received TNFα Inhibitor Treatment) and DISCOVER-2 (Guselkumab in Biologic-Naive Patients with Active Psoriatic Arthritis) phase 3 trials.[14,18] These trials compared guselkumab 100 mg every 4 weeks, every 8 weeks (after 2 induction doses), and placebo in patients who had failed standard treatment and who also had psoriasis. Patients were required to have at least 4 months of apremilast and at least 3 months of non-biologic disease-modifying antirheumatic drugs (DMARDs) or NSAIDs. About 30% of the participants can have received 1 or 2 TNFα inhibitors. The primary endpoint was ACR 20%

improvement. No serious adverse events occurred in the every-4-week group, 4 adverse events in the every-8-week group, and 5 patients receiving placebo.

1. The approved dose is 100 mg subcutaneously at weeks 0, 4, and then every 8 weeks.
2. Guselkumab is superior to placebo and adalimumab 40 mg subcutaneously every 2 weeks at 16 weeks.
3. Guselkumab was effective in participants who had previously failed 1 or 2 TNFα inhibitors.

SAFETY ISSUES

The serious adverse events were comparable between the guselkumab and the placebo groups.[16]

CONCLUSION

Guselkumab is an effective therapy in patients who have contraindications to other drug classes or those who have failed anti-TNFα therapy. It also has FDA approval for psoriasis.

RISANKIZUMAB (SKYRIZI)

Risankizumab is a humanized immunoglobulin G1 monoclonal antibody that inhibits IL-23 by binding to the p19 subunit. It was approved by the FDA for use in moderate to severe plaque psoriasis in 2019.

EFFICACY

FDA approval for risankizumab was obtained in 2022 on the basis of KEEPsAKE 1 (A Study Comparing Risankizumab to Placebo in Participants with Active Psoriatic Arthritis who have a History of Inadequate Response to or Intolerance to at Least One DMARD Therapy) and 2 (A Study Comparing Risankizumab to Placebo in Participants With Active Psoriatic Arthritis Including Those Who Have a History of Inadequate Response or Intolerance to Biologic Therapy[ies]) trials.[19,20] The KEEPsAKE 1 trial evaluated the safety and efficacy in active psoriatic arthritis in patients who had been on at least 1 conventional synthetic DMARD (csDMARD) and the KEEPsAKE 2 trial included patients who had previously been on at least 1 or 2 biologic agents. The primary endpoint was ACR20. The patients were randomized to risankizumab versus placebo.

1. The approved dose is 150 mg subcutaneously at weeks 0, 4, and then every 12 weeks

SAFETY ISSUES

Rates of opportunistic infections were low, consistent with prior studies and not elevated over placebo dosing.

CONCLUSION

Risankizumab works better than placebo for patients who have failed csDMARDs and may be helpful for dactylitis and enthesitis. It is also approved for psoriasis.

UPADACITINIB (RINVOQ)

Upadacitinib, a selective JAK1 inhibitor, was approved for psoriatic arthritis in 2021 based on SELECT-PsA 1 (A Study Comparing Upadacitinib (ABT-494) to Placebo and to Adalimumab in Participants With Psoriatic Arthritis Who Have an Inadequate Response to at Least One Non-Biologic Disease Modifying Anti-Rheumatic Drug) and 2 (A Study Comparing Upadacitinib (ABT-494) to Placebo in Participants With Active Psoriatic Arthritis Who Have a History of Inadequate Response to at Least One Biologic Disease Modifying Anti-Rheumatic Drug) trials.[21,22] It was given to patients with active psoriatic arthritis and inadequate response or intolerance to 1 or more non-biologic DMARDs. Patients were randomized to upadacitinib 15 mg or 30 mg daily, abatacept 40 mg subcutaneously every 2weeks, or placebo with the primary endpoint ACR20. In the upadacitinib 15 mg group, 70.6% met ACR20, as did 78.5% of the upadacitinib 30 mg group, 65% with adalimumab, and 36.2% of the placebo group.

EFFICACY

1. The approved dose is 15 mg once daily.
2. Upadacitinib 15 mg daily and 30 mg daily were both superior to placebo.
3. Upadacitinib 30 mg daily was superior to adalimumab 40 mg subcutaneously every 2 weeks.

CONCLUSION

Upadacitinib adds to the available options for treating psoriatic arthritis in patients that have intolerance or inadequate response to non-biologic DMARDs. Upadacitinib is not approved for psoriasis.

RHEUMATOID ARTHRITIS

RA is an inflammatory arthritis that is a chronic and progressive disease resulting in disability when not adequately treated. There are numerous available treatments for RA yet there are many patients who fail to respond to standard therapies. It is one of the most common inflammatory forms of arthritis. The point prevalence of RA was 51/10,000 and period prevelence was 56 per 10,000 people reported in 2021.[23,24]

NEWER THERAPIES
Olokizumab (Artlegia)

Olokizumab is a humanized monoclonal antibody against the IL-6 cytokine. Two IL-6 biologics are already approved for RA: tocilizumab and sarilumab. There are 3 antigenic sites and both of the approved biologics target site 1 of IL-6, whereas olokizumab targets site 3.[25]

EFFICACY

FDA approval has not yet been obtained but is likely forthcoming after favorable phase 2 and 3 trials. There were 2 phase 2 trials showing safety and efficacy in patients that have failed TNF inhibitors and 3 phase 3 trials for patients who were inadequate responders to methotrexate.[23,25–28] The CREDO 1 (Evaluation of the Effectiveness and Safety of Two Dosing Regimens of Olokizumab (OKZ), Compared to Placebo, in Subjects With Rheumatoid Arthritis (RA) Who Are Taking Methotrexate But Have Active Disease) trial, a phase 3 trial, compared olokizumab 64 mg every 2 weeks to 64 mg every 4 weeks and showed benefit over placebo.[23] The CREDO 2 (Evaluation of the Efficacy and Safety of

Two Dosing Regimens of Olokizumab (OKZ), Compared to Placebo and Adalimumab, in Subjects With Rheumatoid Arthritis (RA) Who Are Taking Methotrexate But Have Active Disease) trial showed that in patients who had an inadequate response to methotrexate after 12 weeks, olokizumab and methotrexate was superior to placebo and methotrexate and noninferior to adalimumab and methotrexate.[28] The CREDO 3 (Evaluation of the Efficacy and Safety of Two Dosing Regimens of Olokizumab (OKZ), Compared to Placebo, in Subjects With Rheumatoid Arthritis (RA) Who Were Taking an Existing Medication Called a Tumour Necrosis Factor Alpha Inhibitor But Had Active Disease) study (phase 3) compared olokizumab 64 mg subcutaneously every 2 weeks versus every 4 weeks in patients with TNFα inhibitor failures and found that in these patients both doses of olokizumab were superior to placebo but the study was unable to compare the differences in doses. Additionally, there were some clinical outcomes that did not show improvement at week 12.[25]

SAFETY ISSUES

There were some serious infections in olokizumab when given every 2 weeks and none in patients on olokizumab every 4 weeks. Elevations in liver enzymes occurred at a higher rate than in patients taking TNFα inhibitors.

CONCLUSION

Olokizumab is awaiting FDA approval after phase 3 trials and has shown to be superior to placebo in RA in patients that have failed TNFα or methotrexate.

SCLERODERMA

Scleroderma is a relatively rare fibrosing autoimmune disease with an annual incidence of 19 cases per million. Women are overrepresented as with other autoimmune diseases.

TOCILIZUMAB (ACTEMRA)

Tocilizumab was approved for scleroderma (systemic sclerosis)-associated interstitial lung disease (SSc-ILD) in December 2022. Tocilizumab binds to both soluble and membrane-bound IL-6, an important cytokine in scleroderma. It was previously approved for RA, systemic juvenile idiopathic arthritis, and giant-cell arteritis. Approval was based on 2 randomized double-blind trials both of 48 week durations termed faSScinate (Safety and Efficacy of Subcutaneous Tocilizumab in Adults with Systemic Sclerosis) and focuSSced (A Study of the Efficacy and Safety of Tocilizumab in Participants with Systemic Sclerosis) and an extension trial of 96 weeks.[29–32]

EFFICACY

1. Dosing is 162 mg subcutaneous weekly.
2. Over 48 weeks, tocilizumab significantly slowed decline in % forced vital capacity (FVC) in patients with SSc-ILD compared to placebo. This same %FVC preservation was noted in an extension trial at 96 weeks.
3. Tocilizumab appears to impact %FVC decline no matter the degree of ILD at baseline.
4. Tocilizumab also impacts high-resolution chest computed tomography (HRCT) progression of fibrosis.
5. The randomized trials did not show a significant benefit on skin disease.

SAFETY

SEs are primarily infections. Tocilizumab can also elevate lipids, liver function tests, reduce the neutrophil count, and may increase the risk of colonic perforation in patients with diverticulitis. It has also been reported to reactivate hepatitis B so that carrier status should be ascertained prior to use.

CONCLUSION

Tocilizumab is a welcome addition to the armamentarium for treating SSc-ILD. Its ability to slow ILD progression in early and advanced disease makes it particularly useful. Its effect on HRCT progression of ILD is an important additional marker of efficacy.

SYSTEMIC LUPUS ERYTHEMATOSUS

Systemic lupus erythematosus (SLE) is an autoimmune rheumatic disease characterized by multiorgan involvement, specific autoantibodies, and female predominance.

ANIFROLUMAB (SAPHNELO)

Anifrolumab is a monoclonal antibody directed against the type 1 interferon receptor. Type 1 interferons are an important group of cytokines that drive both the innate and adaptive immune systems in SLE. It was approved in August 2021 in the United States for moderate to severe SLE as an add-on to standard therapy in patients needing additional disease control. Approval was based on 2 phase III trials TULIP (Treatment of Uncontrolled Lupus via the Interferon Pathway) 1 and 2 of 52 weeks duration each.[33,34] An in-depth review of these trials plus a phase II trial (MUSE) was done by Yoshiya and colleagues[35]

EFFICACY

1. Dose is 300 mg intravenously infused every 4 weeks over 30 minutes so a relatively rapid infusion time.
2. Anifrolumab exhibited greater than 16% differences versus placebo on a composite SLE activity score (BILAG [British Isles Lupus Assessment Group]).
3. Anifrolumab was superior to placebo in steroid reduction, skin disease improvement, and flare reduction.

SAFETY

The safety profile is similar to placebo with a slight excess of upper respiratory illness in patients on anifrolumab and a greater incidence of herpes zoster (7%) versus placebo (2%) in the trials. There are also rare hypersensitivity reactions to anifrolumab. No premedication is needed for infusion in most cases and status of hepatitis B or tuberculosis does not need to be determined prior to beginning anifrolumab.

CONCLUSION

Anifrolumab and other recently approved medication for SLE have been studied and subsequently approved as add-on therapy. We do not know the true power of these agents as they are given to patients with some degree of treatment resistance. Patients with severe lupus nephritis (LN) or neuropsychiatric SLE were excluded from the trials so there are no data for these manifestations.

VOCLOSPORIN (LUPKYNIS)

Voclosporin is a calcinurin inhibitor similar to cyclosporin. It was approved in January 2021 for the treatment of LN in conjunction with background immunosuppression.

EFFICACY

Approval was based on the results of a phase II and phase III (AURORA1 [Efficacy and Safety of Voclosporin Versus Placebo for Lupus Nephritis]) trial of voclosporin of 48 and 52 weeks, respectively, in patients with active LN (class III, IV, V) with the endpoint being a complete renal response compared to placebo.[36,37] Complete renal response was defined as a reduction in proteinuria as measured by a protein/creatinine ratio less than 0.5 mg/mg, need for only low-dose steroids, and stability or improvement of estimated glomerular filtration rate (GFR).

1. Dose is 23.7 mg twice a day with adjustment for GFR and liver disease.
2. Between the 2 studies, approximately 40% of patients randomized to voclosporin achieved a complete renal response compared to 23% taking placebo.
3. Patients on voclosporin showed improved renal response rates across all 3 classes of LN.

SAFETY

Like other calcineurin inhibitors, voclosporin can cause renal insufficiency, hypertension, hyperkalemia, and hypomagnesemia.[38] Rare reactivation of cytomegalovirus and herpes zoster can occur. Voclosporin is a cytochrome P450 3A substrate and when given with other medications that inhibit this enzyme can elevate the level of voclosporin. Voclosporin is also an inhibitor of P-glycoprotein as such may elevate levels of medications such as colchicine or digoxin leading to significant toxicity. Unlike cyclosporin or tacrolimus, voclosporin does not affect glucose levels, lipids, or mycophenolate levels.[38] No therapeutic drug monitoring is needed for voclosporin.

CONCLUSION

Voclosporin is a consideration in combination with mycophenolate for patients with LN who need additional therapy.

VASCULITIS

There are many different vasculitides, typically categorized into small, medium, and large vessel vasculitis. Two new therapies were FDA approved for vasculitis: avacopan for antineutrophil cytoplasmic antibody (ANCA) vasculitis and apremilast for Behcet's syndrome.

AVACOPAN (TAVENOS)

Avacopan was approved in 2021 by the FDA as an add-on treatment for ANCA vasculitis. The rationale is that the alternative complement pathway is important in ANCA vasculitis. Avacopan is a small-molecule C5a receptor antagonist that blocks the C5a receptor.

EFFICACY

Three trials were the basis for approval, 2 phase II trials and 1 phase III trial, the ADVO-CATE (A Phase 3 Clinical Trial of CCX168 (Avacopan) in Patients With ANCA-Associated

Vasculitis) trial.[39–41] The ADVOCATE trial investigated whether or not avacopan could replace glucocorticoid tapering in ANCA vasculitis. Avacopan 30 mg twice daily versus placebo was combined with standard cyclophosphamide or rituximab therapy for 52 weeks in patients with microscopic polyangiitis or granulomatosis with polyangiitis. The primary endpoints were clinical remission by week 26 and successful glucocorticoid taper by week 22. Avacopan was found to be noninferior to glucocorticoids but was also not found to be superior with respect to remission at week 26 or sustained remission at week 52. Steroid-related adverse events were 33% higher in the steroid group.

SAFETY ISSUES

No cases of *Neisseria meningitidis* occurred, a concern with inhibition of complement. There were more serious adverse events, including death, as well as infections in the prednisone group. 5.4% of patients on avacopan had elevated liver enzymes as compared to 3.7% in the prednisone group.

CONCLUSION

Avacopan has similar efficacy to glucocorticoids when combined with standard therapy and less adverse events.

APREMILAST (OTEZLA)

Painful ulcerations are frequent in Behcet's syndrome and may be the first manifestation. Apremilast is an oral small-molecule phosphodiesterase-4 inhibitor that decreases the production of pro-inflammatory cytokines and increases the production

Table 1
Summary of newer medications to treat rheumatologic disease

Medication	Newest Indication	Target	Utilization
Upadacitinib	AS, NrSpA, PsA	JAK 1 enzyme	Second-line agent for all new indications
Canakinumab	Gout flares	IL-1	Indicated for patients who cannot tolerate usual flare therapy
Sarilumab	PMR	IL-6	Used for patients who cannot tolerate prednisone taper
Guselkumab	PsA	IL-23	Active PsA
Risankizumab	PsA	IL-23	Active PsA
Olokizumab	RA	Il-6	On verge of approval for active RA
Tociluzimab	Scleroderma-ILD	IL-6	Active scleroderma-ILD
Anifrolumab	Active SLE	Type 1 interferon receptor	Add on SLE therapy when standard therapy is insufficient
Voclosporin	SLE nephritis	Calcineurin inhibitor	Added to standard therapy in active SLE nephritis
Avacopan	ANCA vasculitis	C5a receptor	Used in active ANCA vasculitis in place of corticosteroids
Apremilast	Behcet disease	PD4 inhibitor	Oral ulcers in Behcet disease

Abbreviations: ANCA, antineutrophil cytoplasmic antibody; AS, axial spondylitis; IL, interleukin; ILD, interstitial lung disease; JAK, Janus kinase; NrSpA, non-radiographic spondyloarthritis; PD4, phosphodiesterase-4; PMR, polymyalgia rheumatica; PsA, psoriatic arthritis; RA, rheumatoid arthritis; SLE, systemic lupus erythematosus.

of anti-inflammatory mediators through preventing degradation of cyclic adenosine monophosphate.[42]

EFFICACY

Apremilast FDA approval in 2019 was based on a phase II trial that showed apremilast was effective at reducing the overall disease activity, number of ulcers, and pain with ulcerations.[42] The phase III trial investigated patients that had failed treatment with a non-biologic agent.[43] The study showed greater reduction of oral ulcers as compared to placebo in patients not previously given a biologic. 53% of patients given apremilast and 22% of placebo patients were free from oral ulcers at 12 weeks. Long-term results shown with the phase III RELIEF (Reflux Assessment and Quality of Life Improvement with Micronized Flavonoids in Chronic Venous Insufficiency [CVI]) study showed sustained benefits up to 64 weeks with continued treatment (**Table 1**).[44]

SAFETY ISSUES

The most common SEs are gastrointestinal with abdominal pain, nausea, and vomiting. Headache and upper respiratory illnesses were also common SEs. Apremilast carries a black box warning for depression and an increased risk of suicidality.

SUMMARY

Apremilast reduces oral ulcerations in patients with Behcet's syndrome who have not been previously on a biologic.

CLINICS CARE POINTS

- Many, if not all, of these medications are best instituted in conjunction with specialist input.
- Cost will impact many of these agents and will in most cases be utilized after less expensive more familiar agents have been tried.
- They do represent a step forward in options for therapy and with time and experience will likely find a firm place in the treatment paradigm.

REFERENCES

1. van der Heijde D, Song IH, Pangan AL, et al. Efficacy and safety of upadacitinib in patients with active ankylosing spondylitis (SELECT-AXIS 1): a multicentre, randomised, double-blind, placebo-controlled, phase 2/3 trial. Lancet 2019; 394(10214):2108–17.
2. Deodhar A, Van den Bosch F, Poddubnyy D, et al. Upadacitinib for the treatment of active non-radiographic axial spondyloarthritis (SELECT-AXIS 2): a randomised, double-blind, placebo-controlled, phase 3 trial. Lancet 2022; 400(10349):369–79.
3. Burmester GR, Cohen SB, Winthrop KL, et al. Safety profile of upadacitinib over 15 000 patient-years across rheumatoid arthritis, psoriatic arthritis, ankylosing spondylitis and atopic dermatitis. RMD Open 2023;9(1).
4. Chakraborty A, Van LM, Skerjanec A, et al. Pharmacokinetic and pharmacodynamic properties of canakinumab in patients with gouty arthritis. J Clin Pharmacol 2013;53(12):1240–51.

5. Schlesinger N, De Meulemeester M, Pikhlak A, et al. Canakinumab relieves symptoms of acute flares and improves health-related quality of life in patients with difficult-to-treat Gouty Arthritis by suppressing inflammation: Results of a randomized, dose-ranging study. Arthritis Res Ther 2011;13(2):1–13.

6. Schlesinger N, Alten RE, Bardin T, et al. Canakinumab for acute gouty arthritis in patients with limited treatment options: Results from two randomised, multicentre, active-controlled, double-blind trials and their initial extensions. Ann Rheum Dis 2012;71(11):1839–48.

7. Schlesinger N, Mysler E, Lin HY, et al. Canakinumab reduces the risk of acute gouty arthritis flares during initiation of allopurinol treatment: Results of a double-blind, randomised study. Ann Rheum Dis 2011;70(7):1264–71.

8. Schlesinger N, Pillinger MH, Simon LS, et al. Interleukin-1β inhibitors for the management of acute gout flares: a systematic literature review. Arthritis Res Ther 2023;25(1):1–16.

9. Espígol-Frigolé G, Dejaco C, Mackie SL, et al. Polymyalgia Rheumatica. Lancet 2023;S01.

10. Dejaco C, Singh YP, Perel P, et al. Recommendations for the Management of Polymyalgia Rheumatica: A European League Against Rheumatism/American College of Rheumatology Collaborative Initiative. Arthritis Rheumatol 2015;67(10): 2569–80.

11. Devauchelle-Pensec V, Carvajal-Alegria G, Dernis E, et al. Effect of Tocilizumab on Disease Activity in Patients with Active Polymyalgia Rheumatica Receiving Glucocorticoid Therapy: A Randomized Clinical Trial. JAMA 2022;328(11): 1053–62.

12. Bonelli M, Radner H, Kerschbaumer A, et al. Tocilizumab in patients with new onset polymyalgia rheumatica (PMR-SPARE): A phase 2/3 randomised controlled trial. Ann Rheum Dis 2022;838–44.

13. Spiera RF, Unizony S, Warrington KJ, et al. Sarilumab for Relapse of Polymyalgia Rheumatica during Glucocorticoid Taper. N Engl J Med 2023;389(14):1263–72.

14. Deodhar A, Helliwell PS, Boehncke WH, et al. Guselkumab in patients with active psoriatic arthritis who were biologic-naive or had previously received TNFα inhibitor treatment (DISCOVER-1): a double-blind, randomised, placebo-controlled phase 3 trial. Lancet 2020;395(10230):1115–25.

15. Reich K, Armstrong AW, Foley P, et al. Efficacy and safety of guselkumab, an anti-interleukin-23 monoclonal antibody, compared with adalimumab for the treatment of patients with moderate to severe psoriasis with randomized withdrawal and retreatment: Results from the phase III, double-blind, placebo- and active comparator–controlled VOYAGE 2 trial. J Am Acad Dermatol 2017;76(3):418–31.

16. Blauvelt A, Papp KA, Griffiths CEM, et al. Efficacy and safety of guselkumab, an anti-interleukin-23 monoclonal antibody, compared with adalimumab for the continuous treatment of patients with moderate to severe psoriasis: Results from the phase III, double-blinded, placebo- and active comparator–controlled VOYAGE 1 trial. J Am Acad Dermatol 2017;76(3):405–17.

17. Langley RG, Tsai TF, Flavin S, et al. Efficacy and safety of guselkumab in patients with psoriasis who have an inadequate response to ustekinumab: results of the randomized, double-blind, phase III NAVIGATE trial. Br J Dermatol 2018; 178(1):114–23.

18. Mease PJ, Rahman P, Gottlieb AB, et al. Guselkumab in biologic-naive patients with active psoriatic arthritis (DISCOVER-2): a double-blind, randomised, placebo-controlled phase 3 trial. Lancet 2020;395(10230):1126–36.

19. Kristensen LE, Keiserman M, Papp K, et al. Efficacy and safety of risankizumab for active psoriatic arthritis: 24-week results from the randomised, double-blind, phase 3 KEEPsAKE 1 trial. Ann Rheum Dis 2022;81(2):225–31.

20. Östör A, Van Den Bosch F, Papp K, et al. Efficacy and safety of risankizumab for active psoriatic arthritis: 52-week results from the KEEPsAKE 2 study. Rheumatol (United Kingdom) 2023;62(6):2122–9.

21. McInnes IB, Anderson JK, Magrey M, et al. Trial of Upadacitinib and Adalimumab for Psoriatic Arthritis. N Engl J Med 2021;384(13):1227–39.

22. Mease PJ, Lertratanakul A, Anderson JK, et al. Upadacitinib for psoriatic arthritis refractory to biologics: SELECT-PsA 2. Ann Rheum Dis 2021;80(3):312–20.

23. Nasonov E, Fatenejad S, Feist E, et al. Olokizumab, a monoclonal antibody against interleukin 6, in combination with methotrexate in patients with rheumatoid arthritis inadequately controlled by methotrexate: efficacy and safety results of a randomised controlled phase III study. Ann Rheum Dis 2022;81(4):469–79.

24. Almutairi KB, Nossent JC, Preen DB, et al. The prevalence of rheumatoid arthritis: A systematic review of population-based studies. J Rheumatol 2021;48(5): 669–76.

25. Feist E, Fatenejad S, Grishin S, et al. Olokizumab, a monoclonal antibody against interleukin-6, in combination with methotrexate in patients with rheumatoid arthritis inadequately controlled by tumour necrosis factor inhibitor therapy: efficacy and safety results of a randomised controlled pha. Sovrem Revmatol 2023;17(2):23–36.

26. Genovese MC, Fleischmann R, Furst D, et al. Efficacy and safety of olokizumab in patients with rheumatoid arthritis with an inadequate response to TNF inhibitor therapy: outcomes of a randomised Phase IIb study. Ann Rheum Dis 2014; 73(9):1607–15.

27. Takeuchi T, Tanaka Y, Yamanaka H, et al. Efficacy and safety of olokizumab in Asian patients with moderate-to-severe rheumatoid arthritis, previously exposed to anti-TNF therapy: Results from a randomized phase II trial. Mod Rheumatol 2016;26(1):15–23.

28. Smolen JS, Feist E, Fatenejad S, et al. Olokizumab versus Placebo or Adalimumab in Rheumatoid Arthritis. N Engl J Med 2022;387(8):715–26.

29. Khanna D, Denton CP, Jahreis A, et al. Safety and efficacy of subcutaneous tocilizumab in adults with systemic sclerosis (faSScinate): a phase 2, randomised, controlled trial. Lancet 2016;387(10038):2630–40.

30. Khanna D, Lin CJF, Furst DE, et al. Tocilizumab in systemic sclerosis: a randomised, double-blind, placebo-controlled, phase 3 trial. Lancet Respir Med 2020;8(10):963–74.

31. Roofeh D, Lin CJF, Goldin J, et al. Tocilizumab Prevents Progression of Early Systemic Sclerosis–Associated Interstitial Lung Disease. Arthritis Rheumatol 2021; 73(7):1301–10.

32. Khanna D, Lin CJF, Furst DE, et al. Long-Term Safety and Efficacy of Tocilizumab in Early Systemic Sclerosis–Interstitial Lung Disease :Open-Label Extension of a Phase 3 Randomized Controlled Trial. Am J Respir Crit Care Med 2022;205(6): 674–84.

33. Furie RA, Morand EF, Bruce IN, et al. Type I interferon inhibitor anifrolumab in active systemic lupus erythematosus (TULIP-1): a randomised, controlled, phase 3 trial. Lancet Rheumatol 2019;1(4):e208–19.

34. Morand EF, Furie R, Tanaka Y, et al. Trial of Anifrolumab in Active Systemic Lupus Erythematosus. N Engl J Med 2020;382(3):211–21.

35. Tanaka Y, Tummala R. Anifrolumab, a monoclonal antibody to the type I interferon receptor subunit 1, for the treatment of systemic lupus erythematosus: an overview from clinical trials. Mod Rheumatol 2021;31(1):1–12.

36. Rovin BH, Solomons N, Pendergraft WF, et al. A randomized, controlled double-blind study comparing the efficacy and safety of dose-ranging voclosporin with placebo in achieving remission in patients with active lupus nephritis. Kidney Int 2019;95(1):219–31.

37. Rovin BH, Teng YKO, Ginzler EM, et al. Efficacy and safety of voclosporin versus placebo for lupus nephritis (AURORA 1): a double-blind, randomised, multi-centre, placebo-controlled, phase 3 trial. Lancet 2021;397(10289):2070–80.

38. van Gelder T, Lerma E, Engelke K, et al. Voclosporin: a novel calcineurin inhibitor for the treatment of lupus nephritis. Expet Rev Clin Pharmacol 2022;15(5):515–29.

39. Jayne DRW, Merkel PA, Schall TJ, et al. Avacopan for the Treatment of ANCA-Associated Vasculitis. N Engl J Med 2021;384(7):599–609.

40. Jayne DRW, Bruchfeld AN, Harper L, et al. Randomized trial of C5a receptor inhibitor avacopan in ANCA-associated vasculitis. J Am Soc Nephrol 2017;28(9): 2756–67.

41. Merkel PA, Niles J, Jimenez R, et al. Adjunctive treatment with avacopan, an oral c5a receptor inhibitor, in patients with antineutrophil cytoplasmic antibody–associated vasculitis. ACR Open Rheumatol 2020;2(11):662–71.

42. Hatemi G, Melikoglu M, Tunc R, et al. Apremilast for Behçet's Syndrome — A Phase 2, Placebo-Controlled Study. N Engl J Med 2015;372(16):1510–8.

43. Hatemi G, Mahr A, Ishigatsubo Y, et al. Trial of apremilast for oral ulcers in Behçet's Syndrome. N Engl J Med 2019;381(20):1918–28.

44. Hatemi G, Mahr A, Takeno M, et al. Apremilast for oral ulcers associated with active Behçet's syndrome over 68 weeks: Long-term results from a phase 3 randomised clinical trial. Clin Exp Rheumatol 2021;39(5):S80–7.

New Therapies in Outpatient Pulmonary Medicine

Laura Granados, MD[a],[*],[1], Mira John, MD[a],[2],
Jeffrey D. Edelman, MD[a],[b],[3]

KEYWORDS

- BPH • Benign prostate hyperplasia • HoLEP • Enucleation • Aquablation • MIST
- Prostate artery embolization

KEY POINTS

- Biologic therapies can improve control of moderate-to-severe asthma.
- Newer options for patients with chronic obstructive pulmonary disease include updated guidelines, bronchoscopic lung volume reduction, and therapies addressing additional pathways to relieve symptoms and inflammation.
- Antifibrotic agents and inhaled treprostinil have an expanding role in interstitial lung disease treatment.
- Newer medications, combined therapies, and procedures are available for patients with pulmonary hypertension although the majority of treatments focus on groups 1 and 4.
- CFTR modifiers have changed the treatment and outcomes for patients with cystic fibrosis.

ASTHMA

Definition and Classification

Asthma is characterized by inflammation of airways and bronchial hyperresponsiveness that leads to variable airflow obstruction.[1–3] It is a heterogeneous disease that is diagnosed clinically through a detailed history and physical examination.[2,3] Diagnosis can be aided by pulmonary function testing, methacholine challenge, and fractional exhaled nitric oxide (FeNO) when available.[2,3] The most common comorbidities of asthma include rhinitis, sinusitis, gastroesophageal reflux disease, and obstructive sleep apnea,[2,4] and appropriate management includes addressing these comorbidities.

[a] Department of Pulmonary, Critical Care and Sleep Medicine, University of Washington, Seattle, WA, USA; [b] Puget Sound Department of Veterans Affairs, Seattle, WA, USA
[1] Present address. 4337 15th Avenue NorthEast Apartment 406, Seattle, WA 98105.
[2] Present address. 1408 East Union Street, Apartment 619, Seattle WA 98122.
[3] Present address. 3866 43rd Avenue NorthEast, Seattle, WA 98105.
* Corresponding author. Division of Pulmonary, Critical Care and Sleep Medicine, University of Washington School of Medicine, Campus Box 356522, Seattle, WA 98195-6522.
E-mail address: granal@uw.edu

Med Clin N Am 108 (2024) 843–869
https://doi.org/10.1016/j.mcna.2024.03.011
0025-7125/24/© 2024 Elsevier Inc. All rights reserved, including those for text and data mining, AI training, and similar technologies.
medical.theclinics.com

Asthma can be allergic, nonallergic, or both.[1,4,5] Allergy is thought to be important in the pathogenesis of asthma, and therefore, patients with persistent asthma should be evaluated for contributing allergies. Allergen immunotherapy has been shown to reduce asthma symptoms, airway hyperresponsiveness, and the use of asthma medications for patients who are sensitized to inhaled allergens. Pharmacotherapy for asthma includes inhaled corticosteroids (ICSs), inhaled corticosteroid and long-acting ß-agonist combinations (ICS-LABAs), leukotriene antagonists (LTRAs) long-acting muscarinic receptor antagonist (LAMAs), short-acting ß-agonists (SABAs) as well as biologics.[2,3] Here, we will not review the traditional stepwise approach to the first-line management of asthma but instead briefly touch on ICS-containing medication used as needed for symptom control and focus on biologic therapies for patients for whom first-line therapies are not enough to achieve symptom control.

Use of Inhaled Corticosteroid-containing Inhaler for as Needed Symptom Control

Citing safety concerns around risk of severe exacerbations in patients using SABA alone for symptom control, recent 2023 guidelines from the Global Initiative for Asthma management recommend against the use of SABA alone for the treatment of asthma. Instead, the guidelines propose patients should receive ICS-containing treatment regardless of severity and, additionally, suggest ICS-formoterol be used as needed for symptoms control. Patients with mild asthma or steps 1 to 2 can be given low-dose ICS-formoterol to be taken as needed for symptom relief. Patients with moderate-to-severe asthma can use ICS-formoterol as "maintenance and reliever therapy" for regular daily controller treatment as well as for symptom control. This guidance replaces the more traditional approach of prescribing SABA as needed for symptom control for all patients with asthma.[6]

Biologic Therapies

The newest agents for asthma are the biologic therapies. These agents are usually reserved for patients with moderate-to-severe asthma who have not achieved symptom control with consistent use of ICSs or ICS/LABAs plus LTRAs or LAMAs.[7,8] Currently approved biologics for asthma involve anti-immunoglobulin (IgE), anti-interleukin (IL)-5, and anti-IL-4/anti-IL-13, and antiepithelial cytokine antibodies. Before a biologic therapy is initiated, the number of exacerbations in the past year, status with respect to oral glucocorticoid use, biomarkers (blood eosinophil count, FeNO, and serum total and allergen-specific IgE), forced expiratory volume in one second (FEV1), asthma control, and quality of life should be recorded.[2,3,8] Since no data from head-to-head randomized controlled trials (RCTs) comparing the efficacy, real-life effectiveness, and long-term safety of monoclonal antibodies in patients with severe asthma are available, the decision of which agent to choose is based on criteria such as biomarkers, coexisting conditions, and other considerations (dosing frequency, route of administration subcutaneous or intravenous, need for monitoring by health care personnel, insurance coverage, cost, and patient preference).[5,7,9,10] Anti-IgE monoclonal antibody, antibodies against IL-5 and IL-5R, and anti-IL-4 receptor antibody have been previously described and can be found in **Table 1**.

Anti–epithelial cytokine antibodies: Thymic stromal lymphopoietin (TSLP), IL-25, and IL-33 are epithelial cytokines released by airway epithelial cells in response to allergens, air pollutants, and viruses and result in downstream inflammation.[5,26,27] It is thought that by interfering upstream in the inflammatory cascade, biologic agents that target epithelial cytokines may improve asthma outcomes in a broader patient population as compared to the medications previously discussed. Addition of the anti-TSLP human monoclonal antibody tezepelumab to traditional first line therapies

Table 1
Food and Drug Administration-approved biologic therapies for asthma

Class	Medication and Mechanism of Action	Dose	Indication and Evidence	Side Effects
Anti-IgE monoclonal antibody	Omalizumab Binding of free IgE to inhibit activation of mast cells, basophils, and other cells involved in the allergic inflammatory response	Frequency and dosing based on body weight and pretreatment total IgE serum levels	Allergic (evidenced by a positive skin-prick test, serum allergen-specific IgE, elevated total IgE, and a clear history of allergen-provoked symptoms.[5,7,10] Reduces asthma exacerbations and can result in small improvements in quality of life and lung function[11]	Anaphylaxis in 0.1%–0.2% of patients and most frequently with one of the first 3 doses Administer in a health care setting, provide patients with epinephrine autoinjectors
Antibodies against IL-5 and IL-5R	Mepolizumab, reslizumab, and benralizumab Mepolizumab and reslizumab are anti-IL-5 humanized monoclonal antibodies Benralizumab is an anti-IL-5R antibody IL-5 or IL5R binding depletes eosinophils	Mepolizumab: 100 mg subcutaneously once every 4 wk Reslizumab: 3 mg/kg subcutaneously once every 4 wk Benralizumab: 30 mg subcutaneously every 4 wk for the first 3 doses, then once every 8 wk	Approved for use in patients with serum eosinophilia (150–300/ μL).[12,13] Have been shown to reduced exacerbations, reduce hospitalizations, and decrease the need for of systemic[5,7,10] corticosteroids[14–16]	Most common side effects include respiratory infections, headache, and worsening asthma. Among 1028 patients receiving intravenous reslizumab, 3 cases of anaphylaxis were observed, leading to an FDA black-box warning[17,18]

(continued on next page)

Table 1
(continued)

Class	Medication and Mechanism of Action	Dose	Indication and Evidence	Side Effects
Anti–IL-4 receptor antibody	Dupilumab Human monoclonal antibody which inhibits the signaling of both IL-4 and IL-13 (IL-4 and IL-13 are involved in Th2 inflammation) by binding to IL-4Rα[19]	400 or 600 mg once followed by 200 or 300 mg subcutaneously every other wk	Approved for the treatment of atopic dermatitis, chronic rhinosinusitis with nasal polyposis, and severe asthma.[20,21] Has been shown to reduce use of oral corticosteroid, decrease severe asthma exacerbations, improve asthma control and prebronchodilator and postbronchodilator FEV[22]	Most common side effects are injection-site reactions (occurring in 15% of patients) and hypereosinophilia (eosinophil count $\geq$1500/ μL observed in 4%–25% of patients).[22–24] Dupilumab-induced hypereosinophilia is often asymptomatic, but there have been cases of eosinophilic granulomatosis with polyangiitis[25]
Anti–epithelial cytokine antibodies	Tezepelumab Human monoclonal antibody that binds to human TSLP blocking inflammatory cascade	Tezepelumab is dosed subcutaneously at 210 mg once every 4 wk	Reduced exacerbations, improved lung function, asthma control, and quality of life	Arthralgias and back pain were reported

reduced exacerbations, improved lung function, asthma control, and health-related quality of life in patients with allergic asthma, eosinophilic asthma and nonallergic; exacerbation rate decreased by 56% in patients with high blood eosinophils (>300/μL) and among patients with low blood eosinophil (<300/μL) the rate was reduced by 41%. Tezepelumab was also noted to reduce blood eosinophil counts, Feno, serum total IgE levels, and airway hyperresponsiveness to mannitol.[28,29] The safety findings were similar for active treatment and placebo. Addition of Itepekimab, an anti-IL-33 human monoclonal antibody prevented the loss of asthma control and improved lung function in patients who had moderate-to-severe asthma and were reducing their maintenance therapy with ICS-LABAs.52 Astegolimab, a human monoclonal antibody inhibiting the IL-33 receptor reduced exacerbations including those with low eosinophil counts. Astegolimab did not improve lung function.[5] Confirmatory phase 3 RCTs of antibodies against IL-33 in patients with severe asthma, particularly type 2–low, are warranted.

CHRONIC OBSTRUCTIVE PULMONARY DISEASE

Treatment of chronic obstructive pulmonary disease (COPD) is multidisciplinary and includes medications, smoking cessation, immunizations, evaluation for supplemental oxygen, pulmonary rehabilitation (PR), noninvasive positive pressure ventilation, endoscopic or surgical lung volume reduction (LVR), palliative care, and lung transplantation. Recent changes in the treatment of COPD include updated guidelines for use of inhaled medications, newer phosphodiesterase inhibitors, use of biologic agents, development of home-based pulmonary rehab programs, and new devices for endoscopic LVR.

The 2023 global initiative for chronic obstructive lung disease (GOLD 2023) defines COPD as "a heterogeneous lung condition characterized by chronic respiratory symptoms (dyspnea, cough, expectoration and/or exacerbations) due to abnormalities of the airways (bronchitis, bronchiolitis) and/or alveoli (emphysema) that cause persistent, often progressive, airflow obstruction."[30] The recent American Thoracic Society/European Respiratory Society uses lower limit of normal values to define the presence of airflow obstruction and severity of pulmonary impairment.[31] GOLD utilizes a postbronchodilator FEV1/forced vital capacity (FVC) ratio of less than 0.7 to define airflow obstruction and categorizes COPD-based assessment of severity of airflow obstruction (Grades 1–4) combined with symptoms (Group A, B, or E)[31–33] (**Fig. 1**).

Medical Treatment Guidelines for COPD Gold 2023 provides a stepwise framework for COPD based on symptoms and frequency of exacerbations reflecting GOLD groups and treatment response. Initial treatment of group A patients consists of a single mechanism short-acting or long-acting bronchodilator, escalating to LABA or long-acting muscarinic receptor antagonist (LAMA) for persistent symptoms. For group B, a LABA/LAMA combination is recommended. Initial treatment of group E consists of a LABA+LAMA with the addition ICSs if peripheral eosinophil count is 300 cells/μL or greater. Addition of an ICS is recommended for patients with persistent symptoms and an eosinophil count of less than 300 to 100 cells/μL or greater. The use of ICS is not recommended if the eosinophil count is less than 100. Further treatment escalation options for all group E patients include a phosphodiesterase 4 (PDE4) inhibitor (if FEV1 <50% and symptoms of chronic bronchitis) or azithromycin. Inhaled treatment includes numerous options with reference to specific agents, combinations, and delivery mechanisms. Additional considerations include the notion that single combination drug inhaler treatment may be more convenient and that response may be variable to different agents or inhaler mechanisms within the same drug classes. Costs

Spirometrically Confirmed Obstruction
Post-bronchodilator FEV1/FVC <0.7

GRADE	FEV1 % Predicted
GOLD 1	≥80
GOLD 2	50-79
GOLD 3	30-49
GOLD 4	<30

EXACERBATION HISTORY PER YEAR		
≥ 2 moderate exacerbations or ≥ 1 leading to hospitalization	E	
0 or 1 moderate exacerbations (not leading to hospitalization)	A	B
	mMRC[a] 0 -1 CAT[b] <10	mMRC ≥ 2 CAT ≥ 10

Fig. 1. Gold COPD assessment. [a]mMRC, modified Medical Research Council dyspnea score. [b]CAT, COPD assessment test score. (Global Initiative for Chronic Obstructive Lung Disease. Global strategy for prevention, diagnosis and management of COPD: 2023 report. Global Initiative for Chronic Obstructive Lung Disease; 2023. Available from: https://goldcopd. org/2023-gold-report-2/.)

may also be variable and patient education regarding medication use and inhaler techniques is also essential.[32,33]

New Medications

Phosphodiesterase inhibitors

Phosphodiesterase (PDE) 3 and 4 pathways represent a more recent target for COPD treatment. Roflumilast, a PDE4 inhibitor and ensifentrine (currently under Food and Drug Administration [FDA] review) a PDE 3,4 inhibitor have been shown to improve outcomes in COPD. PDE4 inhibition reduces airway inflammation and PDE3 inhibition reduces airway smooth muscle tone. Roflumilast is a once daily oral medication shown to improve lung function and decrease the frequency of acute exacerbations in patients with severe (postbronchodilator FEV1 ≤50% predicted). It is indicated for patients with severe COPD associated with chronic bronchitis and a history of exacerbations. In 2 randomized trials roflumilast reduced the overall frequency of moderate-to-severe exacerbations by 12.3% and severe exacerbations by 16.1%. The frequency was reduced by 34.5% for patients with history of exacerbations requiring hospitalization with eosinophils counts of 150 cells/μL or greater and 42.7% for those with counts of 300 cells/μL or greater.[34,35] Ensifentrine is a twice daily nebulized medication that was evaluated in a couple phase 3 randomized trials for patients with COPD and a post-bronchodilator FEV1 between 30% and 70% predicted. In these studies, treatment with ensifentrine was associated with improved lung function, symptoms, and quality of life along with reduction in moderate-to-severe exacerbations.[36]

Biologic agents

Dupilumab, a monoclonal IL-4, IL-13 receptor blocking antibody is the only biologic agent currently approved for COPD. Patients with symptomatic COPD with chronic bronchitis, peripheral eosinophil count of 300 cells/μL or greater, and postbronchodilator FEV1 of 30% to 70% predicted receiving triple inhaled therapy (ICS, LABA_-LABA), received subcutaneous dupilumab at a dose of 300 mg or placebo every 2 weeks for 52 weeks. Dupilumab was associated with the reduction of the annualized rate of moderate-to-severe exacerbations (0.78 vs 1.30); greater improvement in lung function (160 vs 77 mL); and better quality of life (St. George's Respiratory Questionnaire score) in comparison to placebo.[37]

Home-based Pulmonary Rehabilitation

PR is an established element of COPD care and is recommended for patients with significant symptoms and risk of exacerbations.

PR is associated with an improved exercise capacity, reduced symptoms, improved quality of life, and health cost benefits for patients with COPD. While PR itself is an established aspect of COPD care, the limited availability of PR facilities as well as associated cost and travel burden along with changes in health care delivery associated with the COVID-19 pandemic have led to the development of home-based PR programs (HBPRs). HBPRs have been associated with similar benefits in comparison with traditional facility-based outpatient PR.[38–40]

Lung volume reduction

Lung volume reduction surgery (LVRS) can lead to improvements in lung function, exercise capacity, quality of life in selected patients with significant limitations despite maximal medical therapy. LVRS reduces hyperinflation and improvise lung elastic recoil and respiratory mechanics. LVRS has been an established procedure for selected patients for over 20 years.[41,42] More recently, endobronchial valves have been approved for endoscopic lung volume reduction (ELVR). These 1 way valves accomplish LVR by blocking airflow into diseased regions leading to localized atelectasis. Because ELVR is less invasive than LVRS, it is associated with lower morbidity and mortality and potentially available for a larger group of patients. Two 1-way valves have been approved for ELVR in the United States. Randomized trials utilizing these valves in patients with severe heterogeneous emphysema a low likelihood of collateral ventilation demonstrated improvement in lung function, 6 minute walk distance, and SGRQ score.[43,44]

INTERSTITIAL LUNG DISEASE/DIFFUSE PARENCHYMAL LUNG DISEASE

"Interstitial lung disease" or ILD refers to a group of lung diseases classified together due to similar clinical, radiographic, and pathologic findings and manifestations. Another term used is "diffuse parenchymal lung disease," which more accurately reflects involvement of the alveolar and airway architecture as well as the lung interstitium.

There are many disease patterns that fall within the broad category of "ILD." ILD may be categorized by etiology and associated conditions.

- Occupational: inorganic antigens such as asbestos, silica, beryllium, and organic materials
- Iatrogenic: from medications like methotrexate, amiodarone, chemotherapy, immunotherapy, and radiation
- Substance use including cigarette smoking
- Granulomatous disorders: hypersensitivity pneumonitis and sarcoidosis
- Cystic diseases such as pulmonary Langerhans cell histiocytosis, lymphoid interstitial pneumonia, and lymphangioleiomyomatosis

- Related to other systemic diseases such as connective tissue diseases and vasculitis
- Idiopathic

Disorders without an identified etiology are classified as idiopathic interstitial pneumonias (IIPs) and include the following:[45]

- Idiopathic pulmonary fibrosis (IPF)
- Nonspecific interstitial pneumonia
- Desquamative interstitial pneumonia
- Respiratory bronchiolitis interstitial lung disease
- Cryptogenic organizing pneumonia
- Acute interstitial pneumonia
- Lymphoid interstitial pneumonia
- Idiopathic pleuroparenchymal fibroelastosis
- Unclassifiable IIP

The patterns seen in idiopathic disorders are also seen in association with known causes, and thus, it is important to note both the pattern as well as to delineate whether the condition is idiopathic or related to an underlying exposure or condition. Treatment approaches to pulmonary fibrosis vary by disease etiology and associated conditions. Nonpharmacologic therapies including smoking cessation, immunizations, supplemental oxygen, and PR, should be addressed for all patients. Referral for lung transplantation is a consideration for appropriate patients with more advanced or progressive disease. For ILD associated with collagen vascular disease, hypersensitivity, or sarcoidosis, treatment with immunosuppressive regimens may be utilized with choices based on consensus opinion, historical experience, and small studies, although robust data may be limited. Multidisciplinary consultation and conference review (which may include pulmonary medicine, rheumatology, thoracic radiology, thoracic surgery, occupational medicine, and pathology) should be considered for consensus opinion for evaluation and management of complex cases. The remainder of this section will focus only on new pharmacologic therapies for pulmonary fibrosis.

New Pharmacologic Therapies for Pulmonary Fibrosis

Nintedanib

Nintedanib slows IPF disease progression through acting as a receptor blocker for tyrosine kinases that affect growth factors implicated in fibrosis. It has been shown to slow FVC decline and reduce risk of acute IPF exacerbations as compared to trial placebo.

In addition to IPF, nintedanib is indicated for use in the broader group of patients with ILD and a progressive fibrotic phenotype (independent of etiology or associated condition). Standard adult dosing is usually 150 mg oral tablets twice a day. Liver function tests should be checked before dose initiation, repeated every month for the first 3 months of use, and at 3 month interval checks thereafter. Pregnancy tests should also be checked in patients with potential for pregnancy. Therapy should not be initiated in patients on dialysis. Adverse reactions include elevated LFTs, nausea, vomiting, and diarrhea. Diarrhea is the most common side effect and occurs in up to 60% of patients. Dose reductions are recommended for patients with elevated liver function tests or renal impairment patients on cytochrome P450 inhibitor medications, or those with significant gastrointestinal side effect.[46–49]

Pirfenidone

Pirfenidone slows IPF disease progression through multiple molecular mechanisms aimed to decrease fibrosis formation. Like nintedanib, pirfenidone has also been shown to slow FVC decline in mild–moderate disease. Standard adult dosing starts with 1 capsule of 267 mg tid, with uptitrating to 2 tablets (534 mg) tid on week 2, and then full 3 tablet (801 mg) tablets tid with food. Dose reductions are recommended in patients with elevated LFT and renal impairment along with patients taking cytochrome P450 inhibitor medications. Liver function tests should be checked before dose initiation, repeated every month for the first 6 months of use, and spaced to 3 month interval checks afterward. Therapy should not be initiated for patients on dialysis. Adverse reactions include rash, gastrointestinal (GI) symptoms including nausea, vomiting, diarrhea, dyspepsia, and abdominal discomfort, headache, hyperpigmentation, fatigue, and photosensitivity. Although rare, adverse cutaneous reactions including Stevens–Johnson syndrome and DRESS associated with pirfenidone have been reported. Severe cutaneous and GI symptoms can prompt medication discontinuation. Unlike nintedanib, the pirfenidone is indicated only for patients with progressive fibrotic lung disease due to IPF.[50–52]

Inhaled treprostinil

Pulmonary hypertension (PH) occurs frequently with advanced fibrotic lung disorders. While it is tempting to consider PH therapies for patients in this setting, beneficial effects have not been demonstrated for most agents. Note, however, that patients with connective tissue disease may fall under the World Health Organization (WHO) Group 1 PH category and are thus eligible to receive PH therapies as outlined in the subsequent section discussing WHO Group 1 PH. Outside of this group, inhaled treprostinil is the only indicated treatment of PH associated with ILD (PH–ILD) and has been shown to improve exercise tolerance assessed by 6MWT and lung function assessed by FVC in randomized placebo-controlled trials. The greatest improvements were observed in patients with IIP, particularly IPF. Inhaled treprostinil is administered by pulsed-delivery nebulizer at 6 µg per breath. Dosing is initiated at 3 breaths qid increasing by 1 breath qid at 1 to 2 week intervals up to a maximum of 12 breaths qid. More recently, a dry powder inhaler formulation of treprostinil has been approved with dosing as follows: initial dosage: one 16 mcg cartridge per treatment session, increasing by an additional 16 mcg per treatment session at approximately 1 to 2 week intervals, as tolerated with titration to target maintenance doses of 48 to 64 mcg per treatment session, 4 times daily. Because of the observed improvements in lung function and in vitro antifibrotic properties of treprostinil, randomized trials are ongoing to evaluate the effects of inhaled treprostinil in patients with IPF without PH.[53–60]

PULMONARY HYPERTENSION
Definition and Classification

Classification of the hemodynamics of patients with PH guides diagnosis and therapeutic management. PH has been recently redefined by a mean pulmonary arterial pressure (mPAP) greater than 20 mm Hg at rest.[61–65] Precapillary PH is hemodynamically defined as mPAP 20 mm Hg, pulmonary vascular resistance (PVR) greater than 2 WU, and pulmonary arterial wedge pressure (PAWP) 15 mm Hg or less. Postcapillary PH is hemodynamically defined as mPAP greater than 20 mm Hg and PAWP greater than 15 mm Hg. Patients with postcapillary hemodynamics in whom PVR is also elevated (>2 WU) are thought to have combined postcapillary and precapillary PH. Patients with postcapillary hemodynamics who do not have elevated PVR ($\leq$2 WU) are thought to have isolated postcapillary PH, which is due to left heart disease.[66] PH is classified into groups 1 to 5 based on hemodynamic findings, clinical features, and associated conditions (**Box 1**).[66,68] Risk stratification is another crucial aspect of managing PH as it allows physicians to appropriately tailor treatment plans and monitor disease progression.[66] **Table 2** provides a list of factors that should be considered when assessing disease severity in patients with PH.

Pulmonary Hypertension Therapies

The management of PH includes a comprehensive treatment strategy with multidisciplinary care, which includes supervised exercise programs,[70–73] diuresis and iron supplementation,[74,75] in addition to tailored medical therapy. Pharmacotherapy and interventions specific to PH continue to evolve but the majority of pharmacologic agents for PH is FDA approved only for WHO group 1 PH with the exceptions of inhaled treprostinil for group 1 and 3 PH and riociguat for group 1 and 4 PH (**Table 3**).

Group 1: pulmonary hypertension
Vasoreactivity testing is indicated for specific group 1 PH subgroups and guides the use of calcium channel blockers as first-line therapy in these patients.[66] For patients with non-vasoreactive forms of group 1 PH, initial dual therapy with an endothelin receptor antagonist (ERA) plus a phosphodiesterase 5 inhibitor (PDE5i) is

---

Box 1
Summary of current clinical pulmonary hypertension classification[67]

1. Pulmonary arterial hypertension
   Idiopathic
   Heritable
   Drug and toxin induced
   Connective tissue disease
   HIV infection
   Portal hypertension
   Congenital heart disease
   Schistosomiasis
   Pulmonary veno-occlusive disease/pulmonary capillary hemangiomatosis
   Persistent PH of the newborn

2. PH due to left heart disease
   Heart failure with preserved LVEF
   Heart failure with reduced LVEF
   Valvular heart disease
   Congenital/acquired conditions leading to postcapillary PH

3. PH due to lung disease and/or hypoxia
   Obstructive lung disease
   Restrictive lung disease
   Mixed restrictive/obstructive lung disease
   Hypoventilation syndromes
   Hypoxia without lung disease
   Developmental lung disorders

4. PH due to pulmonary artery obstruction
   Chronic thrombo-embolic PH
   Other pulmonary artery obstructions

5. PH with unclear and/or multifactorial mechanisms
   Hematologic disorders
   Systemic and metabolic disorders
   Chronic renal failure
   Fibrosing mediastinitis
   Pulmonary tumor microangiopathy

Table 2
Risk stratification in pulmonary hypertension[69]

Factors Contributing to 1 y Mortality	Low Risk	Intermediate Risk	High Risk
Clinical signs of right heart failure	Absent	Absent	Present
Symptom progression	Absent	Slow	Rapid
Syncope	Absent	Occasional	Multiple
WHO functional class	I, II	III	IV
6 min walk test distance in meters	>440	165–440	<165
Cardiopulmonary exercise test	>15	11–15	<11
Peak Vo_2% predicted	>65%	35%–65%	<35%
Minute ventilation/carbon dioxide production slope	<36	36–44.9	>45
N terminal pro-BNP serum level (ng/L)	<300	300–1400	>1400
BNP (ng/L)	<50	50–300	>300
Echocardiogram or cardiac MRI			
Right atrial area (cm^2)	<18	18–26	>26
Pericardial effusion	Absent	Absent or minimal	Present
Hemodynamics			
Right atrial pressure (mm Hg)	<8	8–14	>14
Cardiac index (L/min/m^2)	>2.5	2.0–2.4	<2.0
Venous oxygen saturation (%)	>65	60–65	<60

recommended for newly diagnosed patients who present at low–intermediate risk[101,102] and initial triple-combination therapy including oral agents plus an intravenous or subcutaneous prostacyclin analog is recommended for patients presenting at high risk.[103,104]

Treatment escalation and/or referral to a lung transplant center should be considered when patients have inadequate response to treatment despite optimized combination therapy, when patients have a disease variant that is known to respond poorly to medical therapy, and when they have intermediate to high or high risk of death (1 year mortality >10% when estimated with established risk-stratification tools).

New drugs in advanced clinical development. Ralinepag and sotatercept are novel agents. Ralinepag is an oral prostacyclin receptor agonist, which, in a phase 2 RCT improved PVR after 22 weeks of therapy as compared with placebo.[105] Sotatercept, a fusion protein that acts as a ligand for transforming growth factor-β proteins, seeks to restore balance between growth-promoting and growth-inhibiting cellular pathways. It is administered subcutaneously at a target dose of 0.7 mg/kg every 21 days. In a phase 3 RCT, sotatercept improved 6MWD in patients receiving background PH therapy as compared to placebo.[106]

Pulmonary artery denervation. The mechanism of this experimental treatment is not completely understood. PAH is thought to be characterized by sympathetic overdrive. Pulmonary artery denervation (PADN) aims to destroy sympathetic nerves that are located along the PA and potentially mediate vasoconstriction and vascular remodeling.[107] A small multicenter study tested the feasibility of PADN using an intravascular ultrasound catheter in patients receiving dual or triple therapy for PAH, and the procedure was felt to be safe, was associated with a reduction in PVR, and leads to increases in 6MWD and daily activity.[108]

Table 3
Food and Drug Administration-approved pulmonary hypertension medications

Class and Mechanism of Action	Medication	Dose	Evidence	Side effects
Calcium channel blocker (CCBs)	*Nifedipine*	Extended release 30 mg once a day. Target dose range 120–240 mg a day. (Short-acting nifedipine should not be used)	Vasoreactivity is defined as a reduction of mPAP ≥10 mm Hg to reach an absolute value of mPAP ≤40 mm Hg and an increased or unchanged cardiac output. Patients with group 1 vasoreactive PH may respond favorably to initiation of CCB[76,77]	Patients with Group 1 PH who have not had a vasoreactivity study or those with a negative test should not be started on CCBs because of potentially severe hypotension, syncope, and RV failure The most common adverse events are systemic hypotension and peripheral edema
	Diltiazem	60 mg twice a day for target dose of 120–720 a day in 2 divided doses Or 120 mg once a day for a maximum dose of 720 mg once a day		
	Amlodipine	Amlodipine, a long-acting dihydropyridine, is a useful alternative for patients who are intolerant of the other CCB agents		
ERAs Bind endothelin-1 to endothelin receptors A and B on smooth-muscle cells to block vasoconstriction and proliferation [380]	*Ambrisentan*	5 mg or 10 mg once a day orally	Improvement of symptom, exercise capacity, hemodynamics, and time to clinical worsening were seen in patients with group 1 PH[78]	All endothelial receptor antagonists have teratogenic effects and should not be used during pregnancy Increased incidence of peripheral edema with ambrisentan use
	Bosentan	Target dose in adults is 125 mg twice a day orally	Improvement of exercise capacity, hemodynamics, and time to clinical worsening were seen in patients with group 1 PH[79]	Dose-dependent increases in liver transaminases have occurred in ~10% of treated patients, and these changes are reversible after dose reduction or discontinuation. Monthly liver function testing is recommended in patients receiving bosentan

	Macitentan	10 mg once a day orally	Improvement of exercise capacity and a clinical worsening was seen in patients with group 1 PH	Hormonal contraceptives may be unreliable, and there may be lower serum levels of warfarin, sildenafil, and tadalafil due to pharmacokinetic interactions[80-82] A reduction in Hb to ≤8 g/dL was observed in 4.3% of patients receiving 10 mg of macitentan[83]
PDE5is and soluble guanylate cyclase stimulators (sGCs) Phosphodiesterase inhibitors block phosphodiesterase enzymes from degrading cAMP and cGMP, which leads to an increase in intracellular calcium that causes vasodilation and smooth muscle relaxation [388]	Sildenafil	20 mg three times a day orally	Improvement of exercise capacity, symptoms and hemodynamics were seen in patients with group 1 PH[84]	PDE5is must not be combined with nitrates as this can result in systemic hypotension Most side effects of sildenafil are mild to moderate and mainly related to vasodilation such as headache, flushing, and epistaxis
Riociguat, a soluble sGC enhances cGMP production leading to vasodilation [394]	Tadalafil	Up to 40 mg a day orally	Improvement of exercise capacity, symptoms, hemodynamics, and time to clinical worsening were seen in patient with group 1 PH[85]	The side effect profile is similar to that of sildenafil
	Riociguat	2.5 mg three times a day orally	Improvement of exercise capacity, hemodynamics, and time to clinical worsening were seen in patients with group 1 PH[86,87] The first phase 3 RCT in patients with CTEPH showed that riociguat improved 6MWD and reduced PVR by 31% after 16 wk of therapy	The side effect profile is similar to that of PDE5is

(continued on next page)

Table 3
(continued)

Class and Mechanism of Action	Medication	Dose	Evidence	Side effects
Prostacyclin analogs and prostacyclin receptor agonists induce potent vasodilation, inhibit platelet aggregation, and have prevent tissue hyperproliferation [397]	Epoprostenol	Half-life of 3–5 min and therefore needs continuous intravenous administration via permanent tunneled catheter an infusion pump. A thermostable formulation is available to maintain stability up to 48 h Initial dose 1–2 ng/kg/min and titrate to clinical effect over days to weeks. Average effective dose 80 ng/kg/min and target dose ranges from 40 to 150 ng/kg/min depending on patient	Its efficacy has been studied in patients with idiopathic and SSc-associated GROUP 1 PH and has been shown to improved symptoms, exercise capacity, hemodynamics, and mortality[88–90]	The most common adverse events observed with these compounds are related to systemic vasodilation and include headache, flushing, jaw pain, and diarrhea. Serious adverse events related to the delivery system include pump malfunction, local site infection, catheter obstruction, and sepsis
	Iloprost	Inhaled administration 2.5–5 mcg per inhalation, 6 to 9 times a day	Has been studied in patients with GROUP 1 PH and CTEPH and shown to increase exercise capacity and improve symptoms, PVR, and clinical events[91]	Side effects related to systemic vasodilation as discussed earlier
	Treprostinil	Inhaled formulation comes in powder and solution and dosing varies slightly between the two: Generally, initial dose of 16–18 mcg per treatment, 4 treatments a day about 4 h apart while patient awake. Can titrate every 1–2 wk by 16–18 mcg for a target dose of 48–63 mcg (for powder form) and 54 mcg (for solution form) per treatment	Intravenous and subcutaneous treprostinil has been shown to improved exercise capacity, hemodynamics, and symptoms in GROUP 1 PH[92–94] A phase 3 RTC showed that subcutaneous treprostinil improved 6MWD at wk 24 in patients with inoperable CTEPH or those with persistent/recurrent PH after PEA[94]	Infusion-site pain was the most common adverse effect

	Oral formulation: initial dose of 0.125 mg every 8 h to 0.25 mg every 12 h. Increase the dose by 0.125 mg every 8 h or by 0.25 mg every 12 h every 3–4 wk. Target dose of ~8 mg 3 times daily by 12 mo. Avoid abrupt discontinuation Based on its chemical stability, intravenous Treprostinil may be administered via implantable pumps, improving convenience and likely decreasing the occurrence of line infections Subcutaneous or intravenous continuous infusion: initial dose of 1.25 ng/kg/min. Increase dose by 1.25 ng/kg/min every wk for the first month and then by 2.5 ng/kg/min thereafter. Target dose of 40–80 ng/kg/min. Avoid abrupt discontinuation IV formulation available only for patients temporarily unable to take oral formulation	Inhaled treprostinil has been shown to improve the 6MWD, NT-proBNP, and quality of life measures in patients with GROUP 1 PH on background therapy with either Bosentan or sildenafil[30] Inhaled treprostinil has also been shown to improve 6MWD and symptoms for patients with ILD associated PH[54,95,96] Oral treprostinil has been evaluated in patients GROUP 1 PH and showed improved 6MWD in treatment-naïve patients and a reduction of clinical worsening events in patients who were receiving concurrent oral ERAs or PDE5is[97,98]	Side effects related to systemic vasodilation as discussed earlier
Selexipag	200 mcg twice daily orally. Increase by 200 mcg twice daily weekly to maximum tolerated dose 1600 mcg twice daily	Selexipag has been shown to reduce PVR after in patients with GROUP 1 PH receiving concurrent ERA and/or PDE5i therapy and to reduce the relative risk of composite morbidity/mortality events by 40% in patients receiving none, mono or double therapy with an ERA and/or a PDE5i[99,100]	

Group 2: pulmonary hypertension associated with left heart disease (PH-LHD)
Optimized treatment of the underlying cardiac disease is the cornerstone of management of group 2 PH. There is otherwise conflicting evidence for the use of PH specific pharmacotherapies for patients in this group with some medications being potentially detrimental. RTCs on bosentan and other endothelin receptor antagonists showed an increase in fluid retention and adverse events in patients with PH associated with HFrEF and HFpEF.[109-111] On the other hand, small studies have suggested that sildenafil may improve hemodynamics and exercise capacity in PH due to HFrEF or HFpEF with a predominantly CpcPH profile.[112-115] Because RCTs are lacking, society guidelines do not strongly currently recommend the use of PH specific therapies for patients with group 2 PH.[116]

Group 3: pulmonary hypertension associated with lung disease and/or hypoxia
For patients with group 3 PH, fundamental management includes optimizing the treatment of the underlying lung disease, supplemental oxygen and noninvasive ventilation if indicated, as well as enrollment into PR programs. Medical management of PH–ILD is discussed in the previous ILD section.

Group 4: chronic thrombo-embolic pulmonary hypertension
General measures recommended for PH also apply to chronic thrombo-embolic pulmonary hypertension (CTEPH), including supervised exercise training. Lifelong therapeutic anticoagulation is also recommended.[117,118] Depending on the anatomic location of lesions (whether microvascular, distal, and/or proximal), CTEPH treatment requires a multimodal approach of medical therapies, pulmonary endarterectomy (PEA), and/or balloon pulmonary angioplasty (BPA).

Pulmonary endarterectomy. Surgical PEA is the treatment of choice for eligible patients. Patient eligibility is based on accessibility of PA lesions, severity of PH, degree of PA obstructions, and comorbidities. This surgery may normalize pulmonary hemodynamics with ~65% decrease in PVR. Following PEA, about 25% of patients may have persistent or recurrent PH and may benefit from additional medical and/or interventional therapies.[119] For patients with mixed anatomic lesions a combined approach with BPA may be beneficial.[120]

Balloon pulmonary angioplasty. This intervention can potentially improve PVR by as much as 66% and lead to better exercise capacity in cases of inoperable CTEPH,[121] but overall evidence for long-term outcomes is insufficient. BPA is associated with serious complications, including vascular injury due to wire perforation, and lung injury, should be performed in experienced CTEPH centers.[122,123]

Medical therapy. Phase 3 RCTs have shown that riociguat[124] and treprostinil[30] are beneficial for patients with CTEPH with a microvascular component. A phase 2 RCT showed that macitentan 10 mg improved PVR and 6 minute walk distance at 16 and 24 weeks in patients with inoperable CTEPH.[125] A phase 3 RCT to evaluate the safety and efficacy of macitentan 75 mg in inoperable or persistent/recurrent CTEPH is ongoing (NCT04271475).

CYSTIC FIBROSIS
Introduction

Cystic fibrosis (CF) is a genetic disorder caused by mutations in the cystic fibrosis transmembrane conductance regulator (CFTR) gene leading to dysfunctional CFTR protein formation and function and subsequent organ dysfunction from buildup of mucus. Organs involved include pancreas, gut, and lungs. Pulmonary manifestations include frequent pulmonary infections, mucus plugging, air trapping, bronchiectasis, and reactive airway disease. Progressive lung disease is a leading cause of morbidity and mortality for many patients with CF, though rate of progression varies and is dependent on genotype, frequency of exacerbations and infections, and environmental factors. Diagnosis is made through a combination of clinical symptoms, positive newborn screen, or having a sibling with CF along with evidence of CFTR dysfunction; the latter can be detected through genetic testing or sweat chloride testing.[126]

Treatment

CFTR modulators are a new class of oral therapies designed to improve function and production of the malfunctioning CFTR protein. There are currently 4 CFTR modulators available for patients with eligible genetic mutations with specific regimens based upon the type of mutation(s) present.

Elexacaftor/tezacaftor/ivacaftor

Elexacaftor/tezacaftor/ivacaftor (ETI) is recommended for patients with at least 1 copy of F508del mutation or another CFTR mutation responsive to ETI based on clinical trial or in vitro data. Standard adult dosing is usually 2 tablets of elexacaftor 100 mg, tezacaftor 50 mg, and ivacaftor 75 mg in the morning and 1 ivacaftor 150 mg tablet in the evening; both doses are recommended with fat-containing food to improve absorption. Dose reductions are recommended for patients with hepatic impairment or on cytochrome P450 3A inhibitor medications. Adverse reactions noted in clinical trials include headache, abdominal pain, rash, upper respiratory tract symptoms or infections, diarrhea, transaminitis, hyperbilirubinemia, and increase in systolic and diastolic blood pressure. Cataracts have been reported amid pediatric populations. Elevated CPK has also been noted, though no patients in clinical trials permanently discontinued ETI based on this laboratory value.

ETI has been associated with increased survival along and well-being among patients with pulmonary and other manifestations of CF. Clinical trial outcomes associated with ETI include improvement in FEV1 by 10% to 15%, respiratory symptoms, quality-of-life index measurements, radiographic findings (bronchial wall thickening and mucus plugging), body mass index, gastrointestinal absorption, and frequency of exacerbations and pulmonary infections. Studies are currently ongoing to assess the long-term effects of TKI on liver and pancreatic manifestations of CF.[127–131]

Ivacaftor

Ivacaftor is recommend for patients with "gating mutations" or mutations causing malformation to the chloride channel gate within the CFTR protein. Standard adult dosing is 150 mg oral tablets every 12 hours and is to be administered with fat-containing food to improve absorption. Dose reductions are recommended for patients with hepatic impairment or on cytochrome P450 3A inhibitor medications. Liver function test monitoring is recommended every month for the first 3 months. Adverse reactions include elevated liver function tests, headaches, skin rash, abdominal pain, nausea, diarrhea, and upper respiratory tract infections; cataracts have been reported amid pediatric populations.[132–135]

Tezacaftor/ivacaftor

Tezacaftor/ivacaftor (TI) recommended for patients with CF secondary to having 2 copies of the F508del mutation as well as patients with other specified mutations. Tezacaftor assists with CFTR protein formation and transit, while ivacaftor helps with the CFTR protein chloride channel gate functioning. TI is generally used for patients who have mutations responsive to TI but not to ETI. Standard adult dosing is one combination oral tablet of tezacaftor 100 mg and ivacaftor 150 mg in the morning with ivacaftor 150 mg in the evening; both tablets are recommend with fat-containing food to increase absorption. Like ETI and ivacaftor, dose reductions are recommended for patients with hepatic impairment or on cytochrome P450 3A inhibitor medications, and liver function test monitoring is recommended every month for the first 3 months. Adverse effects are similar to ETI.[136–142]

Lumacaftor/ivacaftor

Lumacaftor/ivacaftor (LI) is also recommended for patients with CF secondary to having 2 copies of the F508del mutation. Lumacaftor assists with CFTR protein formation and transit, while ivacaftor helps with the CFTR protein chloride channel gate functioning. Like ETI, dose reductions are recommended for patients with hepatic impairment or on cytochrome P450 3A inhibitor medications. ETI is generally preferred now over LI for adults, as it has fewer side effects and has demonstrated greater improvement in FEV1. Adverse effects attributed to LI include cirrhosis, chest discomfort, dyspnea, bronchospasm, and wheezing.[143–149]

CLINICS CARE POINTS

- In patients with uncontrolled asthma despite the use of first line therapies, biologic therapies can be selected using blood eosinophils and total IgE levels and added to first line regimens to achieve better symptom control.

- In addition to smoking cessation, inhaled bronchodilators and pulmonary rehabilitation remain the best available management tools for patients with COPD.

- Antifibrotics, while side effects can be difficult to tolerate for some patients, have been shown to slow the progression of IPF and are now approved for use in patients with other etiologies of pulmonary fibrosis.

- Most pharmacotherapy available for the management of pulmonary hypertension has been studied in patient's with Group 1 and 4. Therefore, they are currently only approved for these groups with the exception of inhaled Treprostinil which was recently approved for patients with group 3 PH.

- CFTR modulators have dramatically changed the disease outcomes of patients with eligible genetic mutations.

REFERENCES

1. Jarjour NN, Kelly EAB. Pathogenesis of asthma. Med Clin North Am 2002;86(5): 925–36.
2. Bateman ED, Hurd SS, Barnes PJ, et al. Global strategy for asthma management and prevention: GINA executive summary. Eur Respir J 2008;31(1): 143–78.
3. Expert Panel Working Group of the National Heart, Lung, and Blood Institute (NHLBI) administered and coordinated National Asthma Education and Prevention Program Coordinating Committee (NAEPPCC), Cloutier MM, Baptist AP, Blake KV, et al. 2020 Focused updates to the asthma management guidelines: a report from the national asthma education and prevention program coordinating committee expert panel working group. J Allergy Clin Immunol 2020; 146(6):1217–70.

4. Fanta CH. Advances in evaluation and treatment of severe asthma (Part One). Med Clin North Am 2022;106(6):971–86.

5. Brusselle GG, Koppelman GH. Biologic therapies for severe asthma. N Engl J Med 2022;386(2):157–71.

6. Global initiative for asthma, Global strategy for asthma management and prevention, Published online July 2023. Available at: www.ginasthma.org, (Accessed January 1, 2023), 2023.

7. Venkatesan P. 2023 GINA report for asthma. Lancet Respir Med 2023;11(7):589.

8. Holguin F, Cardet JC, Chung KF, et al. Management of severe asthma: a European Respiratory Society/American Thoracic Society guideline. Eur Respir J 2020;55(1):1900588.

9. Krings JG, McGregor MC, Bacharier LB, et al. Biologics for severe asthma: treatment-specific effects are important in choosing a specific agent. J Allergy Clin Immunol Pract 2019;7(5):1379–92.

10. Fanta CH. Advances in evaluation and treatment of severe asthma (Part Two). Med Clin North Am 2022;106(6):987–99.

11. National Institute for Health and Care Excellence. Omalizumab for treating severe persistent allergic asthma. 2013. Available at: https://www.nice.org.uk/guidance/ta278.

12. Haldar Pranabashis, Brightling CE, Hargadon B, et al. Mepolizumab and exacerbations of refractory eosinophilic asthma. N Engl J Med 2009;360(10):973–84.

13. Nair Parameswaran, Pizzichini MMM, Kjarsgaard M, et al. Mepolizumab for prednisone-dependent asthma with sputum eosinophilia. N Engl J Med 2009;360(10):985–93.

14. Chupp Geoffrey L, Bradford ES, Albers FC, et al. Efficacy of mepolizumab add-on therapy on health-related quality of life and markers of asthma control in severe eosinophilic asthma (MUSCA): a randomised, double-blind, placebo-controlled, parallel-group, multicentre, phase 3b trial. Lancet Respir Med 2017;5(5):390–400.

15. Erin S Harvey, Langton D, Katelaris C, et al. Mepolizumab effectiveness and identification of super-responders in severe asthma. Eur Respir J 2020;55(5):1902420.

16. Ortega Hector G, Liu MC, Pavord ID, et al. Mepolizumab treatment in patients with severe eosinophilic asthma. N Engl J Med 2014;371(13):1198–207.

17. Khatri Sumita, Moore W, Gibson PG, et al. Assessment of the long-term safety of mepolizumab and durability of clinical response in patients with severe eosinophilic asthma. J Allergy Clin Immunol 2019;143(5):1742–51.e7.

18. Christian Virchow J, Katial R, Brusselle GG, et al. Safety of reslizumab in uncontrolled asthma with eosinophilia: a pooled analysis from 6 trials. J Allergy Clin Immunol 2020;8(2):540–8.e1. In Practice.

19. Fanta, "Advances in Evaluation and Treatment of Severe Asthma (Part Two)"; Brusselle and Koppelman, "Biologic Therapies for Severe Asthma. Medical Clinics 106, no.6 2022: 987-999.

20. Thaçi D, Simpson EL, Beck LA, et al. Efficacy and safety of dupilumab in adults with moderate-to-severe atopic dermatitis inadequately controlled by topical treatments: a randomised, placebo-controlled, dose-ranging phase 2b trial. Lancet (London, England) 2016;387(10013):40–52.

21. Claus Bachert, Mannent L, Naclerio RM, et al. Effect of subcutaneous dupilumab on nasal polyp burden in patients with chronic sinusitis and nasal polyposis: a randomized clinical trial. JAMA 2016;315(5):469–79.

22. Dupin Clairelyne, Belhadi D, Guilleminault L, et al. Effectiveness and safety of dupilumab for the treatment of severe asthma in a real-life french multi-centre adult cohort. Clin Exp Allergy 2020;50(7):789–98.

23. Eger Katrien, Pet L, Weersink EJM, et al. Complications of switching from anti-il-5 or anti-il-5r to dupilumab in corticosteroid-dependent severe asthma. J Allergy Clin Immunol Pract 2021;9(7):2913–5.

24. Castro Mario, Corren J, Pavord ID, et al. Dupilumab efficacy and safety in moderate-to-severe uncontrolled asthma. N Engl J Med 2018;378(26):2486–96.

25. Eger et al., "Complications of Switching from Anti-IL-5 or Anti-IL-5R to Dupilumab in Corticosteroid-Dependent Severe Asthma.".

26. Porsbjerg CM, Sverrild A, Lloyd CM, et al. Anti-alarmins in asthma: targeting the airway epithelium with next-generation biologics. Eur Respir J 2020;56(5):2000260.

27. Gauvreau GM, Sehmi R, Ambrose CS, et al. Thymic stromal lymphopoietin: its role and potential as a therapeutic target in asthma. Expert Opin Ther Targets 2020;24(8):777–92.

28. Sverrild A, Hansen S, Hvidtfeldt M, et al. The effect of tezepelumab on airway hyperresponsiveness to mannitol in asthma (UPSTREAM). Eur Respir J 2022;59(1):2101296.

29. Diver S, Khalfaoui L, Emson C, et al. Effect of tezepelumab on airway inflammatory cells, remodelling, and hyperresponsiveness in patients with moderate-to-severe uncontrolled asthma (CASCADE): a double-blind, randomised, placebo-controlled, phase 2 trial. Lancet Respir Med 2021;9(11):1299–312.

30. Sadushi-Kolici R, Jansa P, Kopec G, et al. Subcutaneous treprostinil for the treatment of severe non-operable chronic thromboembolic pulmonary hypertension (CTREPH): a double-blind, phase 3, randomised controlled trial. Lancet Respir Med 2019;7(3):239–48.

31. Stanojevic S, Kaminsky DA, Miller MR, et al. ERS/ATS technical standard on interpretive strategies for routine lung function tests. Eur Respir J 2022;60(1):2101499.

32. Agustí A, Celli BR, Criner GJ, et al. Global initiative for chronic obstructive lung disease 2023 report: GOLD executive summary. Am J Respir Crit Care Med 2023;207(7):819–37.

33. Terry PD, Dhand R. The 2023 GOLD report: updated guidelines for inhaled pharmacological therapy in patients with stable COPD. Pulm Ther 2023;9(3):345–57.

34. Calverley PMA, Rabe KF, Goehring UM, et al, M2-124 and M2-125 study groups. Roflumilast in symptomatic chronic obstructive pulmonary disease: two randomised clinical trials. Lancet 2009;374(9691):685–94.

35. Fabbri LM, Calverley PMA, Izquierdo-Alonso JL, et al. Roflumilast in moderate-to-severe chronic obstructive pulmonary disease treated with longacting bronchodilators: two randomised clinical trials. Lancet 2009;374(9691):695–703.

36. Anzueto A, Barjaktarevic IZ, Siler TM, et al. Ensifentrine, a novel phosphodiesterase 3 and 4 inhibitor for the treatment of chronic obstructive pulmonary disease: randomized, double-blind, placebo-controlled, multicenter phase III trials (the ENHANCE Trials). Am J Respir Crit Care Med 2023;208(4):406–16.

37. Bhatt SP, Rabe KF, Hanania NA, et al. Dupilumab for COPD with type 2 inflammation indicated by eosinophil counts. N Engl J Med 2023;389(3):205–14.

38. Spruit MA, Singh SJ, Garvey C, et al. An official American thoracic society/european respiratory society statement: key concepts and advances in pulmonary rehabilitation. Am J Respir Crit Care Med 2013;188(8):e13–64.

39. Mendes Xavier D, Lanza Galvão E, Aliane Fonseca A, et al. Effects of home-based pulmonary rehabilitation on dyspnea, exercise capacity, quality of life and impact of the disease in COPD patients: a systematic review. COPD 2022;19(1):18–46.

40. Stafinski T, Nagase FI, Avdagovska M, et al. Effectiveness of home-based pulmonary rehabilitation programs for patients with chronic obstructive pulmonary disease (COPD): systematic review. BMC Health Serv Res 2022;22(1):557.

41. Fishman A, Martinez F, Naunheim K, et al. A randomized trial comparing lung-volume-reduction surgery with medical therapy for severe emphysema. N Engl J Med 2003;348(21):2059–73.

42. Sciurba FC, Rogers RM, Keenan RJ, et al. Improvement in pulmonary function and elastic recoil after lung-reduction surgery for diffuse emphysema. N Engl J Med 1996;334(17):1095–9.

43. Kemp SV, Slebos DJ, Kirk A, et al. A multicenter randomized controlled trial of zephyr endobronchial valve treatment in heterogeneous emphysema (TRANSFORM). Am J Respir Crit Care Med 2017;196(12):1535–43.

44. Criner GJ, Delage A, Voelker K, et al. Improving lung function in severe heterogenous emphysema with the spiration valve system (EMPROVE). a multicenter, open-label randomized controlled clinical trial. Am J Respir Crit Care Med 2019;200(11):1354–62.

45. Travis WD, Costabel U, Hansell DM, et al. An official american thoracic society/european respiratory society statement: Update of the international multidisciplinary classification of the idiopathic interstitial pneumonias. Am J Respir Crit Care Med 2013;188(6):733–48.

46. Flaherty KR, Wells AU, Cottin V, et al. Nintedanib in progressive fibrosing interstitial lung diseases. N Engl J Med 2019;381(18):1718–27.

47. Richeldi L, du Bois RM, Raghu G, et al. Efficacy and safety of nintedanib in idiopathic pulmonary fibrosis. N Engl J Med 2014;370(22):2071–82.

48. Richeldi L, Kolb M, Jouneau S, et al. Efficacy and safety of nintedanib in patients with advanced idiopathic pulmonary fibrosis. BMC Pulm Med 2020;20(1):3.

49. Nintedanib capsules package insert. Ridgefield CT: Boehringer Ingelheim Pharmaceuticals Inc; 2022.

50. King TEJ, Bradford WZ, Castro-Bernardini S, et al. A phase 3 trial of pirfenidone in patients with idiopathic pulmonary fibrosis. N Engl J Med 2014;370(22):2083–92.

51. Pirfenidone capsules [package insert]. Brisbane CA: Intermune Inc; 2014.

52. Noble PW, Albera C, Bradford WZ, et al. Pirfenidone in patients with idiopathic pulmonary fibrosis (CAPACITY): two randomised trials. Lancet 2011;377(9779):1760–9.

53. Nathan SD, Waxman A, Rajagopal S, et al. Inhaled treprostinil and forced vital capacity in patients with interstitial lung disease and associated pulmonary hypertension: a post-hoc analysis of the INCREASE study. Lancet Respir Med 2021;9(11):1266–74.

54. Waxman A, Restrepo-Jaramillo R, Thenappan T, et al. Inhaled treprostinil in pulmonary hypertension due to interstitial lung disease. N Engl J Med 2021;384(4):325–34.

55. Kolb M, Orfanos SE, Lambers C, et al. The antifibrotic effects of inhaled treprostinil: an emerging option for ILD. Adv Ther 2022;39(9):3881–95.

56. Nathan SD, Behr J, Cottin V, et al. Study design and rationale for the TETON phase 3, randomised, controlled clinical trials of inhaled treprostinil in the

treatment of idiopathic pulmonary fibrosis. BMJ Open Respir Res 2022;9(1). https://doi.org/10.1136/bmjresp-2022-001310.

57. Spikes LA, Bajwa AA, Burger CD, et al. BREEZE: Open-label clinical study to evaluate the safety and tolerability of treprostinil inhalation powder as Tyvaso DPITM in patients with pulmonary arterial hypertension. Pulm Circ 2022;12(2): e12063.

58. Waxman A, Restrepo-Jaramillo R, Thenappan T, et al. Long-term inhaled treprostinil for pulmonary hypertension due to interstitial lung disease: INCREASE open-label extension study. Eur Respir J 2023;61(6). https://doi.org/10.1183/13993003.02414-2022.

59. Treprostinil inhalation solution package insert. Research Triangle Park NC: United Therapeutics Corp; 2023.

60. Treprostinil Inhalation Powder Package Insert. Research Triangle Park NC: United Therapeutics Corp; 2023.; 2023.

61. Kovacs G, Berghold A, Scheidl S, et al. Pulmonary arterial pressure during rest and exercise in healthy subjects: a systematic review. Eur Respir J 2009;34(4): 888–94.

62. Kovacs G, Olschewski A, Berghold A, et al. Pulmonary vascular resistances during exercise in normal subjects: a systematic review. Eur Respir J 2012;39(2): 319–28.

63. Maron BA, Hess E, Maddox TM, et al. Association of Borderline pulmonary hypertension with mortality and hospitalization in a large patient cohort: insights from the veterans affairs clinical assessment, reporting, and tracking program. Circulation 2016;133(13):1240–8.

64. Douschan P, Kovacs G, Avian A, et al. Mild elevation of pulmonary arterial pressure as a predictor of mortality. Am J Respir Crit Care Med 2018;197(4):509–16.

65. Kolte D, Lakshmanan S, Jankowich MD, et al. Mild pulmonary hypertension is associated with increased mortality: a systematic review and meta-analysis. JAHA 2018;7(18):e009729.

66. Humbert M, Kovacs G, Hoeper MM, et al. 2022 ESC/ERS Guidelines for the diagnosis and treatment of pulmonary hypertension. Eur Respir J 2023;61(1): 2200879.

67. Humbert Marc, Kovacs G, Hoeper MM, et al. 2022 ESC/ERS guidelines for the diagnosis and treatment of pulmonary hypertension. Eur Respir J 2023;61(1): 2200879.

68. Simonneau G, Montani D, Celermajer DS, et al. Haemodynamic definitions and updated clinical classification of pulmonary hypertension. Eur Respir J 2019; 53(1). https://doi.org/10.1183/13993003.01913-2018.

69. Benza Raymond L, Gomberg-Maitland M, Miller DP, et al. The REVEAL registry risk score calculator in patients newly diagnosed with pulmonary arterial hypertension. Chest 2012;141(2):354–62.

70. Chan L, Chin LMK, Kennedy M, et al. Benefits of intensive treadmill exercise training on cardiorespiratory function and quality of life in patients with pulmonary hypertension. Chest 2013;143(2):333–43.

71. Ehlken N, Lichtblau M, Klose H, et al. Exercise training improves peak oxygen consumption and haemodynamics in patients with severe pulmonary arterial hypertension and inoperable chronic thrombo-embolic pulmonary hypertension: a prospective, randomized, controlled trial. Eur Heart J 2016;37(1):35–44.

72. Grünig E, MacKenzie A, Peacock AJ, et al. Standardized exercise training is feasible, safe, and effective in pulmonary arterial and chronic thromboembolic

pulmonary hypertension: results from a large European multicentre randomized controlled trial. Eur Heart J 2021;42(23):2284–95.

73. Mereles D, Ehlken N, Kreuscher S, et al. Exercise and respiratory training improve exercise capacity and quality of life in patients with severe chronic pulmonary hypertension. Circulation 2006;114(14):1482–9.

74. Kramer T, Wissmüller M, Natsina K, et al. Ferric carboxymaltose in patients with pulmonary arterial hypertension and iron deficiency: a long-term study. J cachexia sarcopenia muscle 2021;12(6):1501–12.

75. Ruiter G, Manders E, Happé CM, et al. Intravenous iron therapy in patients with idiopathic pulmonary arterial hypertension and iron deficiency. Pulm Circ 2015; 5(3):466–72.

76. Sitbon Olivier, Humbert M, Jaïs X, et al. Long-term response to calcium channel blockers in idiopathic pulmonary arterial hypertension. Circulation 2005; 111(23):3105–11.

77. Rich Stuart, Kaufmann Elizabeth, Levy Paul S. The effect of high doses of calcium-channel blockers on survival in primary pulmonary hypertension. N Engl J Med 1992;327(2):76–81.

78. Galiè Nazzareno, Olschewski H, Oudiz RJ, et al. Ambrisentan for the treatment of pulmonary arterial hypertension: results of the ambrisentan in pulmonary arterial hypertension, randomized, double-blind, placebo-controlled, multicenter, efficacy (ARIES) study 1 and 2. Circulation 2008;117(23):3010–9.

79. Lewis J Rubin, Badesch DB, Barst RJ, et al. Bosentan therapy for pulmonary arterial hypertension. N Engl J Med 2002;346(12):896–903.

80. Gideon A Paul, Gibbs JSR, Boobis AR, et al. Bosentan decreases the plasma concentration of sildenafil when coprescribed in pulmonary hypertension. Br J Clin Pharmacol 2005;60(1):107–12.

81. Weber Cornelia, Banken L, Birnboeck H, et al. Effect of the endothelin-receptor antagonist bosentan on the pharmacokinetics and pharmacodynamics of warfarin. J Clin Pharmacol 1999;39(8):847–54.

82. Wrishko Rebecca E, Dingemanse J, Yu A, et al. Pharmacokinetic interaction between tadalafil and bosentan in healthy male subjects. J Clin Pharmacol 2008; 48(5):610–8.

83. Pulido Tomás, Adzerikho I, Channick RN, et al. Macitentan and morbidity and mortality in pulmonary arterial hypertension. N Engl J Med 2013;369(9):809–18.

84. Sastry BKS, Narasimhan C, Reddy NK, et al. Clinical efficacy of sildenafil in primary pulmonary hypertension: a randomized, placebo-controlled, double-blind, crossover study. J Am Coll Cardiol 2004;43(7):1149–53.

85. Galiè Nazzareno, Brundage BH, Ghofrani HA, et al. Tadalafil therapy for pulmonary arterial hypertension. Circulation 2009;119(22):2894–903.

86. Schermuly Ralph T, Janssen W, Weissmann N, et al. Riociguat for the treatment of pulmonary hypertension. Expet Opin Invest Drugs 2011;20(4):567–76.

87. Ghofrani Hossein-Ardeschir, Galiè N, Grimminger F, et al. Riociguat for the treatment of pulmonary arterial hypertension. N Engl J Med 2013;369(4):330–40.

88. Barst Robyn J, Rubin LJ, Long WA, et al. A comparison of continuous intravenous epoprostenol (prostacyclin) with conventional therapy for primary pulmonary hypertension. N Engl J Med 1996;334(5):296–301.

89. Badesch David B, Tapson VF, McGoon MD, et al. Continuous intravenous epoprostenol for pulmonary hypertension due to the scleroderma spectrum of disease: a randomized, controlled trial. Ann Intern Med 2000;132(6):425.

90. Krowka Michael J, Frantz RP, McGoon MD, et al. Improvement in pulmonary hemodynamics during intravenous epoprostenol (prostacyclin): a study of 15

patients with moderate to severe portopulmonary hypertension. Hepatology 1999;30(3):641–8.

91. Olschewski Horst, Simonneau G, Galiè N, et al. Inhaled iloprost for severe pulmonary hypertension. N Engl J Med 2002;347(5):322–9.

92. Simonneau Gerald, Barst RJ, Galie N, et al. Continuous subcutaneous infusion of treprostinil, a prostacyclin analogue, in patients with pulmonary arterial hypertension: a double-blind, randomized, placebo-controlled trial. Am J Respir Crit Care Med 2002;165(6):800–4.

93. Bourge Robert C, Waxman AB, Gomberg-Maitland M, et al. Treprostinil administered to treat pulmonary arterial hypertension using a fully implantable programmable intravascular delivery system. Chest 2016;150(1):27–34.

94. Richter Manuel J, Harutyunova S, Bollmann T, et al. Long-term safety and outcome of intravenous treprostinil via an implanted pump in pulmonary hypertension. J Heart Lung Transplant 2018;37(10):1235–44.

95. McLaughlin Vallerie V, Benza RL, Rubin LJ, et al. Addition of inhaled treprostinil to oral therapy for pulmonary arterial hypertension. J Am Coll Cardiol 2010; 55(18):1915–22.

96. Nathan Steven D, Tapson VF, Elwing J, et al. Efficacy of inhaled treprostinil on multiple disease progression events in patients with pulmonary hypertension due to parenchymal lung disease in the INCREASE trial. Am J Respir Crit Care Med 2022;205(2):198–207.

97. Zhi-Cheng Jing, Parikh K, Pulido T, et al. Efficacy and safety of oral treprostinil monotherapy for the treatment of pulmonary arterial hypertension: a randomized, controlled trial. Circulation 2013;127(5):624–33.

98. James White R, Jerjes-Sanchez C, Bohns Meyer GM, et al. Combination therapy with oral treprostinil for pulmonary arterial hypertension. a double-blind placebo-controlled clinical trial. Am J Respir Crit Care Med 2020;201(6):707–17.

99. Sitbon Olivier, Channick R, Chin KM, et al. Selexipag for the treatment of pulmonary arterial hypertension. N Engl J Med 2015;373(26):2522–33.

100. Gérald Simonneau, Torbicki A, Hoeper MM, et al. Selexipag: an oral, selective prostacyclin receptor agonist for the treatment of pulmonary arterial hypertension. Eur Respir J 2012;40(4):874–80.

101. Kirtania L, Maiti R, Srinivasan A, et al. Effect of combination therapy of endothelin receptor antagonist and phosphodiesterase-5 inhibitor on clinical outcome and pulmonary haemodynamics in patients with pulmonary arterial hypertension: a meta-analysis. Clin Drug Investig 2019;39(11):1031–44.

102. Badagliacca R, D'Alto M, Ghio S, et al. Risk reduction and hemodynamics with initial combination therapy in pulmonary arterial hypertension. Am J Respir Crit Care Med 2021;203(4):484–92.

103. Sitbon O, Jais X, Savale L, et al. Upfront triple combination therapy in pulmonary arterial hypertension: a pilot study. Eur Respir J 2014;43(6):1691–7.

104. D'Alto M, Badagliacca R, Argiento P, et al. Risk reduction and right heart reverse remodeling by upfront triple combination therapy in pulmonary arterial hypertension. Chest 2020;157(2):376–83.

105. Torres F, Farber H, Ristic A, et al. Efficacy and safety of ralinepag, a novel oral IP agonist, in PAH patients on mono or dual background therapy: results from a phase 2 randomised, parallel group, placebo-controlled trial. Eur Respir J 2019;54(4):1901030.

106. Hoeper MM, Badesch DB, Ghofrani HA, et al. Phase 3 trial of sotatercept for treatment of pulmonary arterial hypertension. N Engl J Med 2023;388(16): 1478–90.

107. Chen SL, Zhang FF, Xu J, et al. Pulmonary artery denervation to treat pulmonary arterial hypertension. J Am Coll Cardiol 2013;62(12):1092–100.
108. Rothman AMK, Vachiery JL, Howard LS, et al. Intravascular ultrasound pulmonary artery denervation to treat pulmonary arterial hypertension (TROPHY1). JACC Cardiovasc Interv 2020;13(8):989–99.
109. Kaluski E, Cotter G, Leitman M, et al. Clinical and Hemodynamic Effects of Bosentan Dose Optimization in Symptomatic Heart Failure Patients with Severe Systolic Dysfunction, Associated with Secondary Pulmonary Hypertension - A Multi-Center Randomized Study. Cardiology 2008;109(4):273–80. https://doi.org/10.1159/000107791.
110. Koller B, Steringer-Mascherbauer R, Ebner CH, et al. Pilot Study of Endothelin Receptor Blockade in Heart Failure with Diastolic Dysfunction and Pulmonary Hypertension (BADDHY-Trial). Heart, Lung and Circulation 2017;26(5):433–41. https://doi.org/10.1016/j.hlc.2016.09.004.
111. Vachiéry Jean-Luc, Delcroix M, Al-Hiti H, et al. Macitentan in Pulmonary Hypertension Due to Left Ventricular Dysfunction. European Respiratory Journal 2018; 51(2). https://doi.org/10.1183/13993003.01886-2017. 1701886.
112. Wu X, Yang T, Zhou Q, et al. Additional Use of a Phosphodiesterase 5 Inhibitor in Patients with Pulmonary Hypertension Secondary to Chronic Systolic Heart Failure: A Meta-analysis. European Journal of Heart Failure 2014;16(4):444–53. https://doi.org/10.1002/ejhf.47.
113. Lewis G, Shah R, Shahzad K, et al. Sildenafil Improves Exercise Capacity and Quality of Life in Patients With Systolic Heart Failure and Secondary Pulmonary Hypertension. Circulation 2007;116(14):1555–62. https://doi.org/10.1161/CIRCULATIONAHA.107.716373.
114. Dumitrescu D, Seck C, Möhle L, et al. Therapeutic Potential of Sildenafil in Patients with Heart Failure and Reactive Pulmonary Hypertension. International Journal of Cardiology 2012;154(2):205–6. https://doi.org/10.1016/j.ijcard.2011.10.064.
115. Kramer T, Dumitrescu D, Gerhardt F, et al. Therapeutic Potential of Phosphodiesterase Type 5 Inhibitors in Heart Failure with Preserved Ejection Fraction and Combined Post- and Pre-Capillary Pulmonary Hypertension. International Journal of Cardiology 2019;283:152–8. https://doi.org/10.1016/j.ijcard.2018.12.078.
116. Humbert M, Kovacs G, Hoeper MM, et al. 2022 ESC/ERS Guidelines for the Diagnosis and Treatment of Pulmonary Hypertension. European Respiratory 2023;61(1). https://doi.org/10.1183/13993003.00879-2022. 2200879.
117. Bunclark K, Newnham M, Chiu Y, et al. A multicenter study of anticoagulation in operable chronic thromboembolic pulmonary hypertension. J Thromb Haemostasis 2020;18(1):114–22.
118. Humbert M, Simonneau G, Pittrow D, et al. Oral anticoagulants (NOAC and VKA) in chronic thromboembolic pulmonary hypertension. J Heart Lung Transplant 2022;41(6):716–21.
119. Hsieh WC, Jansa P, Huang WC, et al. Residual pulmonary hypertension after pulmonary endarterectomy: A meta-analysis. J Thorac Cardiovasc Surg 2018; 156(3):1275–87.
120. Wiedenroth CB, Liebetrau C, Breithecker A, et al. Combined pulmonary endarterectomy and balloon pulmonary angioplasty in patients with chronic thromboembolic pulmonary hypertension. J Heart Lung Transplant 2016;35(5):591–6.
121. Darocha S, Pietura R, Pietrasik A, et al. Improvement in quality of life and hemodynamics in chronic thromboembolic pulmonary hypertension treated with balloon pulmonary angioplasty. Circ J 2017;81(4):552–7.

122. Kim NH, Delcroix M, Jais X, et al. Chronic thromboembolic pulmonary hypertension. Eur Respir J 2019;53(1):1801915.

123. Mahmud E, Behnamfar O, Ang L, et al. Balloon pulmonary angioplasty for chronic thromboembolic pulmonary hypertension. Interventional Cardiology Clinics 2018;7(1):103–17.

124. Ghofrani HA, D'Armini AM, Grimminger F, et al. Riociguat for the treatment of chronic thromboembolic pulmonary hypertension. N Engl J Med 2013;369(4):319–29.

125. Ghofrani HA, Simonneau G, D'Armini AM, et al. Macitentan for the treatment of inoperable chronic thromboembolic pulmonary hypertension (MERIT-1): results from the multicentre, phase 2, randomised, double-blind, placebo-controlled study. Lancet Respir Med 2017;5(10):785–94.

126. Farrell PM, White TB, Ren CL, et al. Diagnosis of cystic fibrosis: consensus guidelines from the cystic fibrosis foundation. J Pediatr 2017;181S:S4–15.e1.

127. Daines CL, Tullis E, Costa S, et al. Long-term safety and efficacy of elexacaftor/tezacaftor/ivacaftor in people with cystic fibrosis and at least one F508del allele: 144-week interim results from a 192-week open-label extension study. Eur Respir J 2023;62(6). https://doi.org/10.1183/13993003.02029-2022.

128. Middleton PG, Mall MA, Dřevínek P, et al. Elexacaftor-tezacaftor-ivacaftor for cystic fibrosis with a single Phe508del allele. N Engl J Med 2019;381(19):1809–19.

129. Heijerman HGM, McKone EF, Downey DG, et al. Efficacy and safety of the elexacaftor plus tezacaftor plus ivacaftor combination regimen in people with cystic fibrosis homozygous for the F508del mutation: a double-blind, randomised, phase 3 trial. Lancet 2019;394(10212):1940–8.

130. Zemanick ET, Taylor-Cousar JL, Davies J, et al. A phase 3 open-label study of elexacaftor/tezacaftor/ivacaftor in children 6 through 11 years of age with cystic fibrosis and at least one F508del allele. Am J Respir Crit Care Med 2021;203(12):1522–32.

131. Elexacaftor tezacaftor. Ivacaftor tablets; ivacaftor tablets), co-packaged for oral use[package insert]. Boston MA: Vertex Pharmaceuticals Inc; 2023.

132. Edgeworth D, Keating D, Ellis M, et al. Improvement in exercise duration, lung function and well-being in G551D-cystic fibrosis patients: a double-blind, placebo-controlled, randomized, cross-over study with ivacaftor treatment. Clin Sci (Lond) 2017;131(15):2037–45.

133. Kerem E, Cohen-Cymberknoh M, Tsabari R, et al. Ivacaftor in people with cystic fibrosis and a 3849+10kb C→T or D1152H residual function mutation. Ann Am Thorac Soc 2021;18(3):433–41.

134. Ivacaftor tablets[package insert]. Boston MA: Vertex Pharmaceuticals Inc; 2023.

135. Accurso FJ, Rowe SM, Clancy JP, et al. Effect of VX-770 in persons with cystic fibrosis and the G551D-CFTR mutation. N Engl J Med 2010;363(21):1991–2003.

136. Davies JC, Moskowitz SM, Brown C, et al. VX-659-tezacaftor-ivacaftor in patients with cystic fibrosis and one or two phe508del alleles. N Engl J Med 2018;379(17):1599–611.

137. Keating D, Marigowda G, Burr L, et al. VX-445-Tezacaftor-ivacaftor in patients with cystic fibrosis and one or two phe508del alleles. N Engl J Med 2018;379(17):1612–20.

138. McKone EF, DiMango EA, Sutharsan S, et al. A phase 3, randomized, double-blind, parallel-group study to evaluate tezacaftor/ivacaftor in people with cystic

fibrosis heterozygous for F508del-CFTR and a gating mutation. J Cyst Fibros 2021;20(2):234–42.

139. Munck A, Kerem E, Ellemunter H, et al. Tezacaftor/ivacaftor in people with cystic fibrosis heterozygous for minimal function CFTR mutations. J Cyst Fibros 2020; 19(6):962–8.

140. Rowe SM, Daines C, Ringshausen FC, et al. Tezacaftor-ivacaftor in residual-function heterozygotes with cystic fibrosis. N Engl J Med 2017;377(21):2024–35.

141. Taylor-Cousar JL, Munck A, McKone EF, et al. Tezacaftor-ivacaftor in patients with cystic fibrosis homozygous for Phe508del. N Engl J Med 2017;377(21):2013–23.

142. Tezacaftor/ivacaftor [package insert]. Boston MA: Vertex Pharmaceuticals Inc; 2023.

143. Berkers G, van der Meer R, Heijerman H, et al. Lumacaftor/ivacaftor in people with cystic fibrosis with an A455E-CFTR mutation. J Cyst Fibros 2021;20(5):761–7.

144. Konstan MW, McKone EF, Moss RB, et al. Assessment of safety and efficacy of long-term treatment with combination lumacaftor and ivacaftor therapy in patients with cystic fibrosis homozygous for the F508del-CFTR mutation (PROGRESS): a phase 3, extension study. Lancet Respir Med 2017;5(2):107–18.

145. Ratjen F, Hug C, Marigowda G, et al. Efficacy and safety of lumacaftor and ivacaftor in patients aged 6-11 years with cystic fibrosis homozygous for F508del-CFTR: a randomised, placebo-controlled phase 3 trial. Lancet Respir Med 2017; 5(7):557–67.

146. Rowe SM, McColley SA, Rietschel E, et al. Lumacaftor/Ivacaftor Treatment of Patients with Cystic Fibrosis Heterozygous for F508del-CFTR. Ann Am Thorac Soc 2017;14(2):213–9.

147. Stahl M, Roehmel J, Eichinger M, et al. Effects of lumacaftor/ivacaftor on cystic fibrosis disease progression in children 2 through 5 years of age homozygous for F508del-CFTR: a phase 2 placebo-controlled clinical trial. Ann Am Thorac Soc 2023;20(8):1144–55.

148. Wainwright CE, Elborn JS, Ramsey BW, et al. Lumacaftor-ivacaftor in patients with cystic fibrosis homozygous for Phe508del CFTR. N Engl J Med 2015;373(3):220–31.

149. Lumacaftor and ivacaftor tablets[package insert]. Boston MA: Vertex Pharmaceuticals Inc; 2023.

Update on Therapies and Treatments in Women's Health

Christine Prifti, MD[a],*, Rachel S. Casas, MD, EdM[b],
Sarah Merriam, MD, MS[c], Emmanuelle Yecies, MD, MS[d],
Judith M.E. Walsh, MD, MPH[e]

KEYWORDS

- Women's health • Menopause • Postpartum depression • Contraception
- Osteoporosis • Vulvovaginal candidiasis • Urinary tract infection
- Hypoactive sexual desire disorder

KEY POINTS

- A number of new therapeutics have been approved in the past decade in nearly every clinical area of Women's Health.
- Many are first-in-class medications, including zuranolone/brexanolone for postpartum depression, bremelanotide for hypoactive sexual desire disorder, fezolinetant for vasomotor symptoms of menopause, and romosozumab for osteoporosis.
- Others are new agents in existing classes that enhance prior offerings, such as otesecozazole for vulvovaginal candidiasis or several new contraceptive formulations.
- There is also new evidence for older medications, such as methenamine hippurate for prevention of urinary tract infections.
- Ongoing work is needed to clarify how some of these agents fit into existing treatment algorithms.

[a] Department of General Internal Medicine, Chobanian and Avedisian School of Medicine, Boston University Medical Center, 801 Massachusetts Avenue, 5th Floor, Suite 5A, Boston, MA 02118, USA; [b] Department of Medicine, Division of General Internal Medicine, Penn State Milton S. Hershey Medical Center, Academic Support Building, 90 Hope Drive, Suite 3200, Mail Code A320, Hershey, PA 17033, USA; [c] Division of General Internal Medicine, University of Pittsburgh School of Medicine, VA Pittsburgh Healthcare System, VA Hospital HJ Heinz, Primary Care, Building 71, 1010 Delafield Road, Pittsburgh, PA 15215, USA; [d] Department of Primary Care and Population Health, Stanford University School of Medicine (affiliated), VA Palo Alto Healthcare System, 3801 Miranda Avenue, Building 5, Palo Alto, CA 94304, USA; [e] School of Medicine, University of California, San Francisco, UCSF Valley Tower, 490 Illinois 8th Floor, Box 0856, San Francisco, CA 94158, USA
* Corresponding author.
E-mail address: christine.prifti@bmc.org
Twitter: @RachelCasas14 (R.S.C.); @SarahMerriamMD (S.M.)

Med Clin N Am 108 (2024) 871–880
https://doi.org/10.1016/j.mcna.2024.03.007
0025-7125/24/© 2024 Elsevier Inc. All rights reserved.

INTRODUCTION

Historic clinical research disproportionally represents male patients. The National Institutes of Health did not mandate inclusion of female individuals in clinical trials until 1994, and diseases that primarily impact this population remain understudied.[1] This general underrepresentation is counteracted by developing new treatments for conditions that primarily affect female patients. New therapies for vasomotor symptoms (VMS), postpartum depression (PPD), contraception, osteoporosis, recurrent yeast infections, acute and recurrent urinary tract infections (UTIs), and female hypoactive sexual desire disorder (HSDD) have notable benefits and side effects. Prescribers should be aware of and discuss novel treatment options with patients as appropriate.

FEZOLINETANT IS A NOVEL NONHORMONAL TREATMENT FOR VASOMOTOR SYMPTOMS

VMS are common, experienced by up to 80% of women during the menopausal transition.[2] About one-third of US women experience moderate-to-heavy symptom burden.[3] VMS may begin before the menopause onset, with a mean total duration of 7.4 years and median of 4.5 years following the final menstrual period. Approximately 10% of women have persistent VMS for up to a decade.[4] Importantly, VMS are associated with a decline in quality of life. Available treatments, such as menopausal hormone therapy (MHT) and available nonhormonal treatments (eg, selective serotonin reuptake inhibitors, serotonin and norepinephrine reuptake inhibitors, and gabapentinods), are not appropriate for all.

Fezolinetant, Food and Drug Administration (FDA) approved in May 2023, is a first-in-class selective neurokinin-3-receptor antagonist and alternative nonhormonal option for the treatment of moderate-to-severe VMS of menopause. Declining estradiol levels during the menopausal transition are associated with hypersecretion of neurokinin B, activation of the hypothalamic thermoregulatory center, and disruption of temperature control resulting in VMS. At a 45 mg dose, fezolinetant demonstrated a clinically meaningful reduction in moderate-to-severe VMS by about 2.5 hot flashes per day versus placebo.[5,6] VMS severity was improved, with a reduction of 0.2 to 0.3 (on a 3 point) scale compared to placebo. While no head-to-head studies have compared fezolinetant to other nonhormonal treatments, its effect size appears to be similar to other available nonhormonal options and smaller than that of MHT.

Overall, fezolinetant was well tolerated up to 52 weeks of follow-up.[5,6] It is recommended to monitor liver function tests (baseline, 3, 5, and 9 months) after initiation or with symptoms of liver dysfunction because elevated hepatic transaminases were deemed an adverse event of interest during clinical development (2.3% fezolinetant 45 mg and 0.8% placebo).[7] Fezolinetant is contraindicated in patients with cirrhosis, severe renal impairment or end-stage renal disease, and in patients on CYP1A2 inhibitors. Fezolinetant may be considered an alternative to other nonhormonal therapies for VMS when there is a contraindication, intolerance, or inadequate response.

ZURANOLONE AND BREXANOLONE: NOVEL, FASTER ACTING AGENTS FOR THE TREATMENT OF POSTPARTUM DEPRESSION

PPD is a prevalent mood disorder, estimated to be present with 12% of births. In 2021, the FDA-approved brexanolone, a neuroactive steroid γ-aminobutyric acid type A receptor modulator. Although a promising novel drug class, this 60 h continuous infusion was logistically challenging in a patient population for whom hospitalization presents a significant barrier to access. In 2023, the FDA evaluated and approved zuranolone, an oral agent in the same class.

The efficacy of zuranolone was evaluated in 2 industry-sponsored randomized, placebo-controlled, double-blind trials.[8,9] Participants were women aged 18 to 45 years with PPD, defined as a major depressive episode beginning in the third trimester or within 4 weeks of delivery. Only those with a Hamilton Rating Scale for Depression score of 26 or greater (severe depression) were included. The studies evaluated 14 day courses of once daily oral zuranolone, taken at night with fat-containing food to promote absorption. Patients had higher rates of remission starting at day 3 with zuranolone (19% vs 5% with placebo). Remission remained high throughout treatment and at 1 month after treatment conclusion (53% vs 30%). No evidence exists comparing zuranolone to usual treatment.

Zuranolone does have important safety considerations. Significant central nervous system (CNS) depressant effects were noted, although discontinuation rates were very low during the trial (1%). Patients should be counseled to avoid driving and may need assistance to care for infants or other children. Zuranolone is not recommended during pregnancy, and patients should be advised to use effective contraception during treatment. Zuranolone has been found in low levels in breastmilk, although there is no evidence on the effects of zuranolone on breastfed infants or milk production. CYP3A4 inducers should not be used concomitantly.

While oral zuranolone circumvents the logistical barriers of brexanolone infusions, the cost and lack of comparison to usual care make its incorporation into treatment algorithms challenging. At this time, we recommend case-by-case consideration for patients with severe PPD.

NEW CONTRACEPTIVES INCLUDE ORAL AGENTS, A DIFFERENT RING AND PATCH, AN ON-DEMAND GEL, AND EVIDENCE FOR USE OF 52 MCG LEVONORGESTROL INTRAUTERINE DEVICES FOR EMERGENCY CONTRACEPTION

All patients of childbearing age who desire contraception should be counseled about available options. Several updated and/or novel contraceptives have entered the market in the past several years: 2 novel oral contraceptives; a vaginal ring that can be used for 1 year; a lower systemic estrogen dose patch; a novel on-demand vaginal gel that works by lowering vaginal pH. In addition, there is evidence that the 52 mg levonorgestrol intrauterine device (IUD) has equal efficacy as the copper IUD for emergency contraception. Insurance coverage for novel methods is variable; coverage for new uses of old methods is typically not a problem.

Two novel oral contraceptives have gained FDA approval: drospirenone–estertrol 3 mg/14.2 mg (Nextstellis) and drospirenone 4 mg (Slynd). Drospirenone–estertrol 3 mg/14.2 mg was approved in April 2021 and includes a novel estrogen. Other combined oral contraceptives contain estradiol that is clinically manufactured from pregnant mare's urine. Estertrol is synthetically derived from plant sources. In animal studies, it had a lower impact on hemostasis biomarkers, triglycerides, and breast tissue.[10] Compared to estradiol, less drug metabolite is excreted in the urine, which is motivating to some environmentally conscious patients. The efficacy and safety profile for drospirenone-estertrol is similar to other combined oral contraceptives. It had a Pearl Index (number of pregnancies per 100 woman-years of exposure) of 2.65 (95% confidence interval [CI]: 1.73–3.88) in a phase 3 trial of 1524 patients. The most common reported adverse events were metrorrhagia 4.4% and headache 3.5%.[11]

While drospirenone is not a new agent, a 4 mg drospirenone tablet was approved as a novel progestin-only pill in May 2019. Previously, the only available progestin-only pill was norethindrone 0.35 mg. The new drospirenone-only pill has better efficacy in the setting of delayed or missed pills, and a more favorable bleeding profile. The missed pill window for drospirenone 4 mg is 24 hours; for norethindrone 0.35 mg, it is 3 hours. In a phase 3 trial of 1864 participants, rates of unscheduled bleeding decreased and amenorrhea increased as the study progressed.[11] Less than 2% of participants discontinued due to bleeding. Drospirenone has mineralocorticoid effects. In studied patients, there were no adverse effects on blood pressure; 0.5% of participants developed asymptomatic hyperkalemia.[12] The Pearl Index was 4.0 (95% CI: 2.3–6.4). Approximately one-third of study participants were obese (body mass index [BMI] $\geq$30.0 kg/m^2); the Pearl Index was not affected by BMI. No cases of venus thromboembolism (VTE) were reported.[11,12] We recommend drospirenone 4 mg for patients with contraindications to estrogen who desire improved efficacy and more regular bleeding compared to norethindrone 0.35 mg. Patients should be monitored for hyperkalemia.

A new vaginal ring (Annovera) was FDA approved in 2018 and can be used for 13 cycles or 1 year. It contains segesterone and ethinyl estradiol and has no appreciable differences in side effect profile compared to monthly rings containing etonogestrel and ethinyl estradiol. The 13 cycle ring is approximately twice as thick (8.4 mm vs 4 mm) as the 1 cycle ring, both rings have a similar diameter. The 13 cycle ring is kept in place for 21 days, removed for 7, then reinserted. During the 21 day use period, it should not be removed for more than 2 hours. Although there is no evidence for 12 months of continuous use, some patients have begun to use it this way off label. The Pearl Index was 2.98 (95% CI: 2·13–4·06), similar to other hormonal contraceptives.[13] There is limited evidence for use in patients with BMI greater than 29 as enrollment for this group was halted after 2 participants had a VTE. There are no head-to-head trials comparing vaginal rings. The new ring may be a good choice for patients who struggle to refill medications at a pharmacy.

A new on-demand contraceptive, a lactic acid and potassium bitartrate vaginal gel (Phexxi) was approved in 2020 and lowers vaginal pH to reduce sperm motility. The nonhormonal, user-controlled gel is inserted into the vagina using a single-dose applicator up to 1 hour prior to intercourse; there is no evidence for use after sex. The Pearl Index was 27.5 (95% CI: 22.4%, 33.5%).[14] The most frequently reported adverse effect was vulvovaginal burning sensation (20.0%)[15]; partners may experience a similar sensation. It requires a prescription and expands options for patients seeking on-demand, hormone-free contraception. It can be used in combination with condoms and diaphragms.

A new ethinyl estradiol and levonorgestrel contraceptive patch (Twirla) entered the market in 2020. Previously, there was only one patch on the market, ethinyl estradiol and norelgestromin (Xulane, the generic of Ortho Evra). Serum levels of ethinyl estradiol for Twirla's are similar to those of a low-dose oral contraceptive; Xulane levels are about 60% higher.[16–18] While the 2 patches have not been compared head-to-head, both are less effective in patients with BMI greater than 30. Unfortunately, the risk of VTE with Twirla was in the same range as other combined hormonal contraceptive methods at 3 to 12 per 10,000 users.[17,19] While there is no current evidence to support it, this method may be used for patients who desire a patch and benefit from lower estrogen exposure.

For emergency contraception, the use of the 52 mcg levonorgestrol IUD was found to be non-inferior to the copper IUD in a study of 711 patients seen at 6 Utah clinics. In the modified intention-to-treat and per-protocol analyses, pregnancy rates were 1 in 317 (0.3%; 95% CI: 0.01–1.7) in the levonorgestrel group and 0 in 321 (0%; 95% CI: 0–1.1) in the copper IUD group.[20] Adverse events resulting in participants seeking medical care in the first month after IUD placement occurred in 5.2% of participants in the levonorgestrel IUD group and 4.9% of those in the copper IUD group. While not FDA approved for this use, clinicians have used this evidence to offer the 52 mcg levonorgestrol IUDs for emergency contraception.

ROMOSOZUMAB IS AN OSTEOPOROSIS TREATMENT FOR PATIENTS AT VERY HIGH FRACTURE RISK, OR WHO CANNOT TOLERATE TRADITIONAL THERAPIES

Romosozumab, a monoclonal anti-sclerostin antibody, is an osteoporosis medication that increases bone formation and decreases bone resorption. It was approved by the FDA in 2019. In an early study, 12 months of monthly subcutaneous romosozumab was compared with placebo in 7,180 women. All received denosumab for the following year. There was a reduction in radiologic vertebral fractures but not nonvertebral fractures in those treated with romosozumab.[21]

In a study of over 4,000 women with osteoporosis and a history of a fragility fracture, women were randomized to receive a monthly subcutaneous injection of romosozumab versus weekly oral alendronate for 1 year. After that year, all received alendronate weekly. After 2 years, among these women, whose median age was 74 years, romosozumab resulted in lower rates of new vertebral fracture, any clinical fracture, and hip fracture than did alendronate.[22]

Although there was no difference in overall serious adverse events, there was a higher rate of serious cardiovascular results among women who received romosozumab.[22] Romosozumab is FDA approved for use for 1 year for postmenopausal women at high fracture risk or in whom other treatments have failed, although the approval includes a warning about higher risk of myocardial infarction, stroke, and cardiovascular death.

The American College of Physicians recommends that bisphosphonates remain the first choice for the treatment of osteoporosis. Denosumab should be a second-line treatment for those who have contraindications to or are unable to tolerate bisphosphonates. Finally, the sclerostin inhibitor (romosozumab) or recombinant parathyroid hormone (PTH) (teriparatide or abaloparatide) followed by bisphosphonate should be used in patients with primary osteoporosis and very high risk of fracture.[23]

OTESECONAZOLE IS AN EFFECTIVE TREATMENT FOR RECURRENT VULVOVAGINAL CANDIDIASIS BUT SHOULD BE AVOIDED IN PATIENTS OF REPRODUCTIVE POTENTIAL

Approximately 75% of women develop vulvovaginal candidiasis (VVC) at least once in their lifetime, with around 5% to 10% developing recurrent vulvovaginal candidiasis (rVVC), defined as 3 or more symptomatic episodes in 12 months.[24] Oteseconazole is an azole metalloenzyme inhibitor for CYP51, a fungal enzyme required for cell-wall synthesis and fungal cell growth. Oteseconazole was approved by the FDA in 2022 after three phase 3 trials demonstrated efficacy in the treatment and prevention of rVVC.

In the 2 VIOLET trials (CL-011 and CL-012), participants received fluconazole induction consistent with current complicated VVC treatment, followed by randomization to either placebo or oteseconazole for maintenance.[25] To be included in the trial, participants had at least 3 acute VVC episodes in the past year. At week 48, 4% or 7% of participants in the oteseconazole arms of each of the 2 trials had recurrence of rVVC compared to 36% or 43% in the placebo arms ($P < .001$). The ultra VIOLET trial compared fluconazole and oteseconazole for induction, with induction failure rates in 4% and 7% of participants, respectively.[26] Rates of adverse events were similar between oteseconazole and placebo and included headaches ($\sim 7\%$) and nausea ($\sim 4\%$).

These 3 double-blind, placebo-controlled randomized controlled trials demonstrated that oteseconazole for maintenance after fluconazole induction was superior to placebo, and oteseconazole induction was non-inferior to fluconazole. There is no evidence comparing fluconazole to oteseconazole for maintenance.

Animal studies suggest that oteseconazole is teratogenic, causing fetal ocular abnormalities. As the half-life is approximately 138 days, this drug is contraindicated in those of reproductive potential. In addition, oteseconazole is not recommended in those with moderate–severe hepatic impairment or with an estimated glomerular filtration rate less than 30.

In conclusion, oteseconazole is a promising new agent available to treat a common condition with low rates of adverse events. However, its potential teratogenic potential combined with its long half-life significantly limits the target population to postmenopausal women or those who have undergone permanent sterilization procedures.

SINGLE-DOSE FOSFOMYCIN MAY BE USED FOR PATIENTS UNABLE TO TOLERATE NITROFURANTOIN FOR ACUTE CYSTITIS

The 2010 IDSA guidelines incorporated nitrofurantoin and fosfomycin as first-line agents for the treatment of UTIs.[27] Fosfomycin is administered as a single dose and is attractive as a treatment option where adherence is of concern. In a recent clinical trial, 513 women with less than 1 symptom of UTI and a positive dipstick were randomized to receive a single 3 g dose of fosfomycin or nitrofurantoin 100 mg tid for 5 days (European dosing). The study found that 70% of patients treated with nitrofurantoin had clinical resolution at 28 days compared with 58% of women treated with fosfomycin, for a 12% absolute difference ($P = .004$). There was no difference in symptom duration or occurrence of pyelonephritis or adverse events.[28]

We recommend that given similar rates of adverse effects and higher rates of cure for nitrofurantoin, fosfomycin may be less efficacious than nitrofurantoin for the treatment of uncomplicated UTI in women. However, if a woman is unable or unwilling to take nitrofurantoin, and/or if adherence is a concern, fosfomycin is a reasonable treatment option.

METHENAMINE HIPPURATE IS A NONANTIBIOTIC ALTERNATIVE FOR TREATMENT OF RECURRENT URINARY TRACT INFECTION

Recurrence occurs in 25% of women after their first UTI. Guidelines recommend daily low-dose antibiotics as prophylaxis in women with recurrent UTI.[29] Although prophylactic antibiotic regimens vary, antibiotic resistance is a potential consequence of all regimens.

Methenamine hippurate is a urinary antiseptic and nonantibiotic alternative that has the potential benefit of not inducing antibiotic resistance. Although methenamine hippurate has been available for UTI prevention since 1967, it has not been commonly used, except in pregnancy.

Methenamine hippurate was compared to antibiotic prophylaxis in a randomized multicenter, open-label, non-inferiority trial.[30] Two hundred and forty adult women with recurrent UTI received methenamine hippurate 1 g twice a day or antibiotic prophylaxis (nitrofurantoin, cefalexin, or trimethoprim). The primary outcome was incidence of symptomatic, antibiotic-treated UTI over 12 months of follow-up. The absolute difference in UTI incidence after 12 month follow-up was 0.49 (015–0.84) episodes per person-year and met the prespecified non-inferiority margin (1 episode per person-year). Participants described the antibiotic regimen as more convenient (once a day vs twice a day dosing).

We recommend methenamine hippurate as an acceptable alternative for antibiotic prophylaxis for recurrent UTI; however, it is not known how it compares to specific antibiotic regimens.

BREMELANOTIDE IS A NOVEL THERAPY FOR FEMALE HYPOACTIVE SEXUAL DESIRE DISORDER

HSDD is an absence or reduction of sexual fantasies or interest in sexual activity that causes significant distress for an individual. Low desire is the most common form of sexual dysfunction in women in the United States, with 10% reporting low desire that causes distress.[31] Despite its prevalence, limited pharmacologic treatment options are available for female HSDD.

Bremelanotide (Vyleesi) was approved by the FDA for the treatment of HSDD in premenopausal women in 2019. While the mechanism of action is not entirely understood, bremelanotide is a melanocortin receptor agonist that stimulates endogenous neuropeptides that are associated with the excitatory pathways in sexual response.[32]

Bremelanotide has been shown to improve sexual desire and decrease distress, but not significantly change satisfying sexual events. This medication was studied in two 24 week randomized, double-blind, placebo-controlled trials with extended open-label following for 52 weeks.[33,34] These studies included healthy, premenopausal women with HSDD for over 6 months. Individuals who were pregnant, nursing, or who had diagnoses of a mental health or substance use disorder were excluded. In surveys of participants, there was statistically significant improvement in self-reported sexual desire and a decrease in distress in the treatment compared to the placebo group after 24 weeks, which persisted in the open-label trial. There was no statistically significant change in the number of satisfying sexual events between the treatment and placebo groups.

Patients considering bremelanotide should be counseled about the delivery, potential side effects, and cost of this medication. Bremelanotide is recommended for use as needed at least 45 minutes (and up to 8–10 hours) before planned sexual activity (maximum 1 dose per 24 hours or 8 doses per month). Delivery is via a prefilled subcutaneous auto-injector (dose 1.75 mg per injection). The most commonly reported side effects include nausea (40%), flushing (30%), and headache (11%).[34,35] Less frequent side effects include transient blood pressure increase, fatigue, skin hyperpigmentation, and delayed gastric emptying. Bremelanotide is contraindicated in women with uncontrolled hypertension or who are at risk for cardiovascular disease.[35] Bremelanotide can decrease the serum concentration of naltrexone and indomethacin and should be used with caution in patients with hepatic and/or renal dysfunction. This medication should be avoided in pregnancy, and data are not available for lactation. Unlike the only other FDA-approved medication for female HSDD (Flibanserin [Addyi]), use of bremelanotide with alcohol is not limited. Cost can be substantial ($286 per auto-injector), although a coupon program is available through the manufacturer.

While bremelanotide is a welcome addition to the pharmacologic options to help women with HSDD, use remains limited by the balance of clinical impact with potential side effects and cost.

CLINICS CARE POINTS

- Fezolinetant is an alternative nonhormonal option for the treatment of moderate-to-severe VMS with similar efficacy to other nonhormonal treatments.

- Zuranolone and brexanolone are a new class of agents to treat PPD.
- Updates in contraception include an estetrol/drospirenone combined oral contraceptive, a drospirenone-only pill, a 13 cycle vaginal ring, a new weekly patch, a pH-altering on-demand vaginal gel, and evidence for the 52 mg levonorgestrol IUD for emergency contraception.
- Romosozumab can be considered for patients with high fracture risk and low cardiovascular risk who cannot use bisphosphonates or denosumab.
- Oteseconazole treats recurrent VVC but should not be used in patients of childbearing potential.
- Single-dose fosfomycin treats cystitis but has a lower cure rate than nitrofurantoin. Methenamine hippurate is a nonantibiotic alternative for prevention of recurrent UTIs.
- Bremelanotide improves sexual desire but not sexually satisfying events in female HSDD.

DISCLOSURE

Dr S. Merriam writes content for ACP MKSAP and is compensated.

REFERENCES

1. Liu KA, Mager NAD. Women's involvement in clinical trials: historical perspective and future implications. Pharm Pract 2016;14(1):708.
2. Gold EB, Colvin A, Avis N, et al. Longitudinal analysis of the association between vasomotor symptoms and race/ethnicity across the menopausal transition: study of women's health across the nation. Am J Publ Health 2006;96(7):1226–35.
3. Nappi RE, Kroll R, Siddiqui E, et al. Global cross-sectional survey of women with vasomotor symptoms associated with menopause: prevalence and quality of life burden. Menopause 2021;28(8):875–82.
4. Avis NECS, Greendale G, Bromberger JT, et al, Study of Women's Health Across the Nation. Duration of menopausal vasomotor symptoms over the menopause transition. JAMA Intern Med 2015;175(4):531–9.
5. Lederman SOF, Cano A, Santoro N, et al. Fezolinetant for treatment of moderate-to-severe vasomotor symptoms associated with menopause (SKYLIGHT 1): a phase 3 randomised controlled study. Lancet (London, England) 2023;401(10382):1091–102.
6. Johnson KAMN, Nappi RE, Neal-Perry G, et al. Efficacy and safety of fezolinetant in moderate to severe vasomotor symptoms associated with menopause: a phase 3 RCT - pubMed. J Clin Endocrinol Metab 2023;108(8):1981–97.
7. Neal-Perry G, Cano A, Lederman S, et al. Safety of fezolinetant for vasomotor symptoms associated with menopause: a randomized controlled trial. Obstet Gynecol 2023;141(4):737–47.
8. Deligiannidis KM, Meltzer-Brody S, Gunduz-Bruce H, et al. Effect of zuranolone vs placebo in postpartum depression. JAMA Psychiatr 2021;78(9):951–9.
9. Deligiannidis KM, Meltzer-Brody S, Maximos B, et al. Zuranolone for the treatment of postpartum depression. Am J Psychiatry 2023;180(9):668–75.
10. Fruzzetti F, Fidecicchi T, Guevara MMM, et al. Estetrol: a new choice for contraception. J Clin Med 2021;10(23):5625.
11. Creinin MD, Westhoff CL, Bouchard C, et al. Estetrol-drospirenone combination oral contraceptive: North American phase 3 efficacy and safety results. Contraception 2021;104(3):222–8.
12. Kimble T, Burke AE, Barnhart KT, et al. A 1-year prospective, open-label, single-arm, multicenter, phase 3 trial of the contraceptive efficacy and safety of the oral

progestin-only pill drospirenone 4 mg using a 24/4-day regimen. Contraception 2020;2:100020.

13. Archer DF, Merkatz RB, Bahamondes L, et al. Efficacy of the 1-year (13-cycle) se-gesterone acetate and ethinylestradiol contraceptive vaginal system: results of two multicentre, open-label, single-arm, phase 3 trials. Lancet Global Health 2019;7(8):e1054–64.

14. Anon. Phexxi Prescribing Information. No Year. Available at: https://www.accessdata.fda.gov/drugsatfda_docs/label/2022/208352s002lbl.pdf.

15. Thomas MA, Chappell BT, Maximos B, et al. A novel vaginal pH regulator: results from the phase 3 AMPOWER contraception clinical trial. Contraception 2020;2:100031.

16. Anon. Ortho Evra Label Supplement. No Year.

17. Baker CC, Chen MJ. New Contraception update — annovera, phexxi, slynd, and twirla. Current Obstetrics And Gynecology Reports 2022;11(1):21–7.

18. Anon. Twirla vs Xulane: how do they compare? no year, Available at: https://www.drugs.com/medical-answers/twirla-xulane-compare-3554507/. Accessed February 26, 2024.

19. Nelson AL, Kaunitz AM, Kroll R, et al. Efficacy, safety, and tolerability of a levonor-gestrel/ethinyl estradiol transdermal delivery system: Phase 3 clinical trial results. Contraception 2021;103(3):137–43.

20. Turok DK, Gero A, Simmons RG, et al. Levonorgestrel vs. copper intrauterine de-vices for emergency contraception. N Engl J Med 2021;384(4):335–44.

21. Cosman F, Crittenden DB, Adachi JD, et al. Romosozumab treatment in postmen-opausal women with osteoporosis. N Engl J Med 2016;375(16):1532–43.

22. Saag KG, Petersen J, Brandi ML, et al. Romosozumab or alendronate for fracture prevention in women with osteoporosis. N Engl J Med 2017;377(15):1417–27.

23. Qaseem A, Hicks LA, Etxeandia-Ikobaltzeta I, et al. Pharmacologic treatment of primary osteoporosis or low bone mass to prevent fractures in adults: a living clin-ical guideline from the American college of physicians. Ann Intern Med 2023;176(2):224–38.

24. Sobel JD. Epidemiology and pathogenesis of recurrent vulvovaginal candidiasis. Am J Obstet Gynecol 1985;152(7 Pt 2):924–35.

25. Sobel JD, Donders G, Degenhardt T, et al. Efficacy and safety of oteseconazole in recurrent vulvovaginal candidiasis. NEJM Evid 2022;1(8). EVIDoa2100055.

26. Martens MG, Maximos B, Degenhardt T, et al. Phase 3 study evaluating the safety and efficacy of oteseconazole in the treatment of recurrent vulvovaginal candidi-asis and acute vulvovaginal candidiasis infections. Am J Obstet Gynecol 2022;227(6):880, e881-e811.

27. Gupta K, Hooton TM, Naber KG, et al. International clinical practice guidelines for the treatment of acute uncomplicated cystitis and pyelonephritis in women: a 2010 update by the infectious diseases society of America and the European so-ciety for microbiology and infectious diseases. Clin Infect Dis 2011;52(5):e103–20.

28. Huttner A, Kowalczyk A, Turjeman A, et al. Effect of 5-day nitrofurantoin vs single-dose fosfomycin on clinical resolution of uncomplicated lower urinary tract infec-tion in women: a randomized clinical trial. JAMA 2018;319(17):1781–9.

29. Anger J, Lee U, Ackerman AL, et al. Recurrent uncomplicated urinary tract infec-tions in women: AUA/CUA/SUFU guideline. J Urol 2019;202(2):282–9.

30. Hoffmann TC, Bakhit M, Mar CD. Methenamine hippurate for recurrent urinary tract infections. BMJ 2022;376.

31. Shifren JL, Monz BU, Russo PA, et al. Sexual problems and distress in United States women: prevalence and correlates. Obstet Gynecol 2008;112(5):970–8.

32. Pfaus JG, Sadiq A, Spana C, et al. The neurobiology of bremelanotide for the treatment of hypoactive sexual desire disorder in premenopausal women. CNS Spectr 2022;27(3):281–9.

33. Kingsberg SA, Clayton AH, Portman D, et al. Bremelanotide for the treatment of hypoactive sexual desire disorder: two randomized phase 3 trials. Obstet Gynecol 2019;134(5):899–908.

34. Simon JA, Kingsberg SA, Portman D, et al. Long-term safety and efficacy of bremelanotide for hypoactive sexual desire disorder. Obstet Gynecol 2019;134(5): 909–17.

35. Mayer D, Lynch SE. Bremelanotide: new drug approved for treating hypoactive sexual desire disorder. Ann Pharmacother 2020;54(7):684–90.

Therapy for Hyperlipidemia

Jennifer Wright, MD[a],*, Savitha Subramanian, MD[b]

KEYWORDS

- ASCVD • Statins • Ezetimibe • Bempedoic acid • PCSK9 inhibitors
- Hypertriglyceridemia • Lipoprotein (a) • Coronary artery calcium

KEY POINTS

- For primary prevention of atherosclerotic cardiovascular disease (ASCVD) risk assessment starts with a non-fasting lipids panel, coronary artery calcium assessment can be useful in cases of clinical uncertainty.
- Statins remain first-line agents for ASCVD risk reduction but in high-risk patients, ezetimibe, proprotein convertase subtilisin kexin-9 inhibitors, and bempedoic acid can be added for further risk reduction.
- In statin-intolerant patients, bempedoic acid monotherapy has been found to reduce cardiovascular risk.
- Adding icosapent ethyl to statin therapy can be considered for further ASCVD risk reduction in high-risk patients with elevated triglycerides.

INTRODUCTION

Atherosclerotic cardiovascular disease (ASCVD) is a major contributor to morbidity and mortality globally. Over the past several decades, significant advances have been made in reducing the risk of ASCVD. It is well established that elevated levels of low-density lipoprotein (LDL) cholesterol are causally associated with adverse cardiovascular events such as myocardial infarction (MI) and ischemic stroke. In addition, reduction in LDL cholesterol is associated with a decrease in risk of atherosclerotic events. Here, the authors discuss current assessment of individual cardiovascular risk and review appropriate therapies to mitigate risk.

INDICATIONS FOR LIPID MANAGEMENT

Based on the approach outlined in the 2018 American College of Cardiology/American Heart Association (ACC/AHA) Multisociety cholesterol management guides,[1] the major risk groups include as follows:

[a] Division of General Internal Medicine, Department of Medicine, University of Washington, Seattle, WA, USA; [b] Division of Metabolism, Endocrinology and Nutrition, University of Washington, RR-512 Health Sciences Building, Box 356420, 1959 NE Pacific Street, Seattle, WA 98195-6420, USA
* Corresponding author.
E-mail address: sonic@uw.edu

Med Clin N Am 108 (2024) 881–894
https://doi.org/10.1016/j.mcna.2024.03.005
medical.theclinics.com

1. Secondary prevention: Individuals with a personal history of ASCVD including angina or myocardial infarction, interventions for coronary atherosclerosis, cerebrovascular accident (CVA), and peripheral artery disease.
2. Primary prevention, LDL cholesterol ≥190 mg/dL: Individuals with genetic lipid disorders, such as familial hypercholesterolemia, who are at a very high risk of ASCVD.
3. Primary prevention, patients with diabetes: All individuals over the age of 40 with diabetes are at an intermediate-high risk of ASCVD.
4. Primary prevention in the absence of LDL ≥190 mg/dL or diabetes: Patients without any of the aforementioned conditions but with elevated ASCVD risk based on established risk estimators.

LIPID TESTING

Conventional lipid testing is a fundamental part of ASCVD risk assessment in all individuals. A standard lipid panel reports total cholesterol (TC), triglycerides (TG), high-density lipoprotein cholesterol (HDL-C), and calculated LDL-C. Non-fasting lipid panels are acceptable, as postprandial lipids do reflect a patient's cardiovascular risk, [2] and offer convenience. When non-fasting TG are >400 mg/dL, a fasting lipid panel is recommended.

BEYOND THE LIPID PANEL

The Pooled Cohort Equation is the risk estimator predominately used in the United States. Variables included in this risk estimator include age, sex, race, lipid values (TC and HDL-C), and risk factors including tobacco use, hypertension, and diabetes. A new risk estimator in development called Predicting Risk of Cardiovascular Events (PREVENT) removes race but includes other risk factors including kidney function (estimated glomerular filtration rate).[3] The AHA/ACC 2018 multisociety guidelines recommend treatment with a statin in patients with a 10-year estimated risk of ASCVD ≥7.5% (**Table 1**). Patients with risk of 5% to 7.5% are considered borderline cardiovascular risk and risk enhancers not included in the Pooled Cohort Equation, such as family history of premature ASCVD and presence of comorbid conditions (see **Table 1**) can be helpful in risk stratification. Additional blood tests such as lipoprotein(a) (Lp(a)), apolipoprotein-B (apoB), and high-sensitivity C-reactive protein (hs-CRP), or CT imaging for coronary artery calcification (CAC) can help further stratify risk. Initiating moderate-intensity statin therapy for primary ASCVD prevention should be considered in borderline risk patients when risk enhancers are present and strongly encouraged in all intermediate (≥7.5%–19.9% 10-year risk) and high (>20% 10-year)-risk patients.

LIPOPROTEIN (A)

Lp (a) measurement can be helpful in patients with a family history of premature ASCVD. Lp (a) is a modified LDL particle and levels are genetically determined without influence from diet and physical activity.[4] Plasma concentrations are highly variable, and high levels are seen in up to 20% of the global population. Studies have demonstrated that high lipoprotein (a) levels are a risk factor for ASCVD[5] but trials have not demonstrated that reducing high Lp(a) levels decreases incidence of ASCVD. A level of ≥125 nmol/L or 50 mg/dL is considered risk-enhancing. Since Lp (a) levels are genetically determined, it only needs to be tested once. In a patient with borderline or intermediate ASCVD risk, elevated Lp (a) levels should prompt initiation of statin therapy or pursuit of additional testing such as a CAC score.

Table 1
General risk assessment, risk enhancers to consider, and risks specific to women

Atherosclerotic Cardiovascular Disease (ASCVD) Risk Assessment Based on 10-y Predicted Risk	Risk Enhancers	Risks Specific to Women
<5% Low 5%–7.49% Borderline 7.5%–19.9% Intermediate >20% High	Family history of premature ASCVD (males <55 year old, females <65 year old) Persistently elevated low-density lipoprotein (LDL) (>/ = 160 mg/dL) Metabolic syndrome Chronic kidney disease Chronic inflammatory disorders (rheumatoid arthritis, human immunodeficienc virus [HIV] disease)	History of preclampsia Premature menopause Polycystic ovarian syndrome

Adapted from Grundy SM. AHA/ACC/AACVPR/AAPA/ABC/ACPM/ADA/AGS/APhA/ASPC/NLA/PCNA guideline on the management of blood cholesterol: a report of the American College of Cardiology/American Heart Association Task Force on Clinical Practice Guidelines. Circulation, 2019. 139(25): p. e1082-e1143.

CARDIAC COMPUTED TOMOGRAPHY FOR CORONARY CALCIUM

A non-contrast chest computed tomography (CT) is used to assess for CAC, a surrogate marker for atherosclerosis. Recent studies have confirmed that CAC scoring in Agatston units (AU) is predictive of ASCVD risk.[6] When considered in combination with the calculated risk based on the Pooled Cohort Equation, in borderline-intermediate risk patients, a CAC of 0 AU implies very low ASCVD risk over 10 years and statin therapy can be deferred. **Table 2** provides details on interpretation of CAC score results. In patients with scores of 0 who are in the borderline-intermediate risk category, repeating the test every 3 to 5 years is reasonable.[7] Of note, statin therapy is recommended for all patients with CAC scores of ≥100 AU or greater than the 75th percentile for the patient's age/sex/race group; the Multi-Ethnic Study of Atherosclerosis (MESA) study[6] found that these findings corelated with a 10-year ASCVD risk of >7.5%. This test is often not covered by medical insurance; out of pocket cost varies but is typically in the range of $100 to 200.

Coronary artery calcifications are also frequently noted as an incidental finding on chest CT imaging ordered for other indications. Radiologic societies recommend that radiologists offer quantitative (AU) or qualitative interpretations of the coronary calcium burden, describing it as mild, moderate, or heavy/severe.[8] Moderate to heavy/severe calcifications correspond with a CAC score of >100 AU and are an indication for statin therapy.

LIPID TREATMENT TO REDUCE ATHEROSCLEROTIC CARDIOVASCULAR DISEASE RISK
Lifestyle Management

The AHA/ACC guidelines make general recommendations regarding diet to reduce ASCVD risk with the highest-level recommendation being for Mediterranean and vegetarian diets based on studies finding evidence of reduction in cardiovascular endpoints within groups on these diets[9,10] Observational studies support physical

Table 2
Additional tests to help assess cardiovascular risk

Test	Interpretation
Lipoprotein (a)	Levels ≥50 mg/dL or 125 nmol/L enhance risk and favor statin therapy when risk is borderline-intermediate.
Coronary Artery Calcium Scan	0 Agatston units (AU) = statin therapy can be deferred 1–99 AU and <75th percentile for the patient's age/sex/race group = favor statin therapy, especially in patients ≥55 y ≥100 AU or ≥75th percentile for the patient's age/sex/race group = statin therapy indicated.
Apolipoprotein B ≥130 mg/dL High-sensitivity C-reactive protein ≥2.0 mg/L Ankle-brachial index <0.9	Favor statin therapy in intermediate-risk patients.

Adapted from Grundy SM. AHA/ACC/AACVPR/AAPA/ABC/ACPM/ADA/AGS/APhA/ASPC/NLA/PCNA guideline on the management of blood cholesterol: a report of the American College of Cardiology/American Heart Association Task Force on Clinical Practice Guidelines. Circulation, 2019. 139(25): p. e1082-e1143.

activity as a means to reduce the risk of cardiovascular disease with a dose-response relationship; the greatest benefits are associated with increasing from a low to a moderate level of activity.[11]

Medication Management

Statins
Statins have an extensive body of research establishing their benefit in reducing risk of ASCVD and are considered first-line therapy for primary and secondary prevention (**Table 3**). They act by inhibiting hydroxy-methylglutaryl (HMG) coenzyme-A reductase, the rate limiting enzyme in hepatic cholesterol synthesis, leading to upregulation of cell surface LDL receptors, and lowering plasma LDL-C levels.

Common concerns around statin therapy include side effects including myopathy, myalgias, and development of diabetes. The risk of frank myopathy with elevated creatine kinase (CK) levels is very low (<1 in 1000) being mindful of drug interactions leading to an increase in statin level will reduce a patient's risk, see **Table 4**.[1,12,13] There is controversy regarding the statin-induced myalgias without CK elevations reported by many patients. It has been suggested that these symptoms are a nocebo effect, that is, an individual may be prone to experiencing the symptom based on the expectation of it rather than a physiologic change.[12]

The risk of developing diabetes is very low, ~ 0.2% per year, and greatly outweighed by the overall benefits of statins. New-onset diabetes is more common in patients with high-intensity statin dosing and with risk factors for diabetes such as higher body mass index (BMI), features of the metabolic syndrome, and hypertension.[12]

Non-statins therapies
While current guidelines are not based on treating to targets, there are LDL-C goals that are recommended based on individual ASCVD risk (**Table 5**). If these goals are not achieved through treatment with statin at the maximum tolerated dose, then addition of non-statin medications should be considered. Non-statin agents should also be considered in individuals intolerant of statins.

Table 3
Medications targeting low-density lipoprotein cholesterol -C

Medication Name/Class	Indication	Approximate Degree of Low-Density Lipoprotein Cholesterol (LDL-C) Reduction	Side Effects
Statins	Secondary prevention of ASCVD Primary prevention: Low density lipoprotein (LDL) ≥190 mg/dL ≥40 year old with diabetes ≥40 year old with • ASCVD risk 5%–7.49% + risk-enhancing factors • ASCVD risk of ≥7.5%	High-intensity dosing ≥50%. Moderate-intensity dosing 30%–50%.	Myopathy/myalgia Increased risk of new-onset diabetes
Ezetimibe	Statin add-on therapy in patients not meeting LDL-C goals; Consider in secondary prevention and high-risk patients for primary prevention.	25% additional LDL-C reduction when taken with statins	Abdominal cramps
PCSK9 inhibitors	Statin add-on therapy for secondary prevention when LDL-C goals not met. Statin add-on therapy for primary prevention in patients with baseline LDL-C ≥190 mg/dL not meeting LDL-C goals.	50%–60%	Injection site reactions
Bempedoic Acid	Add on therapy for secondary prevention in patients not meeting LDL-C goals despite statin, ezetimibe, and/or PCSK9 inhibitor therapy. Primary prevention in patients with statin intolerance.	15% additional LDL-C reduction when taken with statins 20% LDL-C reduction as monotherapy	Gout. Cholelithiasis. Tendon rupture

Ezetimibe

Ezetimibe inhibits cholesterol absorption at the intestinal brush border. Ezetimibe is most effective in lowering LDL-C when taken in combination with a statin. The landmark study of ezetimibe was the Improved Reduction of Outcomes: Vytorin Efficacy International Trial (IMPROVE-IT), a secondary prevention trial that compared cardiovascular outcomes in patients on simvastatin and ezetimibe to patients on simvastatin alone.[14] Additional LDL-C lowering with ezetimibe was approximately 25% (53.7 mg/dL simvastatin-ezetimibe vs 69.5 mg/dL simvastatin monotherapy). After 7 years, patients on the combination therapy had a lower rate of the primary composite cardiovascular outcome, (HR 0.94, CI .89–.99; ARR 2%) without a difference in all-cause mortality or cardiovascular mortality. Based largely on this study, the AHA/ACC guidelines recommend the addition of ezetimibe in high-risk patients not meeting LDL-C

Table 4
Comparison of commonly prescribed statin medications

Statin	Intensity, dose range[1]	Drug Interactions,[12] (Note: all Statins should be avoided with gemfibrozil and have potential interactions with protease inhibitors. Those listed below feature differences in other interactions)	Cost ($: <$20/30-day Supply, $$: $20–50/30-day Supply, $$$: $50–100/30-day Supply) Reference: GoodRx.com Accessed 3.3.2024	Other
Lovastatin	Low 20 mg daily; Moderate 40–80 mg daily	Due to cytochrome P450 3A4 (CYP3A4) metabolism has many drug interactions; dose limitations with calcium channel blockers, antiarrhythmics; avoid with azole antifungals, immunosuppressants (eg, tacrolimus), macrolides.	$	
Simvastatin	Low 10 mg daily; Moderate 20–40 mg daily	Due to CYP3A4 metabolism has many drug interactions; dose limitations with calcium channel blockers, antiarrhythmics; avoid with azole antifungals, immunosuppressants (eg, tacrolimus), macrolides.	$	Due to increased risk of side effects overall, doses above 40 mg daily are not recommended and when used in combination with some commonly prescribed medications (eg, amlodipine) further dose reductions are indicated.
Pravastatin	Low 10–20 mg daily; Moderate 40–80 mg daily	Overall much fewer than other statins due to lack of CYP3A4 metabolism; Dose limitations with some immunosuppressants and macrolide antibiotics.	$	

Pitavastatin	Moderate, 1–4 mg daily	Dose limitations with macrolide antibiotics; avoid with immunosuppressants.	$$$	Recent study in patients with HIV disease and low-moderate ASCVD risk (average risk 4.5%) found significant CV RR with pitavastatin compared to placebo.[13]
Atorvastatin	Moderate 10–20 mg daily; High 40–80 mg daily	Moderate CYP3A4 metabolism potential for interactions less so compared to simvastatin; dose limitations recommended with some macrolide antibiotics and immunosuppressants.	$	
Rosuvastatin	Moderate 5–10 mg daily; High 20–40 mg daily	Dose limitations with immunosuppressants (eg, cyclosporin).	$	

Abbreviations: CV, cardiovascular; RR, risk reduction.

Table 5
Low-density lipoprotein cholesterol goals based on risk

ASCVD Risk	LDL-C Goals	Recommended Action if LDL-C Not at Goal on Maximally Tolerated Statin Dose
Very high-risk: History of multiple ASCVD events or a single ASCVD event + multiple high-risk conditions	≥50% LDL-C reduction and LDL-C of <55 mg/dL	Add ezetimibe and/or PCSK9 inhibitor If still not at goal: Consider bempedoic acid
Secondary prevention/patients with history of ASCVD, not considered very-high risk	≥50% LDL-C reduction and LDL-C of <70 mg/dL	Add ezetimibe If still not at goal: Add or replace with PCSK9 inhibitor If still not at goal: Consider bempedoic acid
Primary prevention, LDL-C level ≥190	<100 mg/dL	Add ezetimibe and/or PCSK9 inhibitor If still not at goal: Consider bempedoic acid
Primary prevention, borderline-intermediate ASCVD risk	30%–49% LDL-C reduction and LDL-C <100 mg/dL	Increase to high- intensity/ maximally tolerated statin dose
Primary prevention, high ASCVD risk (≥20%)	≥50% LDL reduction and LDL of <70 mg/dL	In addition to maximally tolerated statin: Add ezetimibe

Adapted from Grundy SM. AHA/ACC/AACVPR/AAPA/ABC/ACPM/ADA/AGS/APhA/ASPC/NLA/PCNA guideline on the management of blood cholesterol: a report of the American College of Cardiology/American Heart Association Task Force on Clinical Practice Guidelines. Circulation, 2019. 139(25): p. e1082-e1143; and Grinspoon, S.K., et al., Pitavastatin to Prevent Cardiovascular Disease in HIV Infection. N Engl J Med, 2023. 389(8): p. 687-699.

goals on statin monotherapy (see **Table 5**). It should be noted that there are no studies of cardiovascular benefits of ezetimibe in primary prevention or used as monotherapy.

Ezetimibe is generally well tolerated with only rare reports of myopathy and no increased risk of diabetes. Concomitant use of cyclosporin and ezetimibe will result in increased levels of both medications. When taken with gemfibrozil, there is a risk of increased biliary cholesterol excretion and in turn an increased risk of cholelithiasis.

Bempedoic acid
Bempedoic acid inhibits ATP citrate lyase, an enzyme upstream of hydroxymethylglutaryl (HMG) Co-A reductase, the target of statins. Therefore, similar to statins, bempedoic acid decreases intrahepatic cholesterol synthesis and up-regulates LDL receptors with increased clearance of LDL from the circulation. Notably, bempedoic acid is a pro-drug that is activated in the liver but not in muscle[15] and thus useful in individuals experiencing myalgias on statins.

Bempedoic acid lowers LDL-C approximately 20% when taken as monotherapy or approximately 15% in combination with a statin.[16],[17] The early Cholesterol Lowering via Bempedoic acid, an ACL-Inhibiting Regimen (CLEAR) trials (Tranquility and Serenity) demonstrated that bempedoic acid monotherapy, in statin-intolerant individuals, was associated with an LDL-C lowering of ~20%.[16],[18] Recently, the CLEAR Outcomes trial evaluated CV outcomes in high-risk patients on bempedoic acid monotherapy due to statin intolerance.[19] This study found a reduction in the composite CV outcome which included death from CVD, nonfatal MI, CVA, and revascularization for patients on bempedoic acid monotherapy compared to placebo, 11.7% versus 13.3%, (HR 0.87, CI 0.79–0.96) without a difference in all-cause mortality or CV mortality (NNT 62 for composite CV outcome).

Side effects identified in the CLEAR Outcomes trial included an increased risk of gout (3.1% vs 2.1%, NNH for gout 100) and cholelithiasis (2.2% vs 1.2%, NNH 100) in addition to small increases in liver enzymes, uric acid, and creatinine. In early studies of bempedoic acid, the risk of tendon rupture was higher in the treatment group than placebo, but this was not seen in the much larger CLEAR Outcomes trial; despite this, a black box warning for tendon rupture remains.[20]

A major barrier to prescribing bempedoic acid is cost and insurance-related barriers such as prior authorization and appeals.[21]

Proprotein convertase subtilisin kexin-9 inhibition

Proprotein convertase subtilisin kexin-9 (PCSK9) is a liver-derived protein that results in degradation of cell surface LDL receptors preventing their recycling resulting in high LDL-C levels. Targeted removal of circulating PCSK9 restores LDL receptor recycling and decreases circulating LDL-C. Two approaches have been developed including human monoclonal antibodies and small interfering RNA (siRNA) described in the following paragraphs.

Monoclonal antibodies

Available PCSK9 inhibitor monoclonal antibodies include alirocumab and evolocumab. The landmark trials of these medications include the Evaluation of Cardiovascular Outcomes After an Acute Coronary Syndrome During Treatment With Alirocumab (ODYSSEY OUTCOMES) trial[22] and the Further Cardiovascular Outcomes Research with PCSK9 Inhibition in Subjects with Elevated Risk (FOURIER) trial of evolocumab.[23] These were both secondary prevention trials in patients with a history of ASCVD on statin therapy. At their full dose, when added to statins, both agents lower LDL-C by > 50%. Both studies found the addition of a PCSK9 inhibitor reduced the primary composite CV endpoint of CHD death, MI, ischemic stroke, or hospitalization for unstable angina (both with HR 0.85). Based on these studies the indication for their use is in high-risk patients with a history of CV disease and in patients with a baseline LDL-C of ≥190. In both cases, they should be considered as add on therapy when there is insufficient lipid lowering on maximum dose statin therapy.[24] See **Table 4** regarding LDL-C goals based on risk category.

Both PCSK9 inhibitors are administered as subcutaneous injections, either every 2 weeks or monthly. They are well tolerated and safe without significant drug-drug interactions. Adverse effects include injection site reactions; hypersensitivity reactions can rarely occur and are the only contraindication. The main barrier in prescribing these medications is cost. Despite a price reduction in 2018 for both alirocumab and evolocumab, financial barriers still exist for many patients, especially for those on Medicare.[25]

Proprotein convertase subtilisin kexin-9 inhibition with small interfering RNAs. RNA interference is a physiologic defense mechanism against viruses and other unwanted RNAs in eukaryotic cells. RNA interference occurs naturally in a cell or exogenously by introducing small interfering RNAs (siRNAs) to silence expression of specific genes. Inclisiran is a novel siRNA that inhibits hepatic PCSK9 synthesis and decreases plasma PCSK9. Inclisiran results in sustained LDL-C reduction by 40% to 50% from baseline.[26] The first dose is administered subcutaneously by a health care professional, followed by another dose at 3 months and subsequently every 6 months.[27] Currently, inclisiran is FDA approved as adjunct to statin therapy for additional LDL-C lowering in adults with ASCVD and heterozygous familial hypercholesterolemia, similar to PCSK9 inhibitor monoclonal antibodies. Treatment appears to be safe, well tolerated, and main adverse effects include mild, transient injection site reactions.[28] Inclisiran can be considered in individuals who prefer lesser injections and adherence to medication can be improved by twice-yearly administration in clinic. Cardiovascular outcomes trials for inclisiran are ongoing (NCT03705234, NCT05030428).

Angiopoietin-like 3 inhibition. Angiopoietin-like 3 (ANGPTL3) is a liver-derived protein that is involved in the metabolism of several lipoproteins. It inhibits removal of triglyceride (TG)-rich lipoproteins thereby increasing circulating triglyceride levels. Individuals with homozygous loss of function variants in ANGPTL3 have significantly reduced plasma levels of both triglyceride and LDL-C.[29] The exact mechanism of how ANGPTL-3 inhibition reduces LDL-C levels is not known. Evinacumab is a human monoclonal antibody developed to inhibit ANGPTL3 resulting in a significant reduction of LDL-C (and TG).[30] Currently, it is only approved for use in individuals over the age of 5 with homozygous familial hypercholesterolemia, a rare genetic condition that results from complete absence of LDL receptors, with resultant very high LDL-C levels and very premature ASCVD. No cardiovascular outcomes trials are ongoing for this agent.

Hypertriglyceridemia

Hypertriglyceridemia (HTG) is very common, and tracks along with prevalence of metabolic syndrome, obesity, and type 2 diabetes. Based on triglyceride levels, HTG can be mild (150–199 mg/dL), moderate (200–499) mg/dL, or severe (>500 mg/dL).[1] The primary risk associated with elevated triglycerides is cardiovascular disease in the long term with mild to moderate HTG and acute pancreatitis in the short term with severe HTG. The role of HTG in relation to CVD, diabetes, and related metabolic conditions is complex. Recent epidemiologic, genetic studies suggest that triglycerides are a risk for CVD.[31] However, the effects of specifically targeting plasma triglyceride levels to address cardiovascular disease have not been fruitful. A list of triglyceride-lowering agents is shown in **Table 6**.

Fibrates

Fibrates such as gemfibrozil and fenofibrate are peroxisome proliferator-activated receptor (PPARa) alpha agonists that are highly efficacious in reducing triglyceride levels by 30% to 50%. However, their benefit in reducing ASCVD risk remains debatable. Studies such as the Fenofibrate Intervention and Event Lowering in Diabetes (FIELD),

Table 6
Triglyceride-lowering drugs

Medication Name/Class	Degree of Triglyceride Lowering	Side Effects
Fibrates- gemfibrozil, fenofibrate	30%–50%	Reversible rise in creatinine, LFT elevation
Omega-3 fish oils-eicosapentanoic acid + docosahexanoic acid mixtures: Omega-3 carboxylic acids (Epanova), Omega 3 ethyl esters (Lovaza, Omacor); EPA only -Icosapent ethyl (Vascepa)	15%–50%	Fishy taste, burping, diarrhea Bleeding and atrial fibrillation risk increased

Abbreviations: LFT, liver function test.

and Action to Control Cardiovascular Risk in Diabetes (ACCORD), also with fenofibrate have failed to demonstrate CVD benefit of fibrates when added to statin therapy.[32,33] Subgroup analyses of the ACCORD trial did show benefit in patients with triglyceride levels >200 mg/dL and low levels of HDL <34 mg/dL.[34] Recently, a novel PPARa modulator called pemafibrate developed in Japan demonstrated a 50% reduction in plasma TG from baseline. This drug was evaluated when added to a statin in individuals with hypertriglyceridemia and low HDL-C, in the Pemafibrate to Reduce Cardiovascular Outcomes by Reducing Triglycerides in Patients with Diabetes (PROMINENT) study.[35] However, the trial was discontinued early due to futility. The results of this recent study may have ended the debate on cardiovascular benefits of adding a fibrate to a statin in individuals with HTG. There is little justification for adding a fibrate to a statin in patients with residual HTG for CVD risk reduction. Fibrates are nevertheless indicated for pancreatitis prevention in individuals with TG >500 mg/dL.[1] When added to a statin, there may be an increased risk of myopathy with fibrate. However, this interaction is dependent upon the specific statin and fibrate used. Gemfibrozil appears to be associated with increased risk of rhabdomyolysis when used in conjunction with a statin due to altered metabolism and resultant increased serum levels of statins. Fenofibrate does not alter statin metabolism and can be used safely in combination with statins.[36]

Omega-3 fatty acids. Omega-3 fatty acids, eicosapentanoic acid (EPA), and docosahexanoic acid (DHA) lower triglycerides and have been recommended for treatment of moderate to severe HTG, although existing data have not demonstrated benefit for primary or secondary cardiovascular prevention. The results of the Reduction of Cardiovascular Events With Icosapent Ethyl–Intervention Trial (REDUCE-IT) trial, where a ~25% risk reduction was observed with addition of purified EPA when added to statins in subjects with residual high triglycerides and ASCVD or diabetes and 2 or more risk factors.[37] This resulted in recommendation of use of EPA alone for cardiovascular risk reduction in appropriate patient populations. Notably, the risk reduction is unrelated to the baseline triglyceride level or the magnitude of triglyceride reduction. However, there is controversy regarding the results of the REDUCE-IT as the placebo group received mineral oil which may have resulted in an increase in LDL-C and C-reactive protein levels. The subsequently published Outcomes Study to Assess STatin Residual Risk Reduction With EpaNova in HiGh CV Risk PatienTs With Hypertriglyceridemia (STRENGTH) trial, failed to show a benefit in CVD risk using combination omega-3 fish oil mixtures of EPA and DHA,[38] which raises the question of whether EPA rather than DHA might be atheroprotective or whether DHA may adversely affect CV risk.[39,40] Overall several trials of fish oil combinations have failed to show a beneficial cardiovascular effect.[41] All trials of high-dose omega-3 fatty acids have demonstrated increased bleeding risk due to platelet inhibition and prolonged bleeding time. Risk of atrial fibrillation was observed in both the REDUCE-IT and STRENGTH trials in the treatment arm using fish oils. OTC supplements of omega-3 fish oil should not be used for ASCVD risk reduction due to lack of evidence of benefit. Nonetheless, at this time, icosapent ethyl is recommended in addition to a statin for residual HTG.

New and emerging therapies. Lp(a) is utilized as a risk enhancer for ASCVD as discussed previously. Nucleic acid therapies targeted at inhibiting the hepatic synthesis of apo(a), the protein on Lp(a), are being developed. Olpasiran is a GalNAc-conjugated siRNA directed against the messenger RNA of the LPA gene, and pelacarsen is a GalNAc-conjugated antisense oligonucleotide (ASO).[42] Clinical efficacy and safety are being evaluated for both; no significant safety signals have emerged for olpasiran.[42]

Triglyceride targeting therapies. ApoC-III is a liver-derived protein that inhibits removal of triglyceride-rich particles from the circulation. ASO and siRNA inhibitors of ApoC3 are in development with the aim of decreasing plasma TGs.[43] Both ASO and monoclonal antibody inhibitors of ANGPTL3 have been also shown to reduce plasma triglyceride levels.

SUMMARY

Significant advances in ASCVD risk stratification and treatment have occurred over the past 10 years. While the lipid panel continues to be the basis of ASCVD risk estimation, imaging for coronary artery calcium is finding widespread use in estimating risk at the individual level. Statins remain the foundation of ASCVD risk reduction but in high-risk patients, newer options can be used in addition to statins to further reduce individual cardiovascular risk. Recent trials of bempedoic acid in statin-intolerant patients offer exciting evidence supporting the benefit of alternative medications. There is not strong evidence to support use of medications targeted at TG lowering for ASCVD risk reduction, but icosapent ethyl can be considered.

CLINICS CARE POINTS

- If after a non-fasting lipid panel, a patient's ASCVD risk is unclear to either the clinician or the patient, order a CT to assess coronary artery calcification.
- If LDL-C lowering is not sufficient with statin therapy alone, add ezetimibe, PCSK9 inhibitors, and/or bempedoic acid as appropriate.
- In statin-intolerant patients, consider bempedoic acid to reduce LDL-C and cardiovascular risk.
- In high-risk patients with elevated triglycerides on maximally tolerated statin therapy, adding icosapent ethyl may further reduce ASCVD risk.

REFERENCES

1. Grundy SM, Stone NJ, Bailey AL, et al. 2018 AHA/ACC/AACVPR/AAPA/ABC/ACPM/ADA/AGS/APhA/ASPC/NLA/PCNA guideline on the management of blood cholesterol: a report of the American College of Cardiology/American Heart Association Task Force on Clinical Practice Guidelines. Circulation 2019;139(25):e1082–143.
2. Langsted A, Nordestgaard BG. Nonfasting versus fasting lipid profile for cardiovascular risk prediction. Pathology 2019;51(2):131–41.
3. Khan SS, Matsushita K, Sang Y, et al. Development and validation of the american heart association predicting risk of cardiovascular disease events (PREVENT) equations. Circulation 2023;149(6):430–49.
4. Kamstrup PR. Lipoprotein(a) and Cardiovascular Disease. Clin Chem 2021;67(1):154–66.
5. Hedegaard BS, Bork CS, Kaltoft M, et al. Equivalent impact of elevated lipoprotein(a) and familial hypercholesterolemia in patients with atherosclerotic cardiovascular disease. J Am Coll Cardiol 2022;80(21):1998–2010.
6. Budoff MJ, Young R, Burke G, et al. Ten-year association of coronary artery calcium with atherosclerotic cardiovascular disease (ASCVD) events: the multiethnic study of atherosclerosis (MESA). Eur Heart J 2018;39(25):2401–8.

7. Orringer CE, Blaha MJ, Blankstein R, et al. The national lipid association scientific statement on coronary artery calcium scoring to guide preventive strategies for ASCVD risk reduction. J Clin Lipidol 2021;15(1):33–60.

8. Munden RF, Carter BW, Chiles C, et al. Managing incidental findings on thoracic CT: mediastinal and cardiovascular findings. a white paper of the ACR incidental findings committee. J Am Coll Radiol 2018;15(8):1087–96.

9. Estruch R, Ros E, Salas-Salvadó J, et al. Primary prevention of cardiovascular disease with a mediterranean diet supplemented with extra-virgin olive oil or nuts. N Engl J Med 2018;378(25):e34.

10. Tharrey M, Mariotti F, Mashchak A, et al. Patterns of plant and animal protein intake are strongly associated with cardiovascular mortality: the adventist health study-2 cohort. Int J Epidemiol 2018;47(5):1603–12.

11. Kyu HH, Bachman VF, Alexander LT, et al. Physical activity and risk of breast cancer, colon cancer, diabetes, ischemic heart disease, and ischemic stroke events: systematic review and dose-response meta-analysis for the Global Burden of Disease Study 2013. BMJ 2016;354:i3857.

12. Newman CB. Safety of statins and nonstatins for treatment of dyslipidemia. Endocrinol Metab Clin North Am 2022;51(3):655–79.

13. Grinspoon SK, Fitch KV, Zanni MV, et al. Pitavastatin to prevent cardiovascular disease in HIV infection. N Engl J Med 2023;389(8):687–99.

14. Cannon CP, Blazing MA, Giugliano RP, et al. Ezetimibe added to statin therapy after acute coronary syndromes. N Engl J Med 2015;372(25):2387–97.

15. Pinkosky SL, Newton RS, Day EA, et al. Liver-specific ATP-citrate lyase inhibition by bempedoic acid decreases LDL-C and attenuates atherosclerosis. Nat Commun 2016;7(1):13457.

16. Laufs U, Banach M, Mancini GBJ, et al. Efficacy and safety of bempedoic acid in patients with hypercholesterolemia and statin intolerance. J Am Heart Assoc 2019;8(7):e011662.

17. Goldberg AC, Leiter LA, Stroes ESG, et al. Effect of bempedoic acid vs placebo added to maximally tolerated statins on low-density lipoprotein cholesterol in patients at high risk for cardiovascular disease: the clear wisdom randomized clinical trial. JAMA 2019;322(18):1780–8.

18. Ballantyne CM, Banach M, Mancini GBJ, et al. Efficacy and safety of bempedoic acid added to ezetimibe in statin-intolerant patients with hypercholesterolemia: A randomized, placebo-controlled study. Atherosclerosis 2018;277:195–203.

19. Nissen SE, Lincoff AM, Brennan D, et al. Bempedoic Acid and Cardiovascular Outcomes in Statin-Intolerant Patients. N Engl J Med 2023;388(15):1353–64.

20. Bays HE, Bloedon LT, Lin G, et al. Safety of bempedoic acid in patients at high cardiovascular risk and with statin intolerance. J Clin Lipidol 2023; S1933-2874(23):00313-6.

21. Warden BA, Cardiology BA, Purnell JQ, et al. Real-world utilization of bempedoic acid in an academic preventive cardiology practice. J Clin Lipidol 2022;16(1):94–103.

22. Schwartz GG, Steg PG, Szarek M, et al. Alirocumab and cardiovascular outcomes after acute coronary syndrome. N Engl J Med 2018;379(22):2097–107.

23. Sabatine MS, Giugliano RP, Keech AC, et al. Evolocumab and clinical outcomes in patients with cardiovascular disease. N Engl J Med 2017;376(18):1713–22.

24. Lloyd-Jones DM, Lloyd-Jones DM, Morris PB, et al. 2022 ACC expert consensus decision pathway on the role of nonstatin therapies for ldl-cholesterol lowering in the management of atherosclerotic cardiovascular disease risk. J Am Coll Cardiol 2022;80(14):1366–418.

25. Smith A, Johnson D, Banks J, et al. Trends in PCSK9 inhibitor prescriptions before and after the price reduction in patients with atherosclerotic cardiovascular disease. J Clin Med 2021;10(17):3828.

26. Fitzgerald K, Frank-Kamenetsky M, Shulga-Morskaya S, et al. Effect of an RNA interference drug on the synthesis of proprotein convertase subtilisin/kexin type 9 (PCSK9) and the concentration of serum LDL cholesterol in healthy volunteers: a randomised, single-blind, placebo-controlled, phase 1 trial. Lancet 2014; 383(9911):60–8.

27. Ray KK, Landmesser U, Leiter LA, et al. Inclisiran in patients at high cardiovascular risk with elevated LDL cholesterol. N Engl J Med 2017;376(15):1430–40.

28. Wright RS, Koenig W, Landmesser U, et al. Safety and tolerability of inclisiran for treatment of hypercholesterolemia in 7 clinical trials. J Am Coll Cardiol 2023; 82(24):2251–61.

29. Raal FJ, Rosenson RS, Reeskamp LF, et al. Evinacumab for homozygous familial hypercholesterolemia. N Engl J Med 2020;383(8):711–20.

30. Gaudet D, Gipe DA, Pordy R, et al. ANGPTL3 Inhibition in Homozygous Familial Hypercholesterolemia. N Engl J Med 2017;377(3):296–7.

31. Farnier M, Zeller M, Masson D, et al. Triglycerides and risk of atherosclerotic cardiovascular disease: An update. Arch Cardiovasc Dis 2021;114(2):132–9.

32. Toth PP. Clinical insights from the Fenofibrate Intervention and Event Lowering in Diabetes study: a community practice perspective. Int J Clin Pract 2009;63(6): 903–11.

33. Ginsberg HN, Ginsberg HN, Elam MB, et al. Effects of combination lipid therapy in type 2 diabetes mellitus. N Engl J Med 2010;362(17):1563–74.

34. Elam MB, Ginsberg HN, Lovato LC, et al. Association of fenofibrate therapy with long-term cardiovascular risk in statin-treated patients with type 2 diabetes. JAMA Cardiol 2017;2(4):370–80.

35. Das Pradhan A, Glynn RJ, Fruchart JC, et al. Triglyceride lowering with pemafibrate to reduce cardiovascular risk. N Engl J Med 2022;387(21):1923–34.

36. Wiggins BS, Saseen JJ, Page RL 2nd, et al. Recommendations for management of clinically significant drug-drug interactions with statins and select agents used in patients with cardiovascular disease: a scientific statement from the american heart association. Circulation 2016;134(21):e468–95.

37. Bhatt DL, Steg PG, Miller M, et al. Cardiovascular risk reduction with icosapent ethyl for hypertriglyceridemia. N Engl J Med 2019;380(1):11–22.

38. Nicholls SJ, Lincoff AM, Garcia M, et al. Effect of high-dose omega-3 fatty acids vs corn oil on major adverse cardiovascular events in patients at high cardiovascular risk: the strength randomized clinical trial. JAMA 2020;324(22):2268–80.

39. Goff ZD, Nissen SE. N-3 polyunsaturated fatty acids for cardiovascular risk. Curr Opin Cardiol 2022;37(4):356–63.

40. Mason RP, Sherratt SCR, Eckel RH. Omega-3-fatty acids: do they prevent cardiovascular disease? Best Pract Res Clin Endocrinol Metab 2023;37(3):101681.

41. Aung T, Halsey J, Kromhout D, et al. Associations of omega-3 fatty acid supplement use with cardiovascular disease risks: meta-analysis of 10 trials involving 77 917 individuals. JAMA Cardiol 2018;3(3):225–34.

42. Chan DC, Watts GF. The promise of PCSK9 and lipoprotein(a) as targets for gene silencing therapies. Clin Ther 2023;45(11):1034–46.

43. Watts GF, Schwabe C, Scott R, et al. RNA interference targeting ANGPTL3 for triglyceride and cholesterol lowering: phase 1 basket trial cohorts. Nat Med 2023; 29(9):2216–23.

Update on Therapies in Older Adults

Sophie Clark, MD[1], Thomas Johnson, MD[2],
Katherine Runkel, MD[3], Jeffrey Wallace, MD, MPH*

KEYWORDS

- Older adults • Dementia • Behaviors • Cognitive impairment • Overactive bladder
- Urinary continence

KEY POINTS

- Memory loss and dementia are among older adults' greatest health fears.
- Physical exercise is an evidenced-based intervention to improve cognitive function for patients with mild cognitive impairment.
- Urinary incontinence is another common problem in older adults that has a major impact on quality of life.

INTERVENTIONS TO PREVENT OR DELAY COGNITIVE DECLINE IN PERSONS AT RISK OF DEMENTIA
Current Management of Mild Cognitive Impairment

Mild cognitive impairment (MCI) is a risk factor for the development of dementia with roughly 10% to 15% of patients with MCI annually progressing to dementia.[1] Patients with MCI have subjective memory problems as well as decreased performance on cognitive tests, but these impairments do not impair daily function. How to prevent the progression of MCI into dementia is a topic of significant public health interest as the American population ages.

For those diagnosed with MCI, current management recommendations include identifying and treating potentially reversible causes of cognitive impairment, including stopping medications with centrally acting side effects, improving sleep quality, treatment of sleep apnea, screening for hypothyroidism or B12 deficiency, and addressing underlying depression or mood disorder. There are no medications currently approved to treat MCI. Nonpharmacologic interventions to reduce the risk of progression to

Division of Geriatric Medicine, University of Colorado School of Medicine, 12631 East 17th Avenue, Box B179, Aurora, CO 80045, USA
[1] Present address: 1715 Ivanhoe Street, Denver CO 80220.
[2] Present address: 8292 East Briarwood Boulevard, Centennial, CO 80112.
[3] Present address: 1122 East 8th Avenue, Denver CO 80218.
* Corresponding author. 12631 East 17th Avenue, Box B179, Aurora, CO 80045.
E-mail address: jeff.wallace@cuanschutz.edu
Twitter: @TMJohnsonMD (T.J.)

Med Clin N Am 108 (2024) 895–910
https://doi.org/10.1016/j.mcna.2024.02.005
medical.theclinics.com

dementia include aerobic and resistance training exercise as well as dietary interventions, such as Mediterranean diet.[2]

New Developments

Tai chi

Tai Chi is a form of low-impact exercise that involves a series of physical movements and postures that integrate breathing control, meditation, and mindfulness. Tai chi is a moderate-intensity aerobic exercise with 4 METS equivalent to a brisk walk.[3] In addition, participation involves learning and memorizing new movements, focusing, and multitasking. This exercise is growing in popularity in the United States, and classes are now commonly offered at community centers.

Health benefits. Over time, the health benefits of tai chi have been increasingly recognized. Previous randomized controlled trials have found tai chi is an effective intervention to decrease falls in community dwelling older adults,[4] as well as to improve cognition and fall risk in older adults with MCI.[5]

Two new randomized controlled trials add to the growing body of evidence supporting the cognitive benefits of tai chi. One study aimed to compare the relative cognitive benefits of tai chi and fitness walking for older adults who had a dual diagnosis of MCI and diabetes.[6] Both intervention groups demonstrated improved performance on the montreal cognitive assessment (MOCA) and in blood sugar control at 24 weeks; however, the tai chi group performed 0.94 points better on average on the MOCA postintervention compared with the brisk walking group at 24 weeks, a cognitive decline benefit of roughly 2 years.[6]

A second trial looked at the effectiveness of a novel form of Tai Ji Quan that integrates cognitive tasks into the standard practice of tai ji quan.[7] The single-blind, parallel group randomized controlled trial explored the benefits of (1) cognitively enhanced tai chi quan; (2) standard tai chi quan; and (3) stretching exercises on global cognition and dual task walking performance task. Participants participated in a twice-weekly, 60-minute exercise class that lasted for 24 weeks with a postintervention observational period up to 48 weeks. Participants were 65 years or older with a self-reported or informant observed memory problem with a mini-mental state examination (MMSE) score greater than24 without any functional impairments. All groups exercised at home via real-time videoconferencing, as the study took place during the COVID-19 pandemic. Both tai ji quan groups experienced a statistically significant improvement in global cognition with the cognitively enhanced tai ji group experiencing a +3.1 point average improvement in MOCA score, and the standard group experiencing a +1.7 point average improvement in MOCA score; no change in MOCA score was observed in the stretching control group. The 1.4-point difference is consistent with a cognitive decline benefit of roughly 3 years. These results were sustained at 48 weeks. This trial provides further support for the cognitive benefits of tai ji quan in those with MCI and suggests that integration of cognitive tasks into the exercise form can further enhance these benefits.

Hearing loss

Background. Observational studies have demonstrated an association between hearing loss and risk of dementia. In a population-based cohort study of more than 16,000 participants, individuals in the cohort that experienced hearing loss were significantly more likely to develop dementia than those without hearing loss.[8] The mechanism of how hearing loss increases dementia risk is not known, although several theories exist, including adverse neuronal health effects of sensory deprivation, and impaired communication increases the risk of social isolation and depressive symptoms.[9]

New data regarding the correction of hearing impairment and cognitive decline. The ACHIEVE (Aging and Cognitive Health Evaluation in Elders) study is the first randomized controlled trial to explore whether correction of hearing impairment can reduce cognitive decline.[10] Study participants were 70 to 84 years old and were cognitively intact. Participants were recruited from 2 distinct groups. Some participants were recruited from healthy volunteers in the community and were considered the de novo population cohort. Other participants were recruited from another ongoing longitudinal study, Atherosclerosis Risk in Communities (ARIC), which aims to understand the relationship between cognitive decline and cardiovascular risk factors. ARIC participants had higher rates of risks factors for dementia compared with de novo participants, including higher amounts of women, lower educational status and income, more participants of Black race, and higher rates of hypertension and diabetes.

The intervention group received bilateral hearing aids, whereas the control group participated in a health education course. At the end of 3 years, there was no difference in scores on the comprehensive neurocognitive battery between the hearing aid and health education course for the entire study population at large. However, subset analysis showed that among the higher-risk ARIC participants, the hearing aid group had a 48% slower rate of 3-year cognitive decline on a neurocognitive battery compared with the health education group. This study provides preliminary evidence that patients with greater risk factors for dementia may benefit the most from the correction of hearing loss.

CLINICS CARE POINTS

- Physical exercise is an evidenced-based intervention to improve cognitive function for patients with mild cognitive impairment.

- There is growing evidence that tai chi confers unique cognitive benefit as an exercise intervention in patients with mild cognitive impairment, especially those who have a concurrent diagnosis of diabetes.

- Correction of hearing loss may help prevent cognitive decline.

NEW BIOLOGICAL MEDICATIONS FOR PERSONS WITH EARLY ALZHEIMER DEMENTIA
Background

There are an estimated 4.7 million individuals 65 years or older with Alzheimer dementia (AD) in the United States, and this number is expected to triple by 2050.[11] Dementia is the second leading cause of death for Medicare beneficiaries, only behind heart failure.[12]

Pharmacologic management of AD has had limited efficacy. Before 2021, the only Food and Drug Administration (FDA)-approved medications for AD were cholinesterase inhibitors and memantine. A Cochrane review found that donepezil demonstrated better outcomes on the Alzheimer's Disease Assessment Scale–Cognitive by a mean of -2.67 on a 0 to 70 point scale,[13] less than the clinically meaningful cutoff of 4 points for this scale.[14] Donepezil did not improve behavioral symptoms, quality of life, or health care resource utilization.[13] A Cochrane review of memantine found similarly small clinical benefits compared with placebo in persons with moderate to severe AD.[15] There was no difference between placebo and memantine for persons with mild dementia.[15] Cholinesterase inhibitors have been associated with important side effects (eg, gastrointestinal symptoms and falls), whereas memantine has been associated with dizziness and headaches.[13,15]

Given the limited benefit of previously available treatments, alternatives have been explored, and 2 novel medications that use monoclonal antibodies to reduce β-amyloid (Aβ) have recently been FDA approved for use in persons with AD: aducanumab in 2021 and lecanemab in 2023.

Definitions

Per the National Institute on Aging-Alzheimer's Association workgroup, a diagnosis of dementia requires a change in function of usual activities; a decline from prior functioning; cognitive impairment established by patient history and objective mental status testing; cognitive impairment involving 2 or more cognitive domains including deficits in learning new information, complex reasoning, visuospatial abilities, language, and personality changes.[16] A diagnosis of AD specifically requires insidious onset, well-defined history of worsening, amnestic presentation, or nonamnestic presentations.[16]

Pharmacology

The amyloid hypothesis of AD was first developed in the 1980s, in part based on the discovery of AD brain pathologic condition in persons with Down syndrome, who have an extra chromosome 21, which contains coding for amyloid precursor protein (APP).[17] APP processing produces Aβ, a peptide that is the main component of brain amyloid plaques that are a pathologic hallmark of AD.[17] The amyloid hypothesis theorizes that amyloid plaques are key to the development of neurofibrillary tangles, vascular damage, and cell loss, all causing a phenotypic presentation of dementia.[17] The current FDA-approved therapies target Aβ in various forms to reduce brain Aβ burden. Aducanumab is a human monoclonal antibody that selectively targets aggregated forms of Aβ, including soluble oligomers and insoluble fibrils.[18] Lecanemab is a humanized monoclonal antibody that binds to Aβ-soluble protofibrils. **Fig. 1** illustrates the mechanism of action for lecanemab.

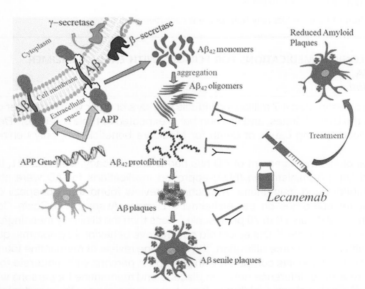

Fig. 1. Mechanism of action of lecanemab. (Chowdhury S, Chowhury NS. Novel anti-amyloid-beta (Aβ) monoclonal antibody lecanemab for Alzheimer's disease: A Systematic Review. Int J Immunopathol Pharmacol 2023; 37. https://doi.org/10.1177/0394632023120.)

Evidence of efficacy

Aducanumab. Two placebo controlled trials, EMERGE and ENGAGE, evaluated aducanumab in patients with AD with MCI or mild dementia stage of disease with confirmed presence of Aβ pathologic condition.[19] Both trials showed a reduction in brain amyloid based on amyloid PET imaging; however, clinical outcome benefits were not demonstrated, and both of these trials were stopped early owing to futility.[20] There has been significant controversy regarding the FDA approval of aducanumab given Aβ burden was not approved as a valid pharmacodynamic biomarker and the questionable clinical benefit of the therapy.[21]

Lecanemab. Lecanemab was evaluated in an 18-month placebo controlled trial in patients with early AD with evidence of brain amyloid on PET imaging or cerebrospinal fluid (CSF) testing. The primary study outcome, the Clinical Dementia Rating–Sum of Boxes (CDR-SOB) score, which was 3.2 in both groups at baseline, demonstrated a statistically significant difference between lecanemab and placebo, 1.21 and 1.66, respectively, with higher scores indicating greater impairment.[22] The CDR-SOB helps to categorize severity of dementia with a score of 0 being normal, a score of 0.5 to 2.5 likely MCI, 3 to 4 very mild, and 4.5 to 9 mild dementia.[23] All secondary outcomes, which included amyloid burden on PET, Alzheimer's Disease Assessment scale, and the Alzheimer's Disease Cooperative Study–Activities of Daily Living Scale for Mild Cognitive Impairment, statistically significantly favored lecanemab over placebo.[22] **Table 1** provides a comparison between aducanumab and lecanemab.

Safety

Amyloid-related imaging abnormalities (ARIAs) have been shown to occur frequently (eg, in 21.5% of persons treated with lecanemab) with both monoclonal antibody treatments.[19,22] ARIAs can present with brain edema (ARIA-E) or increased

Table 1		
Comparison of lecanemab to aducanumab		
	Lecanemab	**Aducanumab**
Drug class	Humanized IgG1 monoclonal antibody	Human IgG1 monoclonal antibody
Mechanism of action	Targets aggregated soluble and insoluble Aβ	
Indication	Mild cognitive impairment, early AD	
Trial primary outcome	Reduction in CDR-SOB scores, 25% less decline in treatment group	Reduction in brain amyloid on PET. Emerge trial found 22% less decline on CDR-SOB at 78 wk after trials stopped due to clinical futility
Safety concerns	ARIA, infusion reactions	ARIA
Before infusion	CSF amyloid measurement or amyloid PET, recent brain MRI, ApoE ε4 status	CSF amyloid measurement or amyloid PET, recent brain MRI
Dosing	10 mg/kg infusion every 2 wk	10 mg/kg every 4 wk after dose uptitration over 6 infusions
Monitoring	Brain MRI before 5th, 7th, 9th, 12th infusions	Brain MRI before 5th, 7th, 14th infusions
Insurance	Medicare will cover if patient meets diagnostic criteria and the prescriber is participating in a qualifying registry	Medicare will only pay if patient is enrolled in qualifying clinical trial

hemosiderin deposits suggestive of microhemorrhage (ARIA-H). Typical symptoms reported with ARIAs include headache, visual disturbance, and confusion.[19,22] No deaths have been attributed to ARIAs for either treatment. ARIAs are more common among patients who are apolipoprotein E ε4 (ApoE ε4) homozygotes.[22] The most common adverse event for lecanemab was infusion-related reactions, occurring in 26.4% of subjects.[22]

Use in practice

Patient assessment. The clinical diagnosis of AD with MCI or early dementia, using accepted criteria, is required, and the presence of central nervous system Aβ should be confirmed by CSF measurement of Aβ or positive amyloid PET imaging before initiating either aducanumab or lecanemab.[24,25] A recent brain MRI, no more than 1 year before first infusion, should be obtained.[24,25] Given higher rates of symptomatic, serious, and severe radiographic ARIAs with ApoE ε4 homozygotes compared with heterozygotes and noncarriers, the patient's ApoE ε4 status should be tested before treatment.[25]

Dosing and monitoring. Total recommended dose for aducanumab is 10 mg/kg infused every 4 weeks, achieved via dose uptitration over the first 6 infusions.[24] Brain MRIs should be obtained before the fifth, seventh, ninth, and 12th infusions for aducanumab.[14] Lecanemab dosage is 10 mg/kg infusions every 2 weeks, and MRI is recommended before the fifth, seventh, and 14th infusions.[25] If ARIAs develop, treatment recommendations are dependent on the type, severity, and presence of symptoms.[24,25]

Cost. Medicare will only cover aducanumab if patients are enrolled in a qualifying clinical trial.[26]

Medicare will cover lecanemab; however, patients must be enrolled in Medicare, meet diagnostic criteria, and have a physician who is participating in a qualifying registry.[27] This is to help collect further evidence on these medications.[27] A Centers for Medicare & Medicaid Services–facilitated registry that is free to access for clinicians requires provider National Provider Identifier, patient Medicare beneficiary ID, provider contact information, clinical diagnosis, testing obtained including cognitive and functional testing, and questions regarding anticoagulation and evidence of ARIA.[28] Requirements include initial submission and submission every 6 months for up to 24 months (5 total assessments).[29]

Lecanemab is covered under Medicare Part B. Patients will pay 0% to 20% for the Medicare-approved amount after they meet their Part B deductible.[30] Eisai has listed the cost of lecanemab at $26,500 per year.[31] A cross-sectional study of total Medicare costs for lecanemab found a per-beneficiary medication cost of $25,851 with $7,330 of additional ancillary costs.[32] They estimated that the coinsurance for this medication would be $6,636 per patient, and the total cost to Medicare would be $2.0 billion to $5.1 billion annually based on currently eligible patients.[32]

CLINICS CARE POINTS

- Aducanumab is the first monoclonal antibody Food and Drug Administration approved for disease-modifying therapy of Alzheimer dementia.
- Efficacy data for aducanumab are mixed and controversial.
- Lecanemab has stronger statistical evidence for supporting its use in patients with early Alzheimer dementia than aducanumab, but data for clinically meaningful benefit remain limited.

- Amyloid-related imaging abnormalities are more severe in ApoE ε4 homozygotes, and genetic testing should be considered before initiating treatment.
- No deaths from amyloid-related imaging abnormalities were reported in initial studies.
- There will be significant burden on the health care system if these therapies are used, widely given the requirements for multiple brain MRIs, frequent infusions, and extensive initial testing.

BEHAVIORAL AND PSYCHOLOGICAL SYMPTOMS OF DEMENTIA
Background

Agitation associated with AD remains one of the most difficult conditions to treat in older adults. Aggressive behaviors are associated with increased rates of institutionalization, significant caregiver distress, and faster cognitive decline.[33] Per the International Psychogeriatric Association consensus criteria, agitation in cognitive disorders is defined as the presence of at least once of these behaviors persisting for at least 2 weeks that causes distress to the individual: (a) excessive motor activity (ie, pacing, repetitive behaviors, and so forth); (b) verbal aggression (ie, using profanity, derogatory remarks, and so forth); (c) physical aggression (ie, hitting others, throwing objects).[33]

Management of Behavioral and Psychological Symptoms of Dementia

For agitation or other behavioral and psychological symptoms of dementia (BPSD), the current standards of care recommend evaluating for reversible causes of aggression first, such as adverse effects of medications, mood disorder, new medical problems, or inadequately treated pain (**Box 1**). Initial management should include implementation of nonpharmacologic treatment strategies, such as caregiver education regarding how they approach the patient, distraction techniques, and newer approaches that might include aromatherapy or music therapy.

Medications may be useful when nonpharmacologic strategies fail to adequately control agitation (**Fig. 2**). Most practitioners choose to implement selective serotonin reuptake inhibitors as first-line medication for agitation, as there is evidence for modest benefit and the side-effect profile is favorable compared with antipsychotics.[34] However, agitation that continues to pose a threat to the safety of the patient or caregivers despite a trial of nonpharmacologic strategies is often treated

---

Box 1
Potential sources of behavioral and psychological symptoms of dementia, the 7 I's

- Iatrogenic—sedatives, anticholinergic agents
- Infection—UTI, pneumonia
- Injury—pain, fracture
- Illness—COPD or CHF exacerbation, metabolic derangement
- Impaction
- Inconsistency—in environment, change in routine
- Is the patient depressed?

Abbreviations: CHF, congestive heart failure; COPD, chronic obstructive pulmonary disease; UTI, urinary tract infection.

Evaluate for delirium, pain, medical, other causes (see 7 "I"s Box 1)
↓

Non-pharmacologic tx → improved
↓ Not improved

Is pt on memantine and/or cholinesterase inhibitor? → no → consider
↓ Not improved

Are there signs/symptoms of depression or anxiety? → yes → SSRI
↓ even if uncertain usually trial SSRI

BPSD persistent and impairing patient care/safety/quality of life
↓

Trial atypical antipsychotic med
-Discuss and document risk/benefit
- Monitor for EPS, sedation, revisit need/taper every 3-6 months

Fig. 2. Management algorithm for behavioral and psychological symptoms of dementia. med, medicine; pt, patient; SSRI, selective serotonin reuptake inhibitor; tx, treatment.

off-label with atypical antipsychotics. Although atypical antipsychotics have shown modest benefit in the treatment of aggression, they are associated with significant side effects, including increased risk of falls, fractures, worsening cognitive decline, cerebrovascular events, and mortality.[35] For these reasons, a black box warning for evidence of increased mortality and risk of cerebrovascular events has been issued for the use of atypical antipsychotics in patients with dementia, along with the statement that, up until now, atypical antipsychotics are not FDA approved for behaviors associated with dementia.

What Is New?

In 2023, brexpiprazole became the first drug that has been FDA approved to treat agitation related to AD.

Pharmacology

Brexpiprazole is an atypical antipsychotic that is also approved to treat schizophrenia and as an adjunct therapy to treat major depressive disorder. The medication is a partial agonist of the serotonin 5-HT1A receptor and the dopamine D2 receptor, as well as an antagonist of several adrenergic receptors.[36]

Brexpiprazole has a side-effect profile similar to that of other atypical antidepressants, including metabolic changes (weight gain, hyperglycemia, and elevated triglycerides), constipation, somnolence, headache, tremor, and dyspepsia. It is also associated with akathisia and extrapyramidal symptoms, although overall risk is less than with first-generation antipsychotics.[37] Somnolence and sedation have a low incidence (all <5%), but rates are still higher than placebo.[38]

Evidence for use

Initial evidence supporting the use of brexpiprazole in AD agitation came from 2 randomized controlled trials that looked at the efficacy of brexpiprazole 1 mg per day, 2 mg per day, and a flexible dose of 0.5 to 2 mg per day. Only the brexpiprazole 2 mg per day group demonstrated statistically significant improvement in Cohen-Mansfield Agitation Inventory (CMAI) scores.[39] CMAI is a well-validated index that measures the frequency of 29 agitated behaviors grading them on a severity of 1 (never occurs) to 7 (occurs a few times per hour) for a range of 29 to 207 total points.[40]

The pivotal randomized controlled trial demonstrating the efficacy of brexpiprazole in reducing agitation related to AD involved 354 patients randomized to one of 3 groups for 12 weeks: (a) control; (b) brexpiprazole 2 mg; or (c) brexpiprazole 3 mg daily.[38] Eligibility criteria included a diagnosis of probable AD supported by an MMSE score of 5 to 22 and MRI or computed tomographic imaging compatible with the diagnosis. All participants had to have persistent agitation despite elimination of reversible causes of agitation and nonpharmacologic treatment approaches. Participants were excluded if taking other antipsychotics, mood stabilizers, or anticonvulsants. Overall, the study group experienced an additional decrease of −5.32 in CMAI score compared with the placebo, which is considered a moderate clinical benefit.[38] The cost of a month's supply of brexpiprazole is about $1600 but is covered by Medicare prescription drug plans.

Safety

Other atypical antipsychotics have been associated with an increased risk of falls, fracture, cerebrovascular accidents, and mortality.[35] In the 3 trials that looked at brexpiprazole use in AD agitation, no increased risk of falls or fractures were seen, but these patients had a mean MMSE score of 15, and approximately 40% resided in nursing homes, possibly representing a cohort with more intact cognition and/or more assistance available than would be seen with real-life use.[41] Across all 3 trials, there were 6 deaths in the treatment group with brexpiprazole compared with one in the placebo group. Although small, these numbers suggest an excess mortality as has been observed with other atypical antipsychotic use in this patient population.[41] In fact, brexpiprazole labeling includes a black box warning stating "Elderly patients with dementia-related psychosis treated with antipsychotic drugs are at increased risk of death. REXULTI is not approved for the treatment of patients with dementia-related psychosis without agitation," emphasizing that the key FDA-approved target behavior for brexpiprazole is agitation rather than psychosis alone.

Dosing

Recommended starting dose is 0.5 mg per day with a target dose of 2 mg per day.[42] This agent is not intended for as-needed, that is, prn, use.

CLINICS CARE POINTS

- Brexpiprazole is the first antipsychotic drug to gain Food and Drug Administration approval for the treatment of agitation in Alzheimer disease.
- Careful evaluation for remediable causes of agitation and nonpharmacologic management are the first-line approaches for behavioral and psychological symptoms of dementia.
- Compared with other atypical antipsychotics, brexpiprazole may be more effective at targeting symptoms of agitation in dementia with an improved safety profile. However, there are still safety concerns regarding its use in this vulnerable population that require further study.
- Like other atypical antipsychotics, brexpiprazole carries a black box warning for increased mortality when used for dementia with psychosis; it is only Food and Drug Administration approved for dementia with agitation.

NEW MEDICATIONS FOR OVERACTIVE BLADDER
Background

Overactive bladder (OAB) is defined by the International Continence Society as urinary urgency, usually with urinary frequency and nocturia, with or without urinary incontinence.[42] The estimated prevalence of OAB symptoms occurring at least "often" is 33% among women and 16% in men.[43] Prevalence estimates increase with age, affecting 35% of men and 43% of women over the age of 75. In addition to being a prevalent condition in older adults, it is significantly associated with falls, depression, and mortality and has a marked negative impact on quality of life.[44]

First-line treatments for OAB include deprescribing of medications that can cause OAB (eg, cholinesterase inhibitors, loop diuretics when possible), limiting alcohol and caffeine, and smoking cessation (chemicals in cigarettes, such as nicotine and tar, can irritate the bladder lining and exacerbate OAB symptoms). Exercise-based interventions include pelvic muscle exercises (eg, Kegel exercises) with or without pelvic floor–specialized physical therapist guidance. Bladder training that includes scheduled voiding every 1 to 2 hours while awake to "beat the bladder to the punch" is a low-risk intervention that is often beneficial.[45] Local estrogen therapy can help reduce OAB symptoms in postmenopausal women with vulvovaginal atrophy.[46] Weight loss in individuals with obesity can be helpful.

When the above first-line approaches do not provide adequate relief of OAB symptoms, it is appropriate to consider adding an antispasmodic agent. It is important to recognize that antispasmodic medications alone have only a marginal benefit on OAB symptoms and should always be used in conjunction with the above nonpharmacologic approaches. The first generation of antispasmodic medications used to treat OAB were muscarinic acetylcholine antagonists. Although these can be efficacious for treating OAB, they are prone to drug interactions and significant side effects, especially in older adults. They are accordingly identified on Beer's list as potentially inappropriate medications.[47]

The beta-3 adrenergic receptor agonists are a newer class of antispasmodic medications for the treatment of OAB. This class includes both mirabegron and vibegron. By using a different mechanism of action, the hope was to develop pharmacotherapeutics that have a more tolerable side-effect profile than the antimuscarinics.

Beta-3 Adrenergic Agonist Pharmacology

Mirabegron and vibegron are both orally available beta-3 adrenergic receptor agonists. They work by inducing detrusor muscle relaxation through decreasing detrusor muscle activity in the storage phase.[48] Mirabegron is metabolized by cytochrome P450 isoenzyme CYP3A4 and CYP2D6.[49] It is also a moderate inhibitor of CYP2D6,[50] which is at least partially responsible for the metabolism of 25% of the drugs in clinical use in the United States.[51] Mirabegron dosing should not exceed 25 mg for patients with renal dysfunction (estimated glomerular filtration rate [eGFR], 15–29 mL per minute) or moderate hepatic impairment (Child-Pugh class B) and is not recommended for use in persons with eGFR <15 mL per minute or in persons with Child-Pugh class C hepatic impairment.[51]

Vibegron, on the other hand, is not an inducer or inhibitor of cytochrome P450; it has higher selectivity for the beta-3 receptor than mirabegron, and it does not require dose changes with renal or hepatic impairment, although it has not been studied in end-stage kidney disease or Child-Pugh class C hepatic impairment.[52]

Evidence for Use

The EMPOWUR double-blind, randomized controlled trial compared vibegron with both placebo and an antimuscarinic antispasmodic, tolterodine.[53] At 12 weeks, patients on vibegron had 1.8 fewer micturitions per day (placebo, 1.3; $P<.001$). Among patients with urge incontinence, incontinent episodes decreased by 2 episodes per day on vibegron versus 1.4 for placebo ($P<.0001$). Vibegron also was superior to placebo in reducing the number of urgency episodes and volume per micturition (P<.01). The following adverse events were noted to be both greater than 2% incidence and higher than placebo: headache (4% vs 2.4%), nasopharyngitis (2.8% vs 1.7%), diarrhea (2.2% vs 1.1), and nausea (2.2% vs 1.1). Vibegron had lower urinary tract infection rates compared with placebo and tolterodine (5.0% vs 6.1% vs 5.8%). There were no differences between hypertension, blood pressure increase, and tachycardia compared with placebo. This trial provides good evidence that vibegron is both efficacious and tolerable.

Vibegron Place in Therapy

The antimuscarinics are oftentimes the medication many providers reach for first when treating OAB in part because of longstanding experience with these older agents and because of the substantially higher cost of newer agents. The EMPOWUR trial did compare vibegron with tolterodine and found no statistically significant difference in efficacy, although it was trending toward improved efficacy in all domains. In a systematic review looking at vibegron versus antimuscarinics,[54] there was no statistically significant differences in efficacy of treating OAB. However, it was noted that vibegron had better safety and tolerance with decreased drug-related treatment-emergent adverse events (OR, 0.63; 95% CI, 0.46–0.87) and dry mouth (OR, 0.17; 95% CI, 0.10–0.31).[54]

Mirabegron Versus Vibegron

In addition to increased potential for drug interactions, mirabegron also has been shown to statistically significantly increase both blood pressure and pulse rate **(Table 2)**.[55] However, this effect is minimal: mirabegron 50 mg was associated with placebo-adjusted mean increases of 0.4 to 0.6 mm Hg in blood pressure and approximately 1 beat per minute in pulse rate, both reversible upon treatment discontinuation. Furthermore, the rate of discontinuation owing to hypertension was similar between mirabegron and tolterodine at 1 year (0.4% in both groups), and the incidence of major adverse cardiovascular events was low and similar across treatment groups.

In a meta-analysis of more than 10,000 patients looking indirectly at mirabegron and vibegron, there was no statistically significant difference between vibegron and placebo, or mirabegron and vibegron in cardiovascular adverse events.[56] In a head-to-head randomized controlled trial of mirabegron and vibegron in women with treatment-naïve OAB, both mirabegron and vibegron were efficacious with no statistically significant difference found in efficacy, safety, or tolerability.[57] Vibegron was found to be superior to mirabegron in some efficacy outcomes in various meta-analyses, including mean voided volume per micturition,[56,58] and total incontinence episodes.[58]

Overall, vibegron is an efficacious treatment option for OAB that is generally well-tolerated. It has minimal drug interactions and does not need to be dose-reduced in moderate renal impairment or hepatic dysfunction. It is just as efficacious as antimuscarinics with improved tolerability. In comparison to mirabegron, it has fewer pharmacologic interactions, may be superior in efficacy in some domains, and has less cardiovascular effects, although the clinical relevance of this is likely minimal. A large consideration for clinicians and their patients is medication cost, so a stepwise approach to management of OAB should always be considered.

Other Approaches

In patients whose symptoms are not controlled with the aforementioned nonpharmacologic and medication options, other advanced therapies include tibial nerve

Table 2
Comparison of beta-3 adrenergic agonists for overactive bladder

	Mirabegron	Vibegron
Dosing	25 mg daily can be increased to 50 mg daily	75 mg daily
Drug interactions	• Moderate inhibitor of CYP2D6 • Metabolized by CYP3A4 and CYP2D6	• Metabolized by CYP3A4
Renal and hepatic dosing considerations	• Maximum dose 25 mg daily for eGFR >15 and <29 mL/min/1.73 m^2 or Child-Pugh class B hepatic impairment • Not recommended in Child-Pugh class C hepatic impairment or if eGFR <15 mL/min/1.73 m^2	• Not recommended in Child-Pugh class C severe hepatic impairment • Not recommended in severe renal impairment with eGFR <15 mL/min/1.73 m^2
Efficacy	• No statistically significant difference compared with antimuscarinics • No statistically significant difference compared with vibegron in overall efficacy for treating OAB	• No statistically significant difference compared with antimuscarinics • May have slight superiority in mean volume voided per micturition and total incontinence episodes compared with mirabegron
Cardiovascular effects	• Placebo-adjusted mean blood pressure increase of 0.4–0.6 mm Hg • Placebo-adjusted mean increase of 1 beat per minute in heart rate	• No difference in rate of discontinuation due to hypertension compared with mirabegron • No difference in major adverse cardiovascular events compared with mirabegron
Other side effects	Nasopharyngitis, headache, diarrhea, nausea, urinary retention, upper respiratory tract infection	Nasopharyngitis, headache, urinary tract infection, urinary retention, constipation

stimulation (percutaneous, transcutaneous, or implanted), botulinum toxin injections, and sacral nerve stimulation devices.[59]

CLINICS CARE POINTS

- The first-line treatments for overactive bladder are pelvic floor exercises and lifestyle and behavioral changes.
- Antimuscarinic agents can have clinically important side effects and are described as potentially inappropriate medications in geriatric medicine.
- Mirabegron and vibegron are both efficacious for pharmacologic management of overactive bladder and are better tolerated than antimuscarinics.
- Mirabegron is a moderate inhibitor of CYP2D6, so drug interactions should come into consideration while prescribing. Vibegron is not an inducer or inhibitor of cytochrome P450.
- Vibegron may be more effective in treating overactive bladder than mirabegron, but more robust head-to-head trials are needed.

- It is unclear how clinically relevant the reductions in nasopharyngeal and cardiovascular side effects are in vibegron when compared with mirabegron; cost may be an important factor to consider when deciding between these 2 agents.

DISCLOSURE

The authors have nothing to disclose.

REFERENCES

1. Langa KM, Levine DA. The diagnosis and management of mild cognitive impairment: a clinical review. JAMA 2014;312(23):2551–61. https://doi.org/10.1001/jama.2014.13806.
2. Chen Y-X, Liang N, Li X-L, et al. Diagnosis and treatment for mild cognitive impairment: A systematic review of clinical practice guidelines and consensus statements. Front Neurol 2021;12.
3. Qi M, Moyle W, Jones C, et al. Tai Chi combined with resistance training for adults aged 50 years and older: A systematic review. J Geriatr Phys Ther 2020;43(1):32–41.
4. Wayne PM, Walsh JN, Taylor-Piliae RE, et al. Effect of Tai Chi on cognitive performance in older adults: Systematic Review and meta-analysis. J Am Geriatr Soc 2014;62(1):25–39.
5. Sungkarat S, Boripuntakul S, Chattipakorn N, et al. Effects of Tai Chi on cognition and fall risk in older adults with mild cognitive impairment: A randomized controlled trial. J Am Geriatr Soc 2016;65(4):721–7.
6. Chen Y, Qin J, Tao L, et al. Effects of Tai Chi Chuan on cognitive function in adults 60 years or older with type 2 diabetes and mild cognitive impairment in China. JAMA Netw Open 2023;6(4).
7. Li F, Harmer P, Eckstrom E, et al. Clinical effectiveness of cognitively enhanced tai ji quan training on global cognition and dual-task performance during walking in older adults with mild cognitive impairment or self-reported memory concerns. Ann Intern Med 2023;176:1498–507.
8. Liu C-M, Lee CT-C. Association of hearing loss with dementia. JAMA Netw Open 2019;2(7). https://doi.org/10.1001/jamanetworkopen.2019.8112.
9. Amieva H, Ouvrard C, Meillon C, et al. Death, depression, disability, and dementia associated with self-reported hearing problems: A 25-year study. J Gerontol: Series A 2018;73(10):1383–9.
10. Lin FR, Pike JR, Albert MS, et al. Hearing intervention versus health education control to reduce cognitive decline in older adults with hearing loss in the USA (achieve): A Multicentre, randomised controlled trial. Lancet 2023;402(10404):786–97.
11. Hebert LE, Weuve J, Scherr PA, et al. Alzheimer disease in the United States (2010-2050) estimated using the 2010 census. Neurology 2013;80(19):1778–83.
12. Tinetti ME, McAvay GJ, Murphy TE, et al. Contribution of individual diseases to death in older adults with multiple diseases. J Am Geriatr Soc 2012;60(8):1448–56.
13. Birks JS, Harvey RJ. Donepezil for dementia due to alzheimer's disease. Cochrane Database Syst Rev 2018;6(6).
14. Rockwood K, Fay S, Gorman M, et al. The clinical meaningfulness of ADAS-COG changes in Alzheimer's disease patients treated with donepezil in an open-label trial. BMC Neurol 2007;7(26).

15. McShane R, Westby MJ, Roberts E, et al. Memantine for dementia. Cochrane Database Syst Rev 2019;3(3).
16. McKhann GM, Knopman DS, Chertkow H, et al. The diagnosis of dementia due to alzheimer's disease: recommendations from the national institute on aging-alzheimer's association workgroups on diagnostic guidelines for alzheimer's disease. Alzheimers Dement 2011;7(3):263–9.
17. Hardy JA, Higgins GA. Alzheimer's disease: the amyloid cascade hypothesis. Science 1992;256(5054):184–5.
18. Sevigny J, Chiao P, Bussière T, et al. The antibody aducanumab reduces aβ plaques in alzheimer's disease. Nature 2016;537(7618):50–6.
19. FDA integrated clinical pharmacology review. Available at: https://www.accessdata.fda.gov/drugsatfda_docs/nda/2021/761178Orig1s000ClinPharm_Redacted.pdf. [Accessed 4 November 2023].
20. Haeberlein SB, Aisen PS, Barkhof F, et al. Two Randomized Phase 3 Studies of Aducanumab in Early Alzheimer's Disease. J Prev Alzheimers Dis 2022;9(2):197–210.
21. van Dyck CH, Swanson CJ, Aisen P, et al. Lecanemab in Early Alzheimer's Disease. N Engl J Med 2023;388(1):9–21.
22. O'Bryant SE, Waring SC, Cullum CM, et al, Texas Alzheimer's Research Consortium. Staging Dementia Using Clinical Dementia Rating Scale Sum of Boxes Scores: A Texas Alzheimer's Research Consortium Study. Arch Neurol 2008;65(8):1091.
23. Alexander GC, Knopman DS, Emerson SS, et al. Revisiting FDA Approval of Aducanumab. N Engl J Med 2021;385(9):769–71.
24. ADUHELM® (aducanumab-avwa) [package insert]. Cambridge, MA: Biogen Inc.; 2023.
25. LEQEMBI® (lecanemab-irmb. [package insert]. Nutley, NJ: Eisaid Inc. and Biogen; 2023.
26. Stephenson J. Medicare to Cover Controversial Alzheimer Disease Drug Only in Clinical Trials. JAMA Health Forum 2022;3(1).
27. Statement: Broader Medicare Coverage of Lequembi Available Following FDA Traditional Approval. CMS. Available at: https://www.cms.gov/newsroom/press-releases/statement-broader-medicare-coverage-leqembi-available-following-fda-traditional-approval. [Accessed 8 January 2024].
28. Alzheimer's CED Registry Resources. CMS. Available at: https://qualitynet.cms.gov/alzheimers-ced-registry/resources. [Accessed 8 January 2024].
29. CMS National patient Registry for New Alzheimer's Drugs: things to know for clinicians. CMS; 2023. Available at: https://www.cms.gov/newsroom/fact-sheets/cms-announces-new-details-plan-cover-new-alzheimers-drugs. [Accessed 8 January 2024].
30. Prescription drugs (outpatient). Medicare.gov. Available at: https://www.medicare.gov/coverage/prescription-drugs-outpatient. [Accessed 8 January 2024].
31. Eisai Co., Ltd. Eisai's Approach to U.S. Pricing for Leqemib™ (Lecanemab), a treatment for early Alzheimer's disease, sets forth our concept of "societal value of medicine" in relation to "price of medicine.". 2023 [News Release]. Available at: https://www.eisai.com/news/2023/news202302.html. . [Accessed 8 January 2023].
32. Arbanas JC, Damberg CL, Leng M, et al. Estimated Annual Spending on Lecanemab and Its Ancillary costs in the US Medicare Program. JAMA Intern Med 2023;183(8):885–9.

33. Sano M, Cummings J, Auer S, et al. Agitation in cognitive disorders: Progress in the International Psychogeriatric Association Consensus Clinical and Research Definition. Int Psychogeriatr 2023;1–13. https://doi.org/10.1017/s1041610222001041.

34. Qasim HS, Simpson MD. A narrative review of studies comparing efficacy and safety of citalopram with atypical antipsychotics for agitation in behavioral and psychological symptoms of dementia (BPSD). Pharmacy 2022;10(3):61.

35. Yunusa I, Alsumali A, Garba AE, et al. Assessment of reported comparative effectiveness and safety of atypical antipsychotics in the treatment of behavioral and psychological symptoms of dementia. JAMA Netw Open 2019;2(3). https://doi.org/10.1001/jamanetworkopen.2019.0828.

36. Maeda K, Sugino H, Akazawa H, et al. Brexpiprazole I: In vitro and in vivo characterization of a novel serotonin-dopamine activity modulator. J Pharmacol Exp Therapeut 2014;350(3):589–604.

37. For Rexulti. highlights of prescribing information rexulti safely. Available at: https://www.otsuka-us.com/sites/g/files/qhldwo8366/files/media/static/Rexulti-PI.pdf. Accessed November 19, 2023.

38. Lee D, Slomkowski M, Hefting N, et al. Brexpiprazole for the treatment of agitation in alzheimer dementia. JAMA Neurol 2023. https://doi.org/10.1001/jamaneurol.2023.3810.

39. Grossberg GT, Kohegyi E, Mergel V, et al. Efficacy and safety of Brexpiprazole for the treatment of agitation in alzheimer's dementia: Two 12-week, randomized, double-blind, placebo-controlled trials. Am J Geriatr Psychiatr 2020;28(4):383–400.

40. Cohen-Mansfield J. Cohen-mansfield agitation inventory. PsycTESTS Dataset 1986. https://doi.org/10.1037/t28576-000.

41. Ballard C. Brexpiprazole for the treatment of agitation and aggression in alzheimer disease. JAMA Neurology 2023. https://doi.org/10.1001/jamaneurol.2023.3967.

42. Abrams P, Cardozo L, Fall M, et al. The standardisation of terminology in lower urinary tract function: report from the standardisation sub-committee of the International Continence Society. Urology 2003;61:37–49.

43. Coyne KS, Sexton CC, Vats V, et al. National community prevalence of overactive bladder in the United States stratified by sex and age. Urology 2011;77(5):1081–7.

44. Coyne KS, Wein A, Nicholson S, et al. Comorbidities and personal burden of urgency urinary incontinence: a systematic review. Int J Clin Pract 2013;67(10):1015–33.

45. Funada S, Yoshioka T, Luo Y, et al. Bladder training for treating overactive bladder in adults. Cochrane Database Syst Rev 2023;10(10):CD013571.

46. Russo E, Caretto M, Giannini A, et al. Management of urinary incontinence in postmenopausal women: an EMAS clinical guide. Maturitas 2020;143:223–30.

47. By the 2023 American Geriatrics Society Beers Criteria® Update Expert Panel. American Geriatrics Society 2023 updated AGS Beers Criteria® for potentially inappropriate medication use in older adults. J Am Geriatr Soc 2023;71(7):2052–81.

48. Takasu T, Ukai M, Sato S, et al. Effect of (R)-2-(2-aminothiazol-4-yl)-4'-{2-[(2-hydroxy-2-phenylethyl)amino]ethyl} acetanilide (YM178), a novel selective beta3-adrenoceptor agonist, on bladder function. J Pharmacol Exp Ther 2007;321(2):642–7.

49. Lee J, Moy S, Meijer J, et al. Role of cytochrome p450 isoenzymes 3A and 2D6 in the in vivo metabolism of mirabegron, a β3-adrenoceptor agonist. Clin Drug Investig 2013;33(6):429–40.

50. Astellas Pharma US Inc, MYRBETRIQ® (mirabegron extended-release tablets). Full prescribing information, 2018, Astellas Pharma US Inc. Available at: https://www.accessdata.fda.gov/drugsatfda_docs/label/2018/202611s011lbl.pdf.

51. Ingelman-Sundberg M. Genetic polymorphisms of cytochrome P450 2D6 (CYP2D6): clinical consequences, evolutionary aspects and functional diversity. Pharmacogenomics J 2005;5(1):6–13.

52. Edmondson SD, Zhu C, Kar NF, et al. Discovery of vibegron: a potent and selective b3 adrenergic receptor agonist for the treatment of overactive bladder. J Med Chem 2016;59:609–23.

53. Staskin D, Frankel J, Varano S, et al. International Phase III, randomized, double-blind, placebo and active controlled study to evaluate the safety and efficacy of vibegron in patients with symptoms of overactive bladder: EMPOWUR. J Urol 2020;204(2):316–24.

54. Su S, Liang L, Lin J, et al. Systematic review and meta-analysis of the efficacy and safety of vibegron vs antimuscarinic monotherapy for overactive bladder. Medicine (Baltim) 2021;100(5):e23171.

55. Nitti VW, Chapple CR, Walters C, et al. Safety and tolerability of the β3-adrenoceptor agonist mirabegron, for the treatment of overactive bladder: results of a prospective pooled analysis of three 12-week randomised Phase III trials and of a 1-year randomised Phase III trial. Int J Clin Pract 2014;68(8):972–85.

56. He W, Zhang Y, Huang G, et al. Efficacy and safety of vibegron compared with mirabegron for overactive bladder: A systematic review and network meta-analysis. Low Urin Tract Symptoms 2023;15(3):80–8.

57. Kinjo M, Masuda K, Nakamura Y, et al. Comparison of mirabegron and vibegron in women with treatment-naive overactive bladder: a randomized controlled study. Urology 2023;175:67–73.

58. Kennelly MJ, Rhodes T, Girman CJ, et al. Efficacy of vibegron and mirabegron for overactive bladder: a systematic literature review and indirect treatment comparison. Adv Ther 2021;38(11):5452–64.

59. Guzman-Negron JM, Goldman HB. New devices and technologies for the management of overactive bladder. Curr Urol Rep 2017;18(12):94.

Newer Treatments for Mood and Anxiety Disorders

Jesse Markman, MD, MBA[*,1], Heidi Combs, MD, MS[2]

KEYWORDS

- Depression • Anxiety • Novel treatments • Antidepressant

KEY POINTS

- First-line pharmacologic agents for the treatment of both major depressive disorder and anxiety disorders remain serotonin reuptake inhibitors and selective serotonin and norepinephrine reuptake inhibitors.
- There are newer novel antidepressants that have less weight gain and/or sexual dysfunction, but are not superior in terms of efficacy.
- Psychotherapy, particularly cognitive behavioral therapy which has the most data supporting efficacy, remains a cornerstone of treatment.
- Data to support the use of psychedelic-assisted psychotherapy are not robust enough to recommend generalized use.

INTRODUCTION

Primary care and family practitioners face some of the most daunting challenges in medicine. They are the first call for the complete gamut of medical maladies and must sort through vague complaints and presentations while staying current on leading treatment strategies. The presentation of mental health concerns during primary care visits can be some of the most challenging as symptoms are often vague and non-specific, but significantly impactful and at times impairing. Reviews on the treatments for major depressive disorder (MDD) and anxiety disorders make clear that these disorders have massive impact and implications on the world stage.[1–23] The World Health Organization has declared that MDD is the single largest contributor to loss of healthy life and anxiety disorders have a 1-year prevalence of up to 20%.[12,21] The primary care provider is positioned on the front line to meet these challenges, but are faced with their own, internal challenge in considering how to stay abreast of current literature and treatment recommendations in a large and rapidly

Department of Psychiatry and Behavioral Sciences, University of Washington School of Medicine, Seattle, WA, USA
[1] Present address: 1660 S. Columbian Way, MS-00-COS, Seattle, WA 98103.
[2] Present address: 325 9th Avenue, Box 359911, Seattle, WA 98104.
* Corresponding author. 1660 South Columbian Way, MS-00-COS, Seattle, WA 98108.
E-mail address: jmarkman@uw.edu

Med Clin N Am 108 (2024) 911–921
https://doi.org/10.1016/j.mcna.2024.03.006
0025-7125/24/Published by Elsevier Inc.

medical.theclinics.com

evolving medical field. This review will summarize the most meaningful advancements in psychiatry over the past 10 years. The authors will focus on the treatment of depression and anxiety disorders given that these are by far and away the most common psychiatric illnesses treated by the primary care provider.

The authors will briefly cover general treatment principles of MDD, anxiety disorders, obsessive-compulsive disorder (OCD), and post-traumatic stress disorder (PTSD) and then review recent treatment advances. Their coverage will focus on pharmacologic therapies, though they acknowledge the place for and necessity of psychotherapy in treatment of all of the discussed diagnoses. Finally, the authors will conclude with a summary digest for the front-line primary care provider, with clinical pearls to guide treatment.

MAJOR DEPRESSIVE DISORDER
General Treatment Principles—Major Depressive Disorder

Over the past 20 to 30 years, first-line treatments of major depressive disorder (MDD) have not seen major advances that have changed recommended treatment guidelines for primary care providers. Pharmacologic treatment continues to be dominated by the use of selective serotonin reuptake inhibitors (SSRIs) and selective serotonin and norepinephrine reuptake inhibitors (SNRIs) as first-line agents.[8,11] Newer antidepressants, some with novel mechanisms of action, have emerged. The authors' Novel Treatment Approaches section will cover these agents and reveal that while novel, these agents have not yet demonstrated to superior treatment efficacy when compared to existing alternatives. This does not mean that these newer agents have no utility for the primary care provider, just that they have not, as of yet, revolutionized the treatment of depression.

Psychotherapy also remains a mainstay of treatment with cognitive behavioral therapy (CBT) and its allegories continuing as the most studied and recommended forms of psychotherapy.[12] This review will only cover the use of psychotherapy as a treatment for MDD in a limited fashion, given primary care providers are rarely engaged as formal psychotherapists. However, the authors will cover the emergence of psychedelics as a pharmacologic enhancement to psychotherapy as the primary care provider is likely to receive questions about this novel treatment approach.

Novel Treatment Approaches

Newer antidepressants

Among oral antidepressants approved for use by the Food and Drug Administration (FDA), levomilnacipran, vilazodone, vortioxetine, and bupropion plus dextromethorphan represent some of the most novel advances in antidepressant treatment over the past 10 years.[1,2,6,10,11,19,23] There are no large, robust, multiagent comparator trials that allow us to compare these agents to the efficacy of older SSRI and SNRI agents. Metanalyses of smaller comparator and non-inferiority trials offer some insight, but only demonstrate non-inferiority.[8,23] Still, they offer some alternatives for consideration for the primary care provider, which the authors will explore after summarizing each agent individually (Table 1).

Levomilnacipran

Levomilnacipran, marketed as the antidepressant Fetzima in the United States, is FDA approved for the treatment of MDD. It is the most active enantiomer of racemic milnacipran, which is FDA approved for the treatment of fibromyalgia, under the brand name Savella.[6] Mechanistically, Levomilnacipran is an SNRI. It distinguishes itself from its SNRI peers by having comparatively more active inhibition of norepinephrine reuptake

Table 1
Newer antidepressants

Medication	Dose	Side Effects	Possible Advantages	Cost[a]
Levomilnacipran (Fetzima)	20 mg–120 mg once daily	Gastrointestinal (GI) side effects; sexual side effects; hypertension (HTN)	Greater potency for norepinephrine reuptake blockade than for serotonin	$540–qty 30 tabs
Vilazodone (Viibryd)	10 mg–40 mg once daily	GI side effects; headaches; sexual side effects	Newer mechanism of action and lower incidence of weight gain and sexual side effects	$95–qty 30 tabs
Vortioxetine (Trintellix)	5 mg–20 mg once daily	GI side effects; headaches; sexual side effects	Unique mechanism of action and lower incidence of weight gain and sexual side effects	$525–qty 30 tabs
Dextromethorphan/ Bupropion (Auvelity)	45 mg/105 mg tabs1 tab once to twice daily	Anxiety; GI side effects; headaches	Novel mechanism of action—reduces glutamate neurotransmission in addition to action of bupropion	$600–qty 30 tabs

[a] Cost quote per Drugs.com.

than serotonin reuptake, particular at lower doses.[6] A metanalysis of studies of levomilnacipran demonstrated similar response rates compared to other SSRIs and SNRIs, though direct comparator trials between levomilnacipran and other antidepressants are lacking.[23] Because of its mechanism of action, levomilnacipran has been theorized to be more effective in providing patients the subjective experience of feeling energized and greater relief from chronic pain. This has not yet been demonstrated in the literature.[6]

Vilazodone

Vilazodone, sold under the brand name Viibryd in the United States, is another FDA approved antidepressant. Mechanistically, vilazodone acts as a traditional SSRI and as a partial agonist at the serotonergic 5-HT1A receptor. The activity as a partial agonist renders it novel compared to traditional SSRIs.[19] A direct comparator trial with citalopram demonstrated similar efficacy between citalopram and vilazodone.[23] Networked metanalyses have demonstrated the same conclusion with other antidepressants.[8,23] Vilazodone can be considered by the primary care provider for patients who have not responded to first-line treatment with an SSRI or SNRI. Vilazodone has also demonstrated lower incidences of sexual side effects and weight gain when compared to traditional SSRIs and SNRIs.[19,20] Given these are common and treatment interfering side effects of SSRIs and SNRIs, vilazodone may have substantial value on that quality alone.

Vortioxetine

Vortioxetine is commercially marketed under the brand name Trintellix in the United States as an FDA-approved antidepressant. The mechanism of vortioxetine is novel as it functions as an SSRI with additional activity as an antagonist at the 5-HT3, 5-HT7, and 5-HT1D receptors, an agonist at the 5-HT1A receptor, and a partial agonist at the 5-HT1B receptor.[23] The impact on efficacy of these additional receptor activities is unclear.[23] Direct comparator trials with duloxetine or venlafaxine XR demonstrated similar efficacy between both agents and vortioxetine.[23] Networked metanalyses have demonstrated the same conclusion with other antidepressants.[8,23] Vortioxetine has distinguished itself in terms of side effect profile, however. In clinical trials, it has demonstrated lower incidence of sexual side effects and weight gain, when compared to traditional SSRIs.[2,20] This sets it apart from most other antidepressants and brings utility for the primary care provider.

Bupropion + Dextromethorphan

Dextromethorphan is a known inhibitor of N-methyl-D-aspartate (NMDA) receptors and has effects at the serotonin and norepinephrine transporters.[1,11] Inhibition of NMDA receptors has been shown to increase release of glutamate from interneurons in the brain, which is theorized to be dysfunctional in patients with depression. Increasing and/or modulating glutamate release is thought to be an important target of future antidepressants.[1,11] In clinical trials, combining dextromethorphan administration with the known antidepressant, bupropion, has had encouraging effects.[1] In 2022, the FDA approved the use of combination bupropion and dextromethorphan for the treatment of MDD in the United States, which is marketed under the brand name Auvelity.[11] At this point, little is known about the comparative efficacy of this combination treatment in the setting of known antidepressants.

Approaches to Treatment-Resistant Depression

Augmentation

The practice of adding an additional agent to a partially effective single antidepressant is not a new concept for most providers. It is not uncommon, however, for primary care providers to be uncomfortable with some or most psychopharmacologic practices in augmentation. Often this is due to limited concrete guidance on how or when to elect an augmentation strategy or which agents to favor over others. A further challenge is presented by the question of when to choose augmentation over switching from 1 antidepressant to any number of alternative agents. While the literature on this topic is somewhat limited, more recent evidence has been generated to help answer some of these questions.

The Veterans Affairs (VA) Augmentation and Switching Treatments for Improving Depression Outcomes (VAST-D) trial was a large, multisite, randomized, single-blind, parallel-assignment trial.[14] In this trial, Veterans Health Administration patients who were unresponsive to at least 1 course of antidepressant treatment were randomized to switch to another antidepressant (bupropion sustained release), augment their current treatment with bupropion sustained release, or augment their current treatment with aripiprazole.[14] Results of the trial demonstrated that participants receiving aripiprazole augmentation had a statistically significant, though modest increase in remission rates compared to the switch group, but not compared to the group receiving augmentation with bupropion.[14] Consideration of response rates (defined as a 50% or greater reduction in ratings on the 16-item Quick Inventory of Depressive Symptomatology-Clinician Rated (QIDS-C$_{16}$)), the augmentation with aripiprazole group was superior to either other treatment arm.[14] None of the 3 treatment groups differed from one another in terms of participant relapse rates, however.[14]

The VAST-D trial is somewhat unique in its size and existence as a direct comparator trial, but metanalyses have attempted to replicate comparisons between agents without the need for large, complex, expensive trials. Though metanalyses are imperfect in design and have limitations themselves, they can offer some insight. Nuñez and colleagues[15] completed a metanalysis comparing 69 studies investigating augmentation strategies and concluded that substantial evidence exists for the use of atypical antipsychotics, other antidepressants (bupropion, mirtazapine, nortriptyline), thyroid hormones, and lithium as augmentation agents. Their study concluded that more head-to-head trials are needed to make firm recommendations on treatment superiority between agents.[15]

Vázquez and collaborators published a metanalysis in 2021 comparing treatment efficacy and tolerability of antidepressants plus atypical antipsychotics versus antidepressants plus esketamine versus antidepressants plus lithium.[22] Their study construction and comparison demonstrated that based on number needed to treat (NNT) and number needed to harm (NNH), studies demonstrate lithium augmentation to be superior (NNT = 5 and NNH = 9) to either augmentation with antipsychotics (NNT = 11 and NNH = 5) or augmentation with esketamine (NNT = 7 and NNH = 5).[22]

The findings of Nuñez and Vázquez and their respective colleagues are somewhat opposite of recent practice patterns concerning use of thyroid hormone and lithium augmentation. Rates of lithium and thyroid augmentation have been lower than other agents.[17,22] The reasons for this change are likely multifactorial. In calculating NNH in their study, Vázquez used the most commonly described side effects, representing tolerability across a population, though this does not reflect the severity of possible side effects.[22] Lithium has a narrow therapeutic window, requires regular monitoring, and can lead to thyroid and kidney toxicity. These side effects can generate anxiety sufficient to cause providers and patients alike to avoid the agent, despite its general tolerability, efficacy, and low incidence of concerning side effects.[22] These concerns mixed with limited commercial marketing could explain the reflection of common practice habits.[22]

For thyroid hormone augmentation, strong data do exist to support this treatment recommendation with more robust results seen in the use of T3 augmentation.[17] Additionally, the tolerability of thyroid supplementation exceeds that of lithium and lacks the long-term cardiometabolic side effects of atypical antipsychotics.[17] The data on this topic are somewhat limited, however, with fewer studies and a lack of data on the long-term impacts and safety of thyroid supplementation for treatment of depression in euthyroid patients. Thyroid hormone augmentation also suffers from commercialization, which may explain partial lack of use in the marketplace.

Ketamine

The utility of ketamine in the treatment of depression has captivated the recent attention of practitioners and the general public alike. Ketamine is a known anesthetic, acting as an NMDA receptor antagonist. Through this activity, ketamine potentiates the activity of glutamate in the CNS, which is known to be dysfunctional in individuals with depression.[11] Ketamine has also been shown to increase the activity of brain-derived neurotrophic factor (BDNF), thought to be a cause of neuroplastic dysfunction in individuals with depression.[11] Ketamine has seen substantial effect in not only the treatment of individuals with depression, but those with treatment-resistant depression.[9,11] The agent can be administered intravenously or intranasally and has been FDA approved for the treatment of depression through either route.[9] While initially only demonstrated to be effective for short-term treatment of depression, additional studies have demonstrated maintenance, or prolonged treatment with ketamine to be an effective strategy in preventing relapse for those individuals also taking a conventional, oral antidepressant.[9]

One of the most attractive aspects of ketamine has been its rapid onset of efficacy. Patients often see improvement within days, which is rarely seen with pharmacologic action of antidepressants.[9,11] Because ketamine must be administered intravenously or intranasally, penetration into the treatment population is somewhat limited. For this reason, practitioners and the medical literature often retain this agent for treatment of those with treatment-resistant depression (TRD).

Both electroconvulsive therapy (ECT) and repetitive transcranial magnetic stimulation (rTMS) are well established treatments for TRD with significant results. Both are known to have significant disadvantages, however. ECT requires general anesthesia and demonstrates cognitive side effects while rTMS requires frequent visits to a clinical setting over several weeks.[3,13] Ketamine presents itself as an attractive alternative, given it can be administered relatively rapidly and requires fewer clinical visits than either ECT or rTMS.[3,13] A number of studies have compared ketamine administration with alternative agents in the treatment of TRD.[3,13] Comparator studies have either demonstrated superiority of ECT over ketamine or non-inferiority of ketamine when compared to ECT.[3,13] In these trials, ketamine demonstrated fewer cognitive side effects when compared with ECT, but greater incidence of dissociation during treatment episodes.[3,13]

ANXIETY DISORDERS, OBSESSIVE-COMPULSIVE DISORDER, AND POST-TRAUMATIC STRESS DISORDER
General Treatment Principles

Pharmacotherapy for anxiety disorders, OCD, and PTSD can be divided into 2 groups of medication with different purposes. The first group consists of agents that function largely to prevent future anxiety, while the second group treat acute anxiety, but do little to decrease future occurrences.

First-line pharmacologic treatment for anxiety disorders, for the purpose of preventing future symptoms, consists of single agent treatment with an SSRI or SNRI.[4,5,21] These agents have been shown to be effective in reduction of symptoms of anxiety in multiple placebo-controlled trials, but no single agent has been shown to be consistently more effective than the others.[4,21] The choice of SSRIs and SNRIs over tricyclic antidepressant (TCA) as first-line therapy is due largely to their lack of anticholinergic side effects and toxicity in overdose.[4] Increased tolerability does not translate to increased efficacy, however, and some experienced primary care providers might find themselves more comfortable with use of TCAs. Unfortunately, these agents can take 4 to 8 weeks to begin to show efficacy and treatment of anxiety disorders typically requires higher doses and longer duration of treatment of these medications than would be needed for treatment of unipolar depression.[20]

Short-acting, anxiolytic medications make up the second set of pharmacologic agents that function to treat acute anxiety, but do little to prevent future occurrence of symptoms. Benzodiazepines have long been used as acute anxiolytic treatment. There are a number of medications in this class allowing for a wide range of choices in terms of onset of action, half-life, and the presence of active metabolites.[4,21] While very effective, care should be taken with these agents as physiologic dependence develops in all users and misuse can be problematic. Additionally, withdrawal from the medications is prolonged and can be dangerous if completed too abruptly. More commonly, and less dangerous, is the rebound anxiety that can accompany reduction in dosing and cessation of use of benzodiazepines. The co-occurrence of a substance use disorder is common with anxiety disorders and should be considered a contraindication to using a benzodiazepine for treatment.[4,21] If anxiolytic agents, that do not have abuse potential, are desired for treatment, the anticholinergic agent hydroxyzine, anticonvulsants gabapentin and pregabalin, and beta blocker propranolol present effective alternatives. Data for these agents are not nearly as robust as for other anxiolytics and they do not have FDA indications for treatment of anxiety disorders, but their common use in practice is significant.[4,5]

Novel Developments in the Pharmacologic Treatment of Anxiety Disorders, Obsessive-Compulsive Disorder, and Post-Traumatic Stress Disorder

There have not been major advances made in the pharmacotherapy of the treatment of anxiety disorders in the past 10 years. The novel antidepressants that were reviewed earlier (vilazodone, vortioxetine, levomilnacipran, and bupropion plus dextromethorphan) do not carry FDA indications for the treatment of anxiety disorders and studies of their efficacy in anxiety disorders have been very limited with mixed or negative results.[4]

Psychotherapy

A number of different modalities of psychotherapy have been shown to be effective in the treatment of anxiety disorders. The modality that has seen the most robust investigation is CBT.[4,5,21] CBT seeks to identify the maladaptive automatic thoughts and behaviors that are present in mental disorders and then to restructure those thoughts and behaviors through the use of therapeutic exercises. In some anxiety disorders, CBT is considered first-line therapy (eg specific phobias, PTSD), but generally, pharmacotherapy and psychotherapy are considered complementary partners in treatment.[4,5,21] Major drawbacks to therapy consist of difficulties with patient engagement (a significant barrier with anxiety disorders) and availability of well-trained therapists. The latter barrier has decreased in recent years, however, as the advent of manualized therapy and computer and smartphone application-based therapy allows for treatment to be delivered without expert therapists or without a therapist at all.[4,5,21] There are limited data on the comparative efficacy of different application-based therapies.

Psychedelics and Psychedelic-Assisted Psychotherapy

One of the most headline-grabbing areas of research in the treatment of depression and anxiety disorders over the past decade has been the use of psychedelics and psychedelic-assisted psychotherapy. These practices are not novel and have existed since the properties of the compounds have been known, but they have received substantial popularization over the past several years.[16] Additionally, the use of these agents has expanded substantially in boutique medical settings, making them much more widely available than previously. For this reason, the authors feel the primary care provider should have general awareness of what may be available to and experienced by their patients, even if the primary care provider is unlikely to partake in the therapy themselves.

Psilocybin

Psilocybin is a plant alkaloid found in a variety of mushroom species. It has been used for spiritual purposes by the people of Central and South America for centuries. Psilocybin is actively metabolized into a serotonin transport inhibitor and serotonin 5-HT_{2A} receptor partial agonist. There has been a resurgence of research on the utility of psilocybin in the treatment of refractory mood and anxiety disorders.[16] In these trials, participants receive doses of psilocybin during sessions with therapists providing nondirective, supportive therapy the experience. Small, open-label trials have been encouraging, though larger trials are needed to better evaluate the efficacy.[16] Psilocybin dosing sessions have also seen promise in small trials of patients with substance use disorder and further trials are ongoing.[16]

Lysergic Acid Diethylamide

LSD is a well-known hallucinogen with effects of partial agonism at the serotonin 5-HT_{2A} receptor, and binding at the 5-HT_{1A}, 5-HT_{2C}, 5-HT_{2B} receptors and binding at the dopamine D2 receptor as well as glutamine release. Recent studies have investigated the potential of LSD dosing sessions for the treatment of substance use disorders as well as mood and anxiety disorders seen in end-of-life care.[16] Results for the treatment of anxiety disorders have not been robust, but treatment of mood symptoms is encouraging.[16] Still, studies are small and larger studies would be needed to demonstrate benefit on a population basis. Microdosing of LSD has also gained recent interest, but there is no clinical evidence to suggest the benefit of this procedure.[16]

3,4-Methylenedioxymethamphetamine

Methylenedioxymethamphetamine (MDMA), commonly referred to as the street drug "ecstasy," causes monoamine release, serotonin and norepinephrine transporter reuptake inhibition, monoamine oxidase inhibition, and partial agonism at multiple serotonin receptors.[16] It creates a euphoric state where the user experiences increase perception of empathy, positive mood, extraversion, trust, and compassion for oneself and others. Additionally, users have demonstrated increased access to emotionally intense material. For these reasons, MDMA has seen multiple studies investigating it as an aid to psychotherapy session. Use of MDMA prior to a session would allow the participant to engage with challenging material during therapy that had previously been too challenging to explore.[16] Small trials of MDMA-assisted psychotherapy have been encouraging, particularly in cases of treatment-resistant PTSD. However, the trials have been too small and lack adequate comparison to draw generalized conclusions, other than that further study is needed.[16]

SUMMARY

Primary care providers are the front line in the detection and treatment of MDD and various anxiety disorders. Given the profound impacts on overall health, effective management of these disorders is paramount. For more than 20 years, the mainstay of treatment for these disorders has been SSRIs and SNIRs. There are newer medications, many with novel mechanisms of action, that have come to market; however, first-line treatments remain the same. Side effect profiles render some of these newer agents appealing and should be considered for select patients. As more data become available, some of these newer agents may become first line, but at this point, there are not advantages sufficient to overcome the greater monetary cost to patients or health systems. There are now more robust data on the use of various augmentation agents in the treatment of MDD. As providers become more familiar with these agents, it is the authors' hope there will be increased comfort it their utilization by primary care providers.

Unlike MDD, there have been no new pharmacologic agents targeting anxiety in the past 10 years. When treating anxiety disorders, it is often necessary to use both agents to prevent future anxiety and agents to treat acute anxiety. In addition to pharmacologic treatment, psychotherapy remains a mainstay of treatment for both depression and anxiety. More recently there has been a marked increase in interest in psychotherapy assisted by psychedelic agents. Currently, however, there is a lack of adequate data to recommend any of these approaches for wide application.

CLINICS CARE POINTS

- First-line pharmacologic agents for the treatment of both MDD and anxiety disorders remain SSRIs and SNRIs.

- There are newer novel agents that have less weight gain and/or sexual dysfunction, but are not superior in terms of efficacy.

- Augmentation is recommended for patients whose depressive symptoms are not adequately treated with an antidepressant alone.

- Augmenting agents should be selected based on patient factors and provider comfort in prescribing.

- Ketamine use should be reserved for patients with treatment-resistant depression, but does not show greater efficacy than known treatments of ETC or rTMS.

- When treating anxiety disorders, utilize both medications to prevent future anxiety and agents to treat acute anxiety.

- Psychotherapy, particularly CBT which has the most data supporting efficacy, remains a cornerstone of treatment.

DISCLOSURE

Neither Dr J. Markman nor Dr H. Combs have any financial conflicts of interest or funding sources to declare.

REFERENCES

1. Akbar D, Rhee TG, Ceban F, et al. Dextromethorphan-Bupropion for the Treatment of Depression: A Systematic Review of Efficacy and Safety in Clinical Trials. CNS Drugs 2023;37(10):867–81.
2. Alvarez E, Perez V, Artigas F. Pharmacology and clinical potential of vortioxetine in the treatment of major depressive disorder. Neuropsychiatr Dis Treat 2014;10: 1297–307.
3. Anand A, Mathew SJ, Sanacora G, et al. Ketamine versus ECT for Nonpsychotic Treatment-Resistant Major Depression. N Engl J Med 2023;388(25):2315–25.
4. Bandelow B, Allgulander C, Baldwin DS, et al. World Federation of Societies of Biological Psychiatry (WFSBP) guidelines for treatment of anxiety, obsessive-compulsive and posttraumatic stress disorders - Version 3. Part I: Anxiety disorders. World J Biol Psychiatr 2023;24(2):79–117.
5. Bandelow B, Allgulander C, Baldwin DS, et al. World Federation of Societies of Biological Psychiatry (WFSBP) guidelines for treatment of anxiety, obsessive-compulsive and posttraumatic stress disorders - Version 3. Part II: OCD and PTSD. World J Biol Psychiatr 2023;24(2):118–34.
6. Bruno A, Morabito P, Spina E, et al. The Role of Levomilnacipran in the Management of Major Depressive Disorder: A Comprehensive Review. Curr Neuropharmacol 2016;14(2):191–9.
7. Caldiroli A, Capuzzi E, Tagliabue I, et al. Augmentative Pharmacological Strategies in Treatment-Resistant Major Depression: A Comprehensive Review. Int J Mol Sci 2021;22(23):13070. https://doi.org/10.3390/ijms222313070.
8. Cipriani A, Furukawa TA, Salanti G, et al. Comparative efficacy and acceptability of 21 antidepressant drugs for the acute treatment of adults with major depressive disorder: a systematic review and network meta-analysis. Lancet 2018; 391(10128):1357–66.
9. Daly EJ, Trivedi MH, Janik A, et al. Efficacy of Esketamine Nasal Spray Plus Oral Antidepressant Treatment for Relapse Prevention in Patients With Treatment-Resistant Depression: A Randomized Clinical Trial. JAMA Psychiatr 2019;76(9): 893–903.
10. Gautam M, Kaur M, Jagtap P, et al. Levomilnacipran: More of the Same? Prim Care Companion CNS Disord 2019;21(5):19nr02475.
11. Marwaha S, Palmer E, Suppes T, et al. Novel and emerging treatments for major depression. Lancet 2023;401(10371):141–53.
12. McIntyre RS, Alsuwaidan M, Baune BT, et al. Treatment-resistant depression: definition, prevalence, detection, management, and investigational interventions. World Psychiatr 2023;22(3):394–412.
13. Menon V, Varadharajan N, Faheem A, et al. Ketamine vs Electroconvulsive Therapy for Major Depressive Episode: A Systematic Review and Meta-analysis [published correction appears in JAMA Psychiatry. 2023 Jun 1;80(6):651]. JAMA Psychiatr 2023;80(6):639–42.
14. Mohamed S, Johnson GR, Chen P, et al. Effect of Antidepressant Switching vs Augmentation on Remission Among Patients With Major Depressive Disorder Unresponsive to Antidepressant Treatment: The VAST-D Randomized Clinical Trial. JAMA 2017;318(2):132–45.
15. Nuñez NA, Joseph B, Pahwa M, et al. Augmentation strategies for treatment resistant major depression: A systematic review and network meta-analysis. J Affect Disord 2022;302:385–400.

16. Reiff CM, Richman EE, Nemeroff CB, et al. Psychedelics and Psychedelic-Assisted Psychotherapy. Am J Psychiatr 2020;177(5):391–410.

17. Rosenthal LJ, Goldner WS, O'Reardon JP. T3 augmentation in major depressive disorder: safety considerations. Am J Psychiatr 2011;168(10):1035–40.

18. Rossano F, Caiazza C, Zotti N, et al. The efficacy, safety, and adverse events of azapirones in anxiety disorders: A systematic review and meta-analysis of randomized controlled trials. Eur Neuropsychopharmacol 2023;76:23–51.

19. Schwartz TL, Siddiqui UA, Stahl SM. Vilazodone: a brief pharmacological and clinical review of the novel serotonin partial agonist and reuptake inhibitor. Ther Adv Psychopharmacol 2011;1(3):81–7.

20. Stahl SM. Prescriber's guide: seventh edition. New York, NY: Cambridge University Press; 2021.

21. Szuhany KL, Simon NM. Anxiety Disorders: A Review. JAMA 2022;328(24):2431–45.

22. Vázquez GH, Bahji A, Undurraga J, et al. Efficacy and Tolerability of Combination Treatments for Major Depression: Antidepressants plus Second-Generation Antipsychotics vs. Esketamine vs. Lithium. J Psychopharmacol 2021;35(8):890–900.

23. Wagner G, Schultes MT, Titscher V, et al. Efficacy and safety of levomilnacipran, vilazodone and vortioxetine compared with other second-generation antidepressants for major depressive disorder in adults: A systematic review and network meta-analysis. J Affect Disord 2018;228:1–12.

Newer Outpatient Diabetes Therapies and Technologies

Nevin Kamal, MD, Kristen Lee, MD, Grazia Aleppo, MD*

KEYWORDS

- GLP-1 receptor agonists • SGLT2 inhibitors • Continuous glucose monitoring
- Connected insulin pens • Automated insulin delivery systems

KEY POINTS

- Glucagon-like peptide-1 receptor agonists (GLP-1 RA) and dual glucose-dependent insulinotropic peptide/GLP-1 RA offer HbA1c reductions, weight loss, and cardiovascular benefits without increasing the risk of hypoglycemia.
- Sodium-glucose cotransporter 2 inhibitors also offer HbA1c reduction, with the advantage of both cardiovascular, renal, and HF benefits also without increasing the risk of hypoglycemia.
- Continuous glucose monitoring (CGM) is a standard of care for all type 1 diabetes individuals, as well as type 2 diabetes persons on any type of insulin regimen.
- Connected insulin pens have emerged as useful tools for insulin dose reminders, memory, and integration with CGM.
- Many automated insulin delivery systems have become available and offer many options to people with type 1 diabetes, reducing HbA1c and improving time in range and quality of life.

INTRODUCTION

Diabetes mellitus is reaching epidemic proportions worldwide, presenting a formidable global health challenge.[1] The journey toward more effective outpatient therapies for type 2 diabetes mellitus (T2DM) and obesity has witnessed remarkable strides in recent years. Central to these advances is the development of new classes such as glucagon-like peptide 1 (GLP-1) receptor agonists (RAs), dual incretin agonists, and sodium-glucose cotransporter 2 (SGLT2) inhibitors in the therapies space, whereas the use of continuous glucose monitoring (CGM) systems, the development of automated insulin delivery (AID) systems as well as connected pens have expanded the field of diabetes technology, transforming the management of both

Division of Endocrinology, Metabolism and Molecular Medicine, Feinberg School of Medicine, Northwestern University, 645 North Michigan Avenue, Suite 530, Chicago, IL, USA
* Corresponding author. Division of Endocrinology, Metabolism and Molecular Medicine, Feinberg School of Medicine, Northwestern University, 645 North Michigan Avenue, Suite 530, Chicago, IL 60611.
E-mail address: aleppo@northwestern.edu

Med Clin N Am 108 (2024) 923–951
https://doi.org/10.1016/j.mcna.2024.03.002
0025-7125/24/© 2024 Elsevier Inc. All rights reserved.
medical.theclinics.com

type 1 diabetes mellitus (T1DM) and T2DM. We embark on an in-depth exploration of these innovative treatments and technologies, providing health care professionals the guidance needed about the most suitable treatment and technology options for their patients.

NEWER OUTPATIENT DIABETES THERAPIES

Traditional therapies, oral medications and insulin, have long served as cornerstones in T2DM management. However, they lack macrovascular benefits and are associated with hypoglycemia, weight gain, and increased heart failure (HF) exacerbations to name a few. The introduction of these newer therapies represents a significant shift toward more targeted, effective, and patient-centric care.

Glucagon-Like Peptide-1 Receptor Agonists

GLP-1 is a hormone produced by the gut in response to meals whose effects increase insulin secretion, decrease glucagon release, and inhibit gastric emptying, leading to lower blood glucose levels, reduction in appetite, and promotion of weight loss.[2] Several GLP-1 RAs have been developed to mimic these effects and are described in **Table 1**. These drugs have demonstrated their glycemic effectiveness in people with T2DM, being highly effective in reducing hemoglobin A1c (HbA1c) levels. In comparative studies, GLP-1 RAs consistently outperformed placebo and other diabetes medications, with HbA1c reductions ranging from 0.55% to 1.38%.[3] Head-to-head trials showed that weekly semaglutide 1 mg was superior to weekly exenatide (−1.5% vs −0.9%, $P < .001$),[4] weekly dulaglutide 1.5 mg (−1.8% vs −1.4%, $P < .001$),[5] and daily liraglutide (1.7% vs 1.0%, $P < .001$)[6] for HbA1c reduction. Numerous trials have established the cardio-renal benefits of several GLP-1 RAs. A meta-analysis of 7 high-quality randomized double-blind placebo-controlled trials (RCTs) with over 56,000 T2DM individuals over a median follow-up of 3 years showed reductions in both major adverse cardiovascular (CV) events (MACEs) and all-cause mortality by 12%, and a broad kidney composite outcome by 17% (mainly driven by reducing albuminuria).[7] Data on prevention of HF hospitalizations are conflicting. Nevertheless, a statistically significant reduction of HF hospitalizations by 9% was seen in meta-analyses.[7] Furthermore, GLP-1 RAs have garnered substantial attention for their weight loss benefits. All GLP-1 RA studies lead to sustained weight loss in a dose-dependent manner even in individuals without diabetes.[8] A review of head-to-head RCTs comparing the various GLP-1 RAs in T2DM for weight loss arranged them in the following order of efficacy: semaglutide > liraglutide > dulaglutide > exenatide XR = exenatide (twice daily) = lixisenatide.[9]

GLP-1 RAs have also been found to have benefits in obesity-related diseases. Insulin resistance is highly prevalent in women with polycystic ovary syndrome (PCOS), with its downstream effects leading to hormonal abnormalities that cascade into weight gain, subfertility, and hyperandrogenism.[10] GLP-1 RAs have demonstrated numerous effects on insulin resistance and its sequelae, increasing glucose transporter expression, reducing oxidative stress and inflammation, and modulating lipid metabolism.[10] In an open-label randomized trial, obese women with PCOS undergoing in vitro fertilization had significantly higher pregnancy rates per embryo transfer if they were on liraglutide in addition to metformin (85.7% vs 28.6%, $P = .03$).[11] Lastly, GLP-1 RAs' benefits have been seen in metabolic dysfunction-associated steatotic liver disease (MASLD) and metabolic dysfunction-associated steatohepatitis, diseases commonly seen in patients with T2DM, and leading causes of cirrhosis in the developed world. One RCT showed that liraglutide led to more frequent resolution

Table 1

Summary of US Food and Drug Administration–approved glucagon-like peptide-1 receptor agonists and glucagon-like peptide-1/glucose-dependent insulinotropic peptide receptor agonists

Brand Name	Molecule	Indication	Route	Frequency	Doses	Dosing titration as Needed to Achieve Goals
Byetta	Exenatide	T2DM	SC	Twice daily	5–10 mcg	5mcg within 1 hr of eating bid, increase to 10mcg after 1 mo
Bydureon	Exenatide (XR/long acting)	T2DM	SC	Weekly	2 mg	2 mg weekly
Adlyxine	Lixisenatide	T2DM	SC	Daily	10–20 mcg	10mcg daily ×14 d, increase to 20mcg daily
Victoza	Liraglutide	T2DM	SC	Daily	0.6–1.2–1.8 mg	0.6 mg daily for >1 wk, increase to 1.2 mg daily for >1 week, then 1.8 mg daily
Saxenda	Liraglutide	Obesity	SC	Daily	0.6–1.2–1.8–2.4-3 mg	0.6 mg daily for 1 wk. Increase up to 3 mg in 0.6 weekly increments
Trulicity	Dulaglutide	T2DM	SC	Weekly	0.75–1.5–3–4.5 mg	0.75 mg weekly, increase dose stepwise in monthly increments
Ozempic	Semaglutide	T2DM	SC	Weekly	0.25–0.5–1–1.7–2.0 mg	Start at 0.25 mg for 4 weeks, increase stepwise up to 2 mg weekly in monthly intervals
Wegovy	Semaglutide	Obesity	SC	Weekly	0.25–0.5–1–1.7–2.4 mg	Start at 0.25 mg for 4 weeks, increase stepwise up to 2.4 mg in monthly intervals.
Rybelsus	Semaglutide	T2DM	PO	Daily	3–7–14 mg	3 mg daily x1 month, increase to 7 mg then 14 mg in monthly intervals
Mounjaro	Tirzepatide (GLP-GIP)	T2DM	SC	Weekly	2.5–5–7.5–10–12.5–15 mg	2.5 mg weekly x4 weeks, increase monthly by 2.5 mg up to 15 mg
Zepbound	Tirzepatide (GLP-GIP)	Obesity	SC	Weekly	2.5–5–7.5–10–12.5–15 mg	2.5 mg weekly x4 weeks, increase monthly by 2.5 mg up to 15 mg

Abbreviations: PO, by mouth; SC, subcutaneous; T2DM, type 1 diabetes mellitus.

of MASLD and reversal of fibrosis on biopsy compared to placebo (39% vs 9%, $P = .017$).[12] Two meta-analyses in T2DM individuals found that GLP-1 RA therapy improved measures of hepatic fat content, body composition, liver biochemistry, inflammatory markers, and lipid parameters compared with insulin therapy and/or other oral antidiabetic agents.[13,14]

Side effects of this drug class include predominantly gastrointestinal symptoms, with incidences ranging from 10% to 50%, often leading to treatment discontinuation.[15] Major side effects[15–17] are summarized in **Table 2**.

Glucagon-Like Peptide-1-Glucose-dependent Insulinotropic Peptide (Dual Incretin) Receptor Agonists

Tirzepatide is a novel dual GIP (glucose-dependent insulinotropic peptide)/GLP-1 RA approved for the management of T2DM and weight loss. In addition to the aforementioned GLP-1 RA effects, GIP activation has an additive benefit on post-prandial insulin secretion and slower gastric emptying. GIP receptors are also expressed in regions of the brain regulating food intake.[18]

The effectiveness of tirzepatide was evaluated in multiple studies, including the SURPASS trials. A recent systematic review and meta-analysis of all the main tirzepatide studies with 6609 participants showed that tirzepatide was superior to semaglutide, liraglutide, and long-acting insulins (glargine and degludec) in lowering HbA1c. Mean differences ranged from −1.62% to −2.06% versus placebo, −0.29% to −0.92% versus other GLP-1 RAs, and −0.7% to −1.09% versus basal insulin.[19] In addition to showing glycemic benefits, the SURPASS trials also showed that all tirzepatide doses were superior to all comparators in body weight reduction; reductions compared to GLP-1 RAs ranged from −1.68 kg with 5 mg dose to −7.16 kg with 15 mg dose. Both tirzepatide and semaglutide led to similar reductions in appetite, although the former caused greater weight loss.[19] The Surmount-1 (Tirzepatide Once Weekly for the Treatment of Obesity) RCT enrolled 2539 non-diabetic individuals with obesity, treated with tirzepatide 5, 10, and 15 mg weekly versus placebo for 72 weeks, and showed a dose-dependent weight loss up to 20.9% from baseline with tirzepatide 15 mg ($P < .0001$), rivaling the efficacy of bariatric surgery.[20] Similarly, the Surmount-2 (Tirzepatide once weekly for the treatment of obesity in people with type 2 diabetes) RCT with 938 participants with obesity and T2DM showed a dose-dependent weight loss of up to 14.7% ($P < .0001$) over 72 weeks treatment with terzipatide.[21]

Tirzepatide has been shown to have several CV benefits, although these were secondary outcomes in all the SURPASS trials and they are described in **Table 3**. Note that CV benefits were secondary outcomes in all the trials. Furthermore, tirzepatide has been shown to reduce intrahepatic triglycerides in T2DM; consequently, it may offer novel treatment options for patients with MASLD. A sub-study of the SURPASS-3 (Effect of tirzepatide versus insulin degludec on liver fat content and abdominal adipose tissue in people with type 2 diabetes, SURPASS-3 MRI) trial using MRI demonstrated that tirzepatide was able to significantly reduce liver fat content, volume of visceral adipose tissue, and abdominal subcutaneous adipose tissue.[22] Like GLP-1 RAs, tirzepatide' s most common adverse effect is gastrointestinal symptoms. The incidence of these side effects was similar between tirzepatide 15 mg and semaglutide 1 mg in SURPASS-2 (Tirzepatide versus Semaglutide Once Weekly in Patients with Type 2 Diabetes) (nausea: 22.1% vs 17.4%, diarrhea: 16.4% vs 11.5%, decreased appetite: 8.9% vs 5.3%), and most cases were during the dose-escalation period. Rare cases of diabetic retinopathy, gallbladder disease, and pancreatitis were noted with tirzepatide (<1%).[23]

Table 2
Glucagon-like peptide-1 receptor agonists' side effects

Side Effect	Description	Frequency	Evidence	Agent(s) with Highest Incidence	Conclusion
GI symptoms	• Predominant side effect • Nausea, vomiting, diarrhea, constipation	Common	Incidence: 10%–50%	All agents	Effects are reduced with longer acting agents, slow dose titration, and with time
Injection sites	• Cellulitis • Abscesses • Necrosis	Rare	More frequently with exenatide (15%–22%) vs liraglutide (2%–8%), semaglutide (0%–2%)	Exenatide Liraglutide Semaglutide	Monitor injection sites regularly
Hypoglycemia	Occurring in 1%–2% in trials that reported it	Rare	Minor hypoglycemic events ranged from 0%–15.9%, with most trials reporting <10% Rates higher when concomitant SU use (11%–20%)	Exenatide Liraglutide	Caution with concomitant SU or insulin, both may need dose reductions upon GLP-1 initiation & dose escalation
GB and biliary disease	• More frequent with weight loss indications, higher doses, and longer duration of use • Post-marketing surveillance reports further support an elevated risk of acute cholecystitis	Rare	Metanalysis of 76 trials showed increased risk of GB and biliary disease	Liraglutide Dulaglutide Semaglutide (≥1.0 mg)	Monitor for signs & symptoms of GB disease
Angioedema and anaphylaxis	Very rare	Very rare	Evidence limited to case reports	Exenatide	A history of anaphylactic reaction to an agent should preclude use of all agents in the class.

(continued on next page)

Table 2
(continued)

Side Effect	Description	Frequency	Evidence	Agent(s) with Highest Incidence	Conclusion
Pancreatitis	Unclear link & insufficient evidence to confirm increased risk	Rare	First noticed in a retrospective study of the FDA adverse event reporting system; OR 10.68 (95% CI: 7.75–15.1, $P < 10^{-16}$) Metanalysis of prospective RCTs on various GLP-1 RAs did not find any increased risk of acute pancreatitis or pancreatic cancer	Exenatide	Given the concern, FDA will continue to monitor. Should avoid GLP-1 RA in patients with history of pancreatitis. Discontinue if patients develop pancreatitis while on therapy.
Medullary thyroid cancer (MTC)	• Insufficient evidence and based on rodent studies only; • Liraglutide, dulaglutide, and exenatide were associated with benign and malignant C cell tumors in rodents. The study also found calcitonin release stimulation mediated through the GLP-1 receptor. But GLP-1 receptor expression in human C cells is very low, and humans have far fewer C cells than rats.	Rare	One short-term human study showed calcitonin levels within normal limits in all patients on exenatide. One case-control study found a slightly increased risk of thyroid cancer in patients on exenatide, liraglutide or dulaglutide, but many key covariates were not controlled, and results possibly influenced by detection bias	Exenatide Dulaglutide Liraglutide	Until further data is available, use is not recommended for individuals with a history of MTC, MEN 2A, or MEN 2B

Aspiration events with general anesthesia (GA)	• Due to slowed gastric motility	Rare	Semaglutide	Case reports linking GLP-1 RAs with regurgitation and aspiration after GA despite adequate fasting	Based on such reports and other observations of increased residuals on ultrasound, some anesthesiologists recommend holding semaglutide for 3 weeks prior to surgery, or undergo rapid sequence intubation to minimize aspiration risk
Thrombocytopenia	• Significant hemorrhage may result	Rare	Exenatide	A case report links exenatide with drug-induced thrombocytopenia due to immunoglobulins directed against platelets, active only when exenatide is present	
Diabetic retinopathy (DR)	• Worsening of diabetic retinopathy	Rare	Semaglutide	In a large, randomized trial comparing semaglutide with placebo, higher rate of DR was noted (HR 1.76, $P < .05$) especially in those with pre-existing DR. In a separate analysis of the trial data, this phenomenon was attributed to the magnitude and rapidity of reduction in hemoglobin A1C during the first 4 months of the trial.	Further studies are needed to further delineate the long-term effects on DR

Abbreviations: FDA, Food and Drug Administration; CI, confidence interval; GB, gall bladder; GI, gastrointestinal; GLP-1, glucagon-like peptide-1; HR, hazard ratio; MEN, multiple endocrine neoplasia; OR, odds ratio; RA, receptor agonists; RCT, randomized controlled trial; SU, sulfonylurea.

Table 3
Effects of tirzepatide on various cardiovascular outcomes[19]

Parameter	Comparator	Effect Size	Notes
BP (ΔSBP/ΔDBP, in mm Hg)	Placebo	−4.7 to −5.2/no difference vs −2.00 mm Hg	SURPASS-1, drug-naïve population
	Semaglutide 1 mg	−4.8/−1.9 (5 mg), −5.3/-2.5 (10 mg), −6.5/-2.9 (15 mg) vs −3.6/-1.0[52]	SURPASS-2, on metformin
	Degludec	−4.9 to −6.6/−1.9 to −2.5 vs no change	SURPASS-3, on metformin ± SGLT2-i
	Glargine	−2.8 to −4.8/−0.80 to −1.0 vs +1.3/+0.7	SURPASS-4, on glargine
	Placebo	−6.1 to −12.6/−2.0 to −4.5 vs −1.7/-2.1	SURPASS-5, all patients on glargine
	Placebo	−7.2/-4.8 vs −1.0/-0.8[54]	SURMOUNT-1
LDL	Semaglutide 1 mg	Decrease by 19.0%, 24.1%, and 24.8% (5, 10, and 15 mg respectively) vs 11.5% with semaglutide 1 mg	SURPASS-2
	Degludec	Decrease by 6.01% (5 mg), 5.70% (10 mg), 6.55% (15 mg) vs 2.71% (P = NS)	SURPASS-3, all patients on metformin ± SGLT2-i
	Glargine	Percent change vs glargine: −8.0% (5 mg), −9.5% (10 mg), −9.2% (15 mg), all P < .0001	SURPASS-4, all T2DM patients inadequately controlled on oral agents
Waist circumference	Semaglutide 1 mg	Decrease by 6.9 cm, 9.6 cm, and 9.9 cm (for 5, 10, and 15 mg respectively) vs 5.6 cm with semaglutide 1 mg	SURPASS-2
	Degludec	Change by −7.1 cm (5 mg), −9.3 cm (10 mg), −10.9 cm (15 mg) vs +1.4 cm (degludec)	SURPASS-3
	Glargine	Change by −8.3 cm (5 mg), −10.5 cm (10 mg), −9.2 cm (15 mg) vs +2.0 cm (glargine), all P > .05 with glargine	SURPASS-4
MACEs	Meta-analysis	RR 0.52 (95% CI: 0.38–0.72, I^2 = 0)	Includes all data from SURPASS and SURMOUNT-1 trials
Cardiovascular death	Meta-analysis	RR 0.51 (95% CI: 0.29–0.89, I^2 = 0)	As earlier
All-cause death	Meta-analysis	RR 0.51 (95% CI: 0.34–0.77, I^2 = 0)	As earlier

Abbreviations: BP, blood pressure; CI, confidence interval; DBP, diastolic blood pressure; LDL, low-density lipoprotein; MACE, major adverse cardiovascular event; RR, relative risk; SBP, systolic blood pressure.

Sodium-Glucose Cotransporter 2 Inhibitors

In the realm of diabetes management, SGLT2 inhibitors have emerged as a transformative class of medications, providing not only improved glycemic outcomes, but also remarkable benefits extending beyond diabetes. SGLT2 inhibitors operate by blocking the SGLT2 cotransporters in the proximal renal tubules, thereby inhibiting renal glucose re-absorption and leading to glucosuria. **Table 4** outlines the available SGLT2 inhibitors and their benefits. In clinical trials, SGLT2 inhibitors have consistently demonstrated their ability to reduce HbA1C levels by 0.6% to 0.9% compared to placebo. The extent of this reduction varies depending on the specific agent and its dose, with the most substantial decrease observed with canagliflozin.[24]

SLGT2 inhibitors have demonstrated a remarkable ability to reduce MACEs in high-risk population with CV disease (CVD) (hazard ratio [HR] 0.89, 95% confidence interval [CI] 0.83–0.96). However, the impact of these medications was further dissected when looking at stratified cohorts. The benefit of reduced MACEs was particularly pronounced in patients with a history of atherosclerotic CVD (ASCVD) events (HR 0.86, 95% CI: 0.80–0.93).[25] Furthermore, the same data have revealed a consistent reduction in HF hospitalizations in high-risk CVD population regardless of prior history of HF.[25] The difference in glycemia between treatment groups in the studies was minimal, suggesting that non-glycemic drug effects were responsible for the CV outcomes. The dual benefits of reducing MACEs and HF hospitalizations underscore the valuable role that SGLT2 inhibitors can play in the management of CVD.

SGLT2 inhibitors have gathered significant attention for their renoprotective properties, even in the absence of diabetes. The mechanism behind the reduction in incidence or worsening nephropathy is likely multifactorial but is thought to be related to a direct renovascular effect irrespective of glycemia. A comprehensive analysis of clinical trials has revealed their ability to reduce composite outcome of worsening renal function, end-stage renal disease, or death from renal causes by a striking 45% ($P < .0001$). Remarkably, this benefit extends to both patients with established ASCVD and those with risk factors but no history of ASCVD event.[25,26] Side effects, including genitourinary (GU) infections, necrotizing fasciitis, volume depletion, amputations, and skeletal fragility,[27–32] are outlined in **Table 5**.

With the rising use of SGLT2 inhibitors, there has been an increased recognition of euglycemic diabetic ketoacidosis (EuDKA) as more cases are reported.[33,34] A comprehensive meta-analysis of 39 RCTs involving more than 60,000 patients with T2DM found that DKA occurred in 0.18% of individuals on SGLT2 inhibitor versus 0.09% of control groups; odds ratio (OR) 2.13 (95% CI 1.38–3.27).[35] A diagnosis of DKA requires a triad of hyperglycemia greater than 250 mg/dL, ketonemia, and metabolic acidosis with elevated anion gap. EuDKA resembles DKA but lacks the classic hyperglycemia component. In EuDKA, blood glucose is generally less than 200 mg/dL, sometimes defined as up to 300 mg/dL.[33] Pathophysiology remains unclear. Theories propose a multifactorial process driven by SLGT2 inhibitors' ability to induce glycosuria, leading to lower blood glucose levels. Relative insulin deficiency leads to increased ketone production despite near-normal blood glucose levels, by allowing for the release of fatty acids from adipose tissue and their conversion to ketones in the liver. Dehydration and volume depletion, along with increased ketone production, contribute to the development of metabolic acidosis and the characteristic symptoms of ketoacidosis. DKA and EuDKA share a similar clinical presentation: nausea, vomiting, fatigue, anorexia, shortness of breath, tachycardia, and abdominal pain.[36,37] However, EuDKA symptoms can develop more gradually than DKA,[37] and

Table 4
US–Food and Drug Administration–approved sodium-glucose cotransporter 2 inhibitors

Brand Name	Molecule	Indication	Route	Frequency	Doses	Cardiovascular Benefits on MACEs	Heart Failure Benefits	Renal Benefits	For Chronic Kidney Disease Benefits
Invokana	Canagliflozin	T2DM	PO	Daily	100, 300 mg	X	X	X	Can initiate/use in people with eGFR ≥ 20 mL/min/1.73 m^2
Farxiga	Dapagliflozin	T2DM	PO	Daily	5, 10 mg		X	X	
Jardiance	Empagliflozin	T2DM	PO	Daily	10, 25 mg	X	X	X	
Steglatro	Ertugliflozin	T2DM	PO	Daily	5, 15 mg		X		

Abbreviations: eGFR, estimated glomerular filtration rate; MACE, major adverse cardiovascular event; PO, by mouth; T2DM, type 1 diabetes mellitus.

Table 5
Side effects of sodium-glucose cotransporter 2 inhibitors

Side Effect	Description	Frequency	Evidence	Agent(s) with Highest Incidence	Observations
Bacterial infection	Urinary tract infections	Common	Incidence: 8%–8.8%	All agents	Increased glucose in the urinary tract, which can serve as a nidus for bacterial infections and fungal overgrowth
Fungal infection	GU fungal infections (vulvovaginal candidiasis and candida balanitis)	Common	Incidence: 3.5% to 10%–15% (women)	All agents	
Necrotizing fasciitis	Fournier's gangrene	Rare	FDA identified 55 cases between 2013 and 2019	All agents	
Volume depletion	• Hypotension • Syncope (Orthostatic hypotension)	Rare	Incidence: 1.1% from 22 RCTs with 4386 subjects on dapagliflozin 10 mg Incidence: 1.2% canagliflozin 100 mg and 1.3 canagliflozin 300 mg (1667 subjects)	Dapagliflozin Canagliflozin	Osmotic diuresis and intravascular volume contraction. In older patient or those on diuretics, initiation of SGLT2i may lead to symptomatic hypotension
Amputations	Very rare	Very rare	CANVAS study HR 1.95	Canagliflozin	High-risk patients with neuropathy, foot issues, vascular disease, or prior foot ulcers should approach SGLT2 inhibitors cautiously. Monitoring for foot ulcerations is essential, and individualized care is crucial.

(continued on next page)

Table 5
(continued)

Side Effect	Description	Frequency	Evidence	Agent(s) with Highest Incidence	Observations
Skeletal fragility	Rare	Rare	Low trauma fractures and greater bone density loss (700 older adults) at hip (0.9% and 1.2% decline on 100 mg and 300 mg respectively), and at the spine (0.3% and 0.7% 100 mg and 300 mg, respectively)	Canagliflozin	Increased postural dizziness and increased falls
DKA and Euglycemic DKA	Common	Common	Overall risk 2.13 (>60,000 subjects, 39 RCTs)	All agents	Dehydration, volume depletion, illness, surgery, nausea/vomiting increase risk of DKA or EuDKA. Hold SGLT2 inhibitors 3–4 d prior to surgery to avoid postoperative DKA

Abbreviations: DKA, diabetic ketoacidosis; EuDKA, euglycemic diabetic ketoacidosis; FDA, Food and Drug Administration; GU, genitourinary; RCT, randomized controlled trial; SGLT2, sodium-glucose cotransporter 2.

notably lack pronounced hyperglycemia, resulting in the absence of osmotic symptoms (polyuria, polydipsia). This masking of symptoms is more pronounced in patients on SGLT2 inhibitors due to renal excretion of glucose.[37] As such, clinicians face diagnostic challenges due to relatively normal or only mildly elevated glucose levels, potentially delaying diagnosis and treatment, leading to poorer outcomes.[37,38] A high clinical suspicion is needed for an accurate diagnosis and timely management.[39] Patients may require extended treatment for DKA when SGLT2 inhibitors are used as there is a high risk of relapse into DKA if the intravenous insulin infusion is stopped prematurely or the dose of basal insulin is inadequate. Therefore, the continuous monitoring of ketones and anion gap should persist for an additional 24 to 72 hours after DKA resolution. Deciding to restart the SGLT2 inhibitor should be an individualized and shared decision. Resumption is possible if an underlying trigger that contributed to DKA was determined, but generally, it is recommended to discontinue SGLT2 inhibitors as a class in patients who develop EuDKA during therapy.[33] Prevention of EuDKA involves intensive patient education including a discussion on 'sick day rules,' where patients should be advised to hold the medication if they are feeling unwell including nausea/vomiting, and should check their blood glucose and ketone levels regularly during that period.[33] Patients should be educated that a normal plasma glucose does not preclude the possibility of EuDKA and should be encouraged to have sufficient fluid and carbohydrate intake along with insulin coverage and correction doses during periods of illness. Expert opinion also suggests stopping SLGT2 inhibitors 3 to 4 days prior to surgery to avoid postoperative DKA.[40]

DIABETES TECHNOLOGY
Continuous Glucose Monitoring

CGM has emerged as a powerful tool to monitor glucose levels and has been shown to be superior to traditional blood glucose monitoring (BGM). CGM systems continuously measure glucose in the interstitial fluid level via a disposable sensor which is placed below the skin into the subcutaneous tissue. The information is forwarded to a transmitter via Bluetooth technology to a receiver or compatible smart device (eg, smartphone, smart watch) that displays the glucose information.[41]

There are 2 CGM categories:

- Professional (diagnostic) CGM
- Personal: real-time CGM (rt-CGM) and intermittently scanned CGM (isCGM)

Professional CGM systems are owned by the clinician's practice, and are worn for a short period (eg, 7–14 days); they can be used blinded (when the user does not see the glucose levels) or unblinded (where the user sees the glucose levels on their smart phone). Once the device is returned to the provider's office, the data are analyzed and reviewed with the person with diabetes and a therapy adjustment plan is made. Professional CGM can be useful in helping clinicians identify glucose trends and patterns especially if facilitated by insulin dose, meal, and physical activity information.[42]

Personal CGM systems are owned by people with diabetes with sensor duration between 7 and 180 days. rt-CGM measures interstitial glucose levels every 1 to 15 minutes and transmits glucose information automatically to a reading device, a smartphone app, or an insulin pump. In contrast, isCGM requires that the user actively scans the sensor/transmitter unit to transfer the glucose information onto the reader or a smartphone app multiple times per day, at least every 8 hours, to avoid gaps in glucose data. CGM systems have achieved such accuracy that users no longer require confirmatory finger stick to make insulin dosing decisions. Furthermore, CGM systems have now been successfully integrated with insulin pumps and connected pens, expanding therapy options for people with diabetes.

The American Diabetes Association (ADA) 2024 Standards of Care recommend that personal CGM be offered to people with diabetes on intensive and non-intensive insulin therapy plans, who can safely use this technology.[43] **Table 6** describes available CGM systems.

The benefits of CGM in T1DM are well established from a wide array of clinical trials with data available since 2008, when the first seminal study from the Juvenile Diabetes Research Foundation established the role of CGM in the management of T1DM.[44] Since then, hundreds of publications have confirmed CGM benefits in this population from pediatric age to seniors,[44–48] with improved HbA1c, decreased hypoglycemia, and improved time in target range (TIR, 70–180 mg/dL) which, as a whole, have made CGM use in T1DM a standard of care.[42,43,49] Today, CGM should be started at diagnosis in people with T1DM, this statement being supported by the literature and by the 2024 ADA Standards of Care.[43,50]

The literature on the benefits of CGM in T2DM has increased dramatically since a prospective, 2-arm randomized trial comparing rt-CGM versus BGM in T2DM not taking mealtime insulin showed that after 12 weeks of intermittent use, the CGM group saw a HbA1c reduction of 1% versus 0.5% in the BGM group ($P = .006$), and the effects were sustained through 40 weeks of follow-up in the CGM group.[51] Subsequently, the Diamond (Multiple Daily Injections and Continuous Glucose Monitoring in Diabetes) 2 trial, an RCT of continued rt-CGM use versus BGM use, showed that in people with T2DM treated with multiple daily insulin injections, the adjusted difference in mean change in HbA1c levels was -0.3% ($P = .022$) in the CGM group at the end of 6 months.[52] Similarly, the REPLACE (An Evaluation of a Novel Glucose Sensing Technology in Type 2 Diabetes) study on 224 subjects with T2DM showed reduction of time spent in hypoglycemia by 43% ($P = .0006$).[53] Additional studies confirmed the benefits of CGM in 2463 T2DM subjects intensively treated with insulin, including decreasing acute diabetes-related events by 61% ($P < .001$) and all-cause inpatient hospitalizations by 32% ($P < .001$), occurring during the first 6 months after initiation of isCGM.[54]

Recently, the data on the clinical benefits of CGM in T2DM non-intensively treated have now grown substantially. The MOBILE (Effect of Continuous Glucose Monitoring on Glycemic Control in Patients With Type 2 Diabetes Treated With Basal Insulin) RCT studied 175 T2DM subjects seen in primary care and treated with basal insulin and combination of oral antihyperglycemic agents with or without GLP-1 RA, and randomized them to CGM versus BGM over 8 months. At study end, the CGM group experienced a mean adjusted decrease in HbA1c of -0.4% ($P = .02$), increase of TIR(70–180 mg/dL) of 15% ($P < .001$), and decrease in time below range (TBR <70 mg/dL) of-0.24% ($P = .002$).[55] The first randomized control trial in 116 adults with T2DM using non-insulin therapies was published in 2023. The IMMEDIATE (Impact of Flash Glucose Monitoring in People with Type 2 Diabetes Using Non-Insulin Antihyperglycemic Therapy) study randomized the participants to isCGM use and diabetes self-management education versus diabetes self-management education alone. At 16-week, the isCGM group had significantly higher mean TIR by 9.9% and less time above range by 8.1% compared to the diabetes self-management education group alone.[56] These data have contributed to the expansion of CGM coverage to Centers of Medicare and Medicaid beneficiaries who are treated with insulin or who have documented problematic hypoglycemia.[57]

Table 6
Available continuous glucose monitoring systems (US-Food and Drug Administration cleared)

	Intermittently Scanned Continuous Glucose Monitoring	Real-Time Continuous Glucose Monitoring					
	Abbott FreeStyle Libre 2 and 2 Plus	Dexcom G6	Dexcom G7	Medtronic Guardian 4	Medtronic Guardian 3	Eversense E3	Abbott FreeStyle Libre 3
Age	>4 y (>2 y for Libre 2 Plus)	>2 y	>2 y	>7 y	>2 y	>18 y	>4 y
Pregnancy use	Yes	Yes	Yes	No	No	No	Yes
Sensor duration	14 d (Libre 2 plus 15 d)	10 d	10 d +12 h grace period	7 d	7 d	180 d	14 d
Calibration	Factory calibrated	Factory calibrated; calibrations optional	Factory calibrated; calibrations optional	No calibrations required, calibrations optional	Every 12 hr	2/day: Day 1-21, 1/day: Day 22-180	Factory calibrated
Pump integration	Yes (Libre 2 plus version) Tandem t:slim x2 with Control IQ, Tandem Mobi	Yes Tandem t:slim x2 with Control IQ, Tandem Mobi, Insulet OmniPod 5, Beta Bionics iLet	Yes Tandem t:slim x2 with Control IQ, Tandem Mobi, Beta Bionics iLet	Yes MiniMed 780G	Yes MiniMed 770G	No	Approved
Alarms	Yes, optional	Yes, predictive Urgent low soon	Yes, predictive Urgent low soon	Yes, predictive	Yes, predictive	Yes, predictive	Yes, optional
Mean absolute relative difference	9.2%	9.9%	8.7%	10.6% (Adults ≥18 y) 11.6% (ages 7-17 y)	10.4%	8.5%	7.9%
Approved locations	Upper arm	Abdomen (age > 2) Upper buttocks (ages 2-17 y)	Back of the upper arm (age > 2) Upper buttocks (ages 2-6 y)	Back of the upper arm	Abdomen, arm (age > 14 y). Abdomen, buttocks (ages 2-6 y)	Upper arm	Upper arm

Table 7
Continuous Glucose Monitoring Metrics and Targets

Continuous Glucose Monitoring Metrics	Adults, Non-Pregnant, Targets	Older[a]/Higher Risk Adult Targets	Pregnancy (Type 1 Diabetes Mellitus) Targets
1 Number of days CGM is worn	14 d	14 d	14 d
2 % CGM active time	>70% (of 14 d)	> 70% (of 14 d)	>70% (of 14 d)
3 Mean glucose	Not standardized	Not standardized	Not standardized
4 Glucose management indicator	Not standardized	Not standardized	Not standardized
5 Glycemic variability (%CV)	≤36%	≤36%	≤36%
6 Time above range (TAR, very high, hyperglycemia level 2)	<5% time at >250 mg/dL	<10% time at >250 mg/dL	N/A
7 Time above range (TAR, high, hyperglycemia level 1)	<25% time at >180 mg/dL of which <5% at >250 mg/dL	<50% time at >180 mg/dL of which <10% at >250 mg/dL	<25% time at >140 mg/dL
8 Time in range (TIR)	>70% time at 70–180 mg/dL	>50% time at 70–180 mg/dL	>70% time at 63–140 mg/dL
9 Time below range (TBR, low, hypoglycemia level 1)	<4% time at <70 mg/dL of which <1% at <54 mg/dL	<1% time at <70 mg.dL	<4% time at <63 mg/dL of which <1% at <54 mg/dL
10 Time below range (TBR very low, hypoglycemia level 2)	<1% time at <54 mg/dL	N/A	<1% time at <54 mg/dL

[a] Older adults defined as aged 60 y or older.

Adapted from Battelino T, Danne T, Bergenstal RM, et al. Clinical targets for continuous glucose monitoring data interpretation: recommendations from the international consensus on time in range. Diabetes Care 2019; 42(8): 1593-1603.

Continuous Glucose Monitoring Metrics and Ambulatory Glucose Profile

The strong evidence of clinical benefits of CGM in T1DM and T2DM has expanded its use in endocrinology and primary care settings. CGM data review has become part of daily clinical practice; this new and updated type of diabetes practice has created the need to standardize CGM metrics and the analysis of specific information during or between office visits. In 2019, an international consensus established 10 key CGM metrics and recommended targets for use in clinical practice. The standards are summarized in **Table 7**. Additionally, the consensus reports recommended that the ambulatory glucose profile (AGP) be used as a template for CGM data visualization (**Fig. 1**). The AGP provides a summary of glucose statistics over the previous 14 days and condenses glycemic patterns into a 24-hour graph.[58,59] Glucose levels are depicted in the AGP as median (50 percentile), the 25 to 75 percentile, and the 5/95 or 10/90 percentiles (see **Fig. 1**). Included on the AGP report is also the glucose management indicator, which represents an estimate of HbA1c based on average sensor glucose over the previous 14 days.[58,60] Finally, TIR are also outlined in the AGP as well as the coefficient of variation, which estimates glycemic variability and gives insight into hypoglycemia risk.[61,62] When analyzing the AGP, it is important to identify areas of concern that is, hypoglycemia or hyperglycemia. Reviewing such abundant data can be overwhelming for the clinician without a systematic, stepped approach to CGM interpretation. Recently, several approaches to CGM interpretation have been published, all aimed to simplify the data interpretation and adjust therapy to minimize excessive glycemic fluctuations, especially hypoglycemia.[59,63]

Insulin Pens, Connected Pens, and Insulin Delivery Devices

Insulin delivery by vial and syringe has been mostly replaced by the use of disposable or reusable insulin pens. They offer simplicity and convenience, and now people with

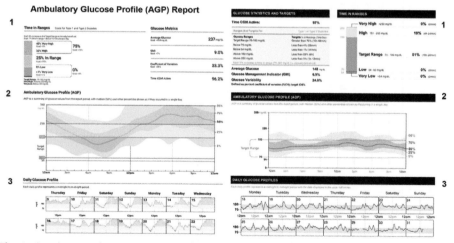

Fig. 1. Continuous glucose monitoring (CGM) report. (*1*). Glucose metrics, mean glucose, standard deviation, CGM use, glucose management indicator (GMI), times in range: time in target range (TIR, 70–180 mg/dL), time above range (TAR, >180 and > 250 mg/dL CGM), time below range (TBR, <70 and < 54 mg/dL). (*2*). Ambulatory glucose profile (AGP) graph with median, 25 to 75 percentile, and 10/90 (Dexcom) or 5/95 (Abbott) percentile. (*3*). Daily glucose profiles. (*Report derived from*: Left AGP Report derived from Dexcom Clarity (Dexcom, San Diego, CA), Right AGP Report derived from Libreview (Abbott Diabetes, Alameda, CA).)

Table 8
Connected pens and pen caps

	InPen (Medtronic Diabetes)	Big Foot Unity (Abbott Diabetes)	Tempo Button and Pen (Eli Lilly)
Description	Reusable smart insulin pen with Bluetooth connection to InPen app, 1 y battery life Can calculate insulin by: • Carbohydrate counting in bolus calculator: insulin to carbohydrate ratio, insulin sensitivity factor, active insulin time and BG target • Fixed dose • Meal size estimation Missed bolus and basal dose reminder Connects with InPen App (Android, iOS)	Smart pen caps system, rechargeable battery Long-acting pen cap (black) • Displays time since last recorded long-acting insulin dose • Alerts for missed doses Short acting pen cap (white) • Displays dose recommendations and CGM values • Captures and uploads glucose and insulin dose time data • Can be used to scan Libre CGM Connect with Unity Mobile App (IOS)	Tempo prefilled insulin pen Tempo button, reusable Bluetooth smart button, 8 mo battery life Tempo button stores and transfers insulin dose data from a Tempo Pen to the Tempo App Tempo system tracks insulin doses Doses reminders Tempo App
Insulin	Eli Lilly Humalog cartridge (U-100) Novo Nordisk Novolog penfill (U-100) Novo Nordisk Fiasp penfill (U-100)	Long-acting prefilled pens • Eli Lilly KwikPen: Basaglar • Sanofi SoloSTAR: Lantus • Sanofi SoloSTAR: Toujeo (U-300) • Sanofi SoloSTAR: Toujeo Max (U-300) • Novo Nordisk FlexTouch: Tresiba (U-100) and (U-200) Short acting prefilled pens • Eli Lilly KwikPen Humalog (U-100) and (U-200) • Eli Lilly KwikPen Lispro • Eli Lilly KwikPen Lyumjev (U-100) and (U-200) • Sanofi SoloSTAR: Apidra • Sanofi SoloSTAR: Admelog	Eli Lilly Humalog (U-100) Tempo Pen Eli Lilly Lyumjev (U-100) Tempo Pen Eli Lilly Basaglar (U-100) Tempo Pen

Integration	Medtronic Guardian 4 CGM	• Novo Nordisk FlexTouch: Fiasp (U-100)	Bluetooth blood glucose meter transmits	Tempo blood glucose meter transmits
	Medtronic Guardian Connect App	• Novo Nordisk FlexPen: NovoLog (U-100)	values to short acting pen cap (White)	values to Tempo Smart App
	Dexcom G6 CGM	• Novo Nordisk FlexPen: ReliOn NovoLog (U-100)	Values stored in the Bigfoot Unity app	Dexcom G6
	Dexcom G6 App	• Novo Nordisk FlexPen: Aspart	Abbott FreeStyle Libre 2 CGM	
	Dexcom Clarity App			

Table 9
US-Food and Drug Administration–cleared automated insulin delivery systems

Brand-Model	Compatible CGM		Features	Food and Drug Administration Approval	CE (Conformité Européenne," or European Conformity) Mark
Medtronic MiniMed 770G	Medtronic Guardian 3	Hybrid closed loop	300 units insulin reservoir Requires carbohydrate entry for meal bolus Manual mode: uses pre-programmed basal rate settings Auto mode: replaces pre-programmed basal settings with adjustments every 5 min	Sensor glucose (SG) target setpoint: 120 mg/dL Temporary target setpoint: 150 mg/dL for up to 12 h Correction bolus (calculated by algorithm in auto mode) SG target:150 mg/dL Correction bolus available based on pre-programmed insulin sensitivity factor in manual mode only	Yes ≥7 y	Yes ≥years
Medtronic MiniMed 780G	Medtronic Guardian 4	Advanced hybrid closed loop	300 units insulin reservoir Requires carbohydrate entry for meal bolus Manual mode: uses pre-programmed basal rate settings Smart guard: replaces pre-programmed basal settings with adjustments every 5 min	SG target set points: 100 mg/dL 110 mg/dL 120 mg/dL Temporary target set point: 150 mg/dL for up to 24 h Auto correction bolus (calculated by algorithm) SG target: 120 mg/dL up to every 5 min	Yes ≥7 y	Yes ≥years

| Tandem t:slim X2 with Control IQ | Advanced hybrid closed loop | Dexcom G6 Dexcom G7 FreeStyle Libre 2 (modified version) | 300 units insulin cartridge Requires carbohydrate entry for meal bolus Extended bolus up to 2 h Works on pre-programmed basal settings based on CGM values Predicts adjustments based on SG values to 30 min | SG: 112.5–160 mg/dL maintains basal rates SG: >160 mg/dL increases basal rates SG: <112.5 mg/dL decreases basal rates SG: < 70 mg/dL stops basal infusion Automatic correction bolus SG:>180 mg/dL up to every 1 h (60% of calculated correction bolus) Manual correction boluses available based on pre-programmed insulin sensitivity factor Sleep activity target SG:112.5–120 mg/dL (no automated correction boluses during sleep activity) Exercise activity target SG: 140–160 mg/dL for up to 8 h with automated correction bolus if SG:> 180 mg/dL | Yes ≥6 y | Yes ≥6 y |

(continued on next page)

Table 9 (continued)				
Brand-Model	Compatible CGM	Features		Food and Drug Administration Approval	CE (Conformité Européenne," or European Conformity) Mark
Tandem MOBI with Control IQ	Dexcom G6 Dexcom G7 FreeStyle Libre 2 (modified version)	Advanced hybrid closed loop	200 units insulin cartridge Requires carbohydrate entry for meal bolus Extended bolus up to 2 h Works on pre-programmed basal settings based on CGM values Predicts adjustments based on SG values to 30 min Fully controlled by smart phone app (IOS) Screenless pump Includes a 5-inch tubing option or regular tubing option Charged wirelessly	SG: 112.5–160 mg/dL maintains basal rates SG > 160 mg/dL increases basal rates SG < 112.5 mg/dL decreases basal rates SG < 70 mg/dL stops basal infusion Automatic correction bolus SG > 180 mg/dL up to every 1 h (60% of calculated correction bolus) Manual correction boluses available based on pre-programmed insulin sensitivity factor Sleep activity target SG: 112.5–120 mg/dL (no automated correction boluses during sleep activity) Exercise activity target SG: 140–160 mg/dL for up to 8 h with automated correction bolus if SG:> 180 mg/dL	Yes ≥6 y

Device	CGM	Mode	Features	Targets		
Insulet OmniPod 5	Dexcom G6	Advanced hybrid closed loop	200 units insulin POD OmniPod 5 Controller or smartphone app (Android, IOS) Requires carbohydrate entry for meal bolus Smart bolus calculator (with CGM Rate of Change Trend Arrows) Manual mode; uses pre-programmed basal settings Automated Mode: replaces pre-programmed basal settings with Smart adjust technology every 5 min Predictive adjustments based on SG values to 60 min	Customizable targets for 24 h or up to 8 segments/day 110 mg/dL 120 mg/dL 130 mg/dL 140 mg/dL 150 mg/dL Activity Mode target: 150 mg/dL up to 24 h, with more conservative basal rates adjustments Automated correction boluses via more aggressive basal rate adjustments every 5 min Manual correction boluses available	Yes ≥2 y	Yes ≥2 y
Beta Bionics iLet	Dexcom G6 Dexcom G7	Advanced hybrid closed loop	160 units insulin cartridge Requires only weight to initialize No manual mode available No programmable basal rates, no programmable bolus calculators Does not require carbohydrate counting/entry for meals Fully automated glucose correction BG- run mode available up to 72 h if CGM not available, after 72 h back up therapy is needed (insulin via multiple daily injections)	Default SG:120 mg/dL Can be shifted by 10 mg/dL "lower" or "higher". (110–130 mg/dL) Qualitative meal estimation: meal type ("Breakfast", "Lunch", "Dinner") meal carb content "Usual for me", "More", "Less" iLet delivers ~75% estimated insulin need, then autonomously adjusts dose No programmable correction boluses No exercise mode available	Yes ≥6 y	No

visual impairment or dexterity issues can dose insulin accurately.[64] In people with T2DM, insulin pen devices are generally preferred with reported improvement in quality-of-life rating scale over vial and syringe.[43,64]

More recently, Bluetooth-connected insulin pens and pen caps have become available. These are described in **Table 8**. Connected pens and pen caps are reusable devices integrated with a smartphone app and carry various features, including insulin dose recording or reminders. The InPen (Medtronic Diabetes, Northridge, CA, USA) also has a bolus calculator to assist with insulin doses either via carbohydrate counting or meal size. These pens usually fit the most common rapid acting insulin cartridges and have a battery duration of about 1 year. The pen caps attach to disposable, prefilled insulin pens, whether long-acting or rapid-acting insulin. Both integrate with traditional BGM or selected CGM systems. These devices also connect with software, and data can be reviewed retrospectively with the clinician.

Newer, mechanical, insulin delivery devices have been developed to enhance adherence to mealtime insulin dosing. The CeQur simplicity (CeQur Corporation, Greenville, SC, USA) is a wearable insulin patch that holds 200 units and delivers rapid-acting insulin for mealtime dosing subcutaneously in 2 units increments. An RCT comparing CeQur to insulin pens showed non-inferiority with HbA1c improvement at 24 weeks in both groups, which was maintained at 44 weeks. In the same study, more subjects preferred the patch to pens.[65] Lastly, the V-Go (MannKind Corporation, Westlake Village, CA, USA) is a wearable 24-hour patch that delivers continuously rapid-acting insulin at preset basal rates (V-Go 20, 0.83 units/h; V-Go 30, 1.25 units/h; V-Go 40, 1.65 units/h), and has an on-demand bolus button to deliver mealtime insulin in 2 units increments.[66] In a multicenter prospective study of 140 patients with T2DM, use of the V-Go patch resulted in a 0.64% decrease in HbA1C from baseline and a total daily dose decrease of insulin by 12 units per day.[67] When comparing the V-Go Patch to insulin multiple daily injections, multiple studies have described improved glycemic outcomes and a decrease in total daily dose of insulin.[68]

Automated Insulin Delivery Systems

Insulin delivery devices have advanced substantially and integration with CGM has allowed the development of AID systems; these systems differ from standard insulin pumps and have generally 3 components: an insulin pump for insulin delivery, a CGM system, and an algorithm that modulates insulin delivery, by increasing, decreasing, or suspending insulin delivery based on CGM values and their rate of change over a pre-specified period of time.[43] The algorithm can be housed on the insulin pump or on a smart app. Users generally need to announce their meals by entering carbohydrate or semiqualitative meal announcements. **Table 9** describes the various types of AID systems available in the United States and their features. In several clinical trials in T1DM individuals aged 2 years and above, AID systems have consistently shown to be safe and effective, not only in lowering HbA1c, but most importantly increasing TIR, lowering hypoglycemia and TBR, and increasing patient satisfaction and quality of life.[69–71] Training and setting expectations remain crucial for the success of AID use in T1DM.[43]

SUMMARY

Diabetes therapy landscape has expanded with the advent of new medication classes such as GLP-1 RAs, GIP/GLP-1 RAs, and SGLT2 inhibitors, providing greater therapeutic options not only for glycemic outcomes but also for cardiorenal-metabolic benefits. Similarly, diabetes technology has rapidly evolved to reach not only T1DM individuals but also T2DM on less-intensive therapies with proven benefits for glycemic outcomes. Connected pens have progressed to integrate with CGM and offer a more personalized approach to insulin therapy for diabetes. Finally, T1DM therapy options have greatly increased with the advent of AID systems; their different and specific features offer multiple opportunities for therapy choices, personalization, and decrease in diabetes distress. Clinicians are tasked with becoming champions of newer therapies and technologies, raising patients' awareness of their many options and connecting them with the appropriate education, and support to successfully implement these advances in therapies and technologies.

CLINICS CARE POINTS

- GLP-1 RAs and GIP/GLP-1 RAs offer many benefits; it is important to start with lowest dose and progress slowly to limit side effects and reduce discontinuation rates.

- SGLT2 inhibitors should be used early in diabetes. Patients are to be informed on the risk of GU infections and other side effects. Importantly, caution should be used in patients with HbA1c over 9% to limit side effects and the risk of developing either DKA or EuDKA.

- CGM should be used in people with diabetes with appropriate training, guiding patients on trouble shooting possible interferences and inaccurate reading, including the concept of lag time in hypoglycemia management.

- Connected pens and pen caps are very useful to decrease the number of missed insulin doses and assist patients with more accurate mealtime insulin dosing.

- AID systems have many variable features; it is critical to choose these systems based on patient ability to safely use them, train the patients, and set realistic expectations of the various algorithms and their limitations for successful and continued use.

DISCLOSURE

N. Kamal and K. Lee have nothing to disclose. G. Aleppo has received consultant fees from Dexcom, Insulet and Medscape. G. Aleppo has received research support to her employer, Northwestern University from Fractyl Health, Insulet, MannKind, Tandem Diabetes, and Welldoc.

REFERENCES

1. International diabetes federation (IDF) atlas. Available at: https://diabetesatlas. org/. [Accessed 2 January 2024].
2. Drucker DJ. Mechanisms of action and therapeutic application of glucagon-like peptide-1. Cell Metab 2018;27(4):740–56.
3. Andreadis P, Karagiannis T, Malandris K, et al. Semaglutide for type 2 diabetes mellitus: A systematic review and meta-analysis. Diabetes Obes Metab 2018; 20(9):2255–63.
4. Ahmann AJ, Capehorn M, Charpentier G, et al. Efficacy and safety of once-weekly semaglutide versus exenatide ER in subjects with type 2 diabetes (SUSTAIN 3): A 56-week, open-label, randomized clinical trial. Diabetes Care 2018; 41(2):258–66.
5. Pratley RE, Aroda VR, Lingvay I, et al. Semaglutide versus dulaglutide once weekly in patients with type 2 diabetes (SUSTAIN 7): a randomised, open-label, phase 3b trial. Lancet Diabetes Endocrinol 2018;6(4):275–86.

6. Capehorn MS, Catarig AM, Furberg JK, et al. Efficacy and safety of once-weekly semaglutide 1.0mg vs once-daily liraglutide 1.2mg as add-on to 1-3 oral antidiabetic drugs in subjects with type 2 diabetes (SUSTAIN 10). Diabetes Metab 2020; 46(2):100–9.

7. Kristensen SL, Rørth R, Jhund PS, et al. Cardiovascular, mortality, and kidney outcomes with GLP-1 receptor agonists in patients with type 2 diabetes: a systematic review and meta-analysis of cardiovascular outcome trials. Lancet Diabetes Endocrinol 2019;7(10):776–85.

8. Iqbal J, Wu HX, Hu N, et al. Effect of glucagon-like peptide-1 receptor agonists on body weight in adults with obesity without diabetes mellitus-a systematic review and meta-analysis of randomized control trials. Obes Rev 2022;23(6): e13435.

9. Trujillo JM, Nuffer W, Smith BA. GLP-1 receptor agonists: an updated review of head-to-head clinical studies. Ther Adv Endocrinol Metab 2021;12. 20420188219 97320.

10. Bednarz K, Kowalczyk K, Cwynar M, et al. The role of Glp-1 receptor agonists in insulin resistance with concomitant obesity treatment in polycystic ovary syndrome. Int J Mol Sci 2022;23(8):4334.

11. Salamun V, Jensterle M, Janez A, et al. Liraglutide increases IVF pregnancy rates in obese PCOS women with poor response to first-line reproductive treatments: a pilot randomized study. Eur J Endocrinol 2018;179(1):1–11.

12. Armstrong MJ, Gaunt P, Aithal GP, et al. Liraglutide safety and efficacy in patients with non-alcoholic steatohepatitis (LEAN): a multicentre, double-blind, randomised, placebo-controlled phase 2 study. Lancet 2016;387(10019):679–90.

13. Ghosal S, Datta D, Sinha B. A meta-analysis of the effects of glucagon-like-peptide 1 receptor agonist (GLP1-RA) in nonalcoholic fatty liver disease (NAFLD) with type 2 diabetes (T2D). Sci Rep 2021;11(1):22063.

14. Wong C, Lee MH, Yaow CYL, et al. Glucagon-like peptide-1 receptor agonists for non-alcoholic fatty liver disease in type 2 diabetes: a meta-analysis. Front Endocrinol 2021;12:1.

15. Trujillo J. Safety and tolerability of once-weekly GLP-1 receptor agonists in type 2 diabetes. J Clin Pharm Ther 2020;45(Suppl 1):43–60.

16. Gulak MA, Murphy P. Regurgitation under anesthesia in a fasted patient prescribed semaglutide for weight loss: a case report. Can J Anaesth 2023;70(8): 1397–400.

17. Vallatharasu Y, Hayashi-Tanner Y, Polewski PJ, et al. Severe, prolonged thrombocytopenia in a patient sensitive to exenatide. Am J Hematol 2019;94(3):E78–80.

18. Bass J, Tschöp MH, Beutler LR. Dual gut hormone receptor agonists for diabetes and obesity. J Clin Invest 2023;133(3):e167952.

19. Karagiannis T, Avgerinos I, Liakos A, et al. Management of type 2 diabetes with the dual GIP/GLP-1 receptor agonist tirzepatide: a systematic review and meta-analysis. Diabetologia 2022;65(8):1251–61.

20. Jastreboff AM, Aronne LJ, Ahmad NN, et al. Tirzepatide once weekly for the treatment of obesity. N Engl J Med 2022;387(3):205–16.

21. Garvey WT, Frias JP, Jastreboff AM, et al. SURMOUNT-2 investigators. Tirzepatide once weekly for the treatment of obesity in people with type 2 diabetes (SURMOUNT-2): a double-blind, randomised, multicentre, placebo-controlled, phase 3 trial. Lancet 2023 19;402(10402):613–26.

22. Gastaldelli A, Cusi K, Fernández Landó L, et al. Effect of tirzepatide versus insulin degludec on liver fat content and abdominal adipose tissue in people with type 2 diabetes (SURPASS-3 MRI): a substudy of the randomised, open-label, parallel-

group, phase 3 SURPASS-3 trial. Lancet Diabetes Endocrinol 2022;10(6): 393–406.

23. Mishra R, Raj R, Elshimy G, et al. Adverse events related to tirzepatide. J Endocr Soc 2023;7(4):bvad016.

24. Fonseca-Correa JI, Correa-Rotter R. Sodium-glucose cotransporter 2 inhibitors mechanisms of action: a review. Front Med (Lausanne) 2021;8:777861.

25. Zelniker TA, Wiviott SD, Raz I, et al. SGLT2 inhibitors for primary and secondary prevention of cardiovascular and renal outcomes in type 2 diabetes: a systematic review and meta-analysis of cardiovascular outcome trials. Lancet 2019; 393(10166):31–9.

26. Baigent C, Emberson JR, Haynes R, et al. Impact of diabetes on the effects of sodium glucose co-transporter-2 inhibitors on kidney outcomes: collaborative meta-analysis of large placebo-controlled trials. Lancet 2022;400(10365):1788–801.

27. Li D, Wang T, Shen S, et al. Urinary tract and genital infections in patients with type 2 diabetes treated with sodium-glucose co-transporter 2 inhibitors: A meta-analysis of randomized controlled trials. Diabetes Obes Metab 2017; 19(3):348–55.

28. Nyirjesy P, Zhao Y, Ways K, et al. Evaluation of vulvovaginal symptoms and Candida colonization in women with type 2 diabetes mellitus treated with canagliflozin, a sodium glucose co-transporter 2 inhibitor. Curr Med Res Opin 2012; 28(7):1173–8.

29. Bersoff-Matcha SJ, Chamberlain C, Cao C, et al. Fournier gangrene associated with sodium-glucose cotransporter-2 inhibitors: a review of spontaneous postmarketing cases. Ann Intern Med 2019;170(11):764–9.

30. Johnsson K, Johnsson E, Mansfield TA, et al. Osmotic diuresis with SGLT2 inhibition: analysis of events related to volume reduction in dapagliflozin clinical trials. Postgrad Med 2016;128(4):346–55.

31. Inzucchi SE, Iliev H, Pfarr E, et al. Empagliflozin and assessment of lower-limb amputations in the empa-reg outcome trial. Diabetes Care 2018;41(1):e4–5.

32. Bilezikian JP, Watts NB, Usiskin K, et al. Evaluation of bone mineral density and bone biomarkers in patients with type 2 diabetes treated with canagliflozin. J Clin Endocrinol Metab 2016;101(1):44–51.

33. Chow E, Clement S, Garg R. Euglycemic diabetic ketoacidosis in the era of SGLT-2 inhibitors. BMJ Open Diabetes Res Care 2023;11(5):e003666.

34. Douros A, Lix LM, Fralick M, et al. Sodium-glucose cotransporter-2 inhibitors and the risk for diabetic ketoacidosis : a multicenter cohort study. Ann Intern Med 2020;173(6):417–26.

35. Liu J, Li L, Li S, et al. Sodium-glucose co-transporter-2 inhibitors and the risk of diabetic ketoacidosis in patients with type 2 diabetes: A systematic review and meta-analysis of randomized controlled trials. Diabetes Obes Metab 2020; 22(9):1619–27.

36. Ahmed M, McKenna MJ, Crowley RK. Diabetic ketoacidosis in patients with type 2 diabetes recently commenced on SGLT-2 inhibitors: an ongoing concern. Endocr Pract 2017;23(4):506–8.

37. Barski L, Eshkoli T, Brandstaetter E, et al. Euglycemic diabetic ketoacidosis. Eur J Intern Med 2019;63:9–14.

38. Modi A, Agrawal A, Morgan F. Euglycemic diabetic ketoacidosis: a review. Curr Diabetes Rev 2017;13(3):315–21.

39. Rawla P, Vellipuram AR, Bandaru SS, et al. Euglycemic diabetic ketoacidosis: a diagnostic and therapeutic dilemma. Endocrinol Diabetes Metab Case Rep 2017;2017:17–0081.

40. Nasa P, Chaudhary S, Shrivastava PK, et al. Euglycemic diabetic ketoacidosis: A missed diagnosis. World J Diabetes 2021;12(5):514–23.

41. Adolfsson P, Parkin CG, Thomas A, et al. Selecting the appropriate continuous glucose monitoring system - a practical approach. Eur Endocrinol 2018; 14(1):24–9.

42. Friedman JG, Cardona Matos Z, Szmuilowicz ED, et al. Use of continuous glucose monitors to manage type 1 diabetes mellitus: progress, challenges, and recommendations. Pharmgenomics Pers Med 2023;16:263–76.

43. American Diabetes Association Professional Practice Committee. 7. diabetes technology: standards of care in diabetes-2024. Diabetes Care 2024;47(Suppl 1):S126–44.

44. Tamborlane WV, Beck RW, Bode BW, et al. Continuous glucose monitoring and intensive treatment of type 1 diabetes. N Engl J Med 2008;359:1464–76.

45. Prahalad P, Ding VY, Zaharieva DP, et al. Teamwork, targets, technology, and tight control in newly diagnosed type 1 diabetes: the pilot 4T study. J Clin Endocrinol Metab 2022;107(4):998–1008.

46. Pratley RE, Kanapka LG, Rickels MR, et al. Wireless innovation for seniors with diabetes mellitus (WISDM) study group. effect of continuous glucose monitoring on hypoglycemia in older adults with type 1 diabetes: a randomized clinical trial. JAMA 2020;323(23):2397–406.

47. Miller KM, Kanapka LG, Rickels MR, et al. Benefit of continuous glucose monitoring in reducing hypoglycemia is sustained through 12 months of use among older adults with type 1 diabetes. Diabetes Technol Therapeut 2022;24(6): 424–34.

48. Leelarathna L, Evans ML, Neupane S, et al. Intermittently scanned continuous glucose monitoring for type 1 diabetes. N Engl J Med 2022;387(16):1477–87.

49. Friedman JG, Coyne K, Aleppo G, et al. Beyond A1C: exploring continuous glucose monitoring metrics in managing diabetes. Endocr Connect 2023;12(7): e230085.

50. Champakanath A, Akturk HK, Alonso GT, et al. Continuous glucose monitoring initiation within first year of type 1 diabetes diagnosis is associated with improved glycemic outcomes: 7-year follow-up study. Diabetes Care 2022;45(3):750–3.

51. Vigersky RA, Fonda SJ, Chellappa M, et al. Short- and long-term effects of real-time continuous glucose monitoring in patients with type 2 diabetes. Diabetes Care 2012;35(1):32–8.

52. Beck RW, Riddlesworth TD, Ruedy K, et al. Continuous glucose monitoring versus usual care in patients with Type 2 diabetes receiving multiple daily insulin injections: a randomized trial. Ann Intern Med 2017;167:365–74.

53. Haak T, Hanaire H, Ajjan R, et al. Flash glucose-sensing technology as a replacement for blood glucose monitoring for the management of insulin-treated Type 2 diabetes: a multicenter, open-label randomized controlled trial. Diabetes Therapy: Research, Treatment and Education of Diabetes and Related Disorders 2017;8:55–73.

54. Bergenstal RM, Kerr MSD, Roberts GJ, et al. Flash CGM Is associated with reduced diabetes events and hospitalizations in insulin-treated type 2 diabetes. J Endocr Soc 2021;5(4):bvab013.

55. Martens T, Beck RW, Bailey R, et al. Effect of continuous glucose monitoring on glycemic control in patients with Type 2 diabetes treated with basal insulin: a randomized clinical trial. JAMA 2021;325:2262–72.

56. Aronson R, Brown RE, Chu L, et al. IMpact of flash glucose Monitoring in pEople with type 2 Diabetes Inadequately controlled with non-insulin Antihyperglycaemic

ThErapy (IMMEDIATE): A randomized controlled trial. Diabetes Obes Metab 2023;25(4):1024–31.

57. Center for medicare and medicaid (CMS) LCD - glucose monitors (L33822). Availabe at: https://cms.gov. [Accessed 26 December 2023].

58. Battelino T, Danne T, Bergenstal RM, et al. Clinical targets for continuous glucose monitoring data interpretation: recommendations from the international consensus on time in range. Diabetes Care 2019;42(8):1593–603.

59. Szmuilowicz ED, Aleppo G. Stepwise approach to continuous glucose monitoring interpretation for internists and family physicians. Postgrad Med 2022;134(8): 743–51.

60. Bergenstal RM, Beck RW, Close KL, et al. Glucose management indicator (GMI): A new term for estimating A1C from continuous glucose monitoring. Diabetes Care 2018;41(11):2275–80.

61. Monnier L, Colette C, Wojtusciszyn A, et al. Toward defining the threshold between low and high glucose variability in diabetes. Diabetes Care 2017;40(7): 832–8.

62. Umpierrez GE, B PK. Glycemic variability: how to measure and its clinical implication for type 2 diabetes. Am J Med Sci 2018;356(6):518–27.

63. Isaacs D, Cox C, Schwab K, et al. Technology integration: the role of the diabetes care and education specialist in practice. Diabetes Educ 2020;46(4):323–34.

64. Singh R, Samuel C, Jacob JJ. A Comparison of insulin pen devices and disposable plastic syringes - simplicity, safety, convenience and cost differences. Eur Endocrinol 2018;14(1):47–51.

65. Bergenstal RM, Peyrot M, Dreon DM, et al. Implementation of basal-bolus therapy in type 2 diabetes: a randomized controlled trial comparing bolus insulin delivery using an insulin patch with an insulin pen. Diabetes Technol Therapeut 2019; 21(5):273–85.

66. Sutton D, Higdon CD, Nikkel C, Hilsinger KA. Clinical Benefits Over Time Associated with Use of V-Go Wearable Insulin Delivery Device in Adult Patients with Diabetes: A Retrospective Analysis. Adv Ther 2018;35(5):631–43.

67. Grunberger G, Rosenfeld CR, Bode BW, et al. Effectiveness of V-Go® for Patients with Type 2 Diabetes in a Real-World Setting: A Prospective Observational Study. Drugs Real World Outcomes 2020;7(1):31–40.

68. Meade LT, Battise D. Evaluation of Clinical Outcomes With the V-Go Wearable Insulin Delivery Device in Patients With Type 2 Diabetes. Clin Diabetes 2021;39(3): 297–303.

69. Weissberg-Benchell J, Vesco AT, Shapiro J, et al. Psychosocial Impact of the Insulin-Only iLet Bionic Pancreas for Adults, Youth, and Caregivers of Youth with Type 1 Diabetes. Diabetes Technol Ther 2023;25(10):705–17.

70. Amigó J, Ortiz-Zúñiga Á, de Urbina AMO, et al. Switching from treatment with sensor augmented pump to hybrid closed loop system in type 1 diabetes: Impact on glycemic control and neuropsychological tests in the real world. Diabetes Res Clin Pract 2023;201:110730.

71. Polonsky WH, Hood KK, Levy CJ, et al. How introduction of automated insulin delivery systems may influence psychosocial outcomes in adults with type 1 diabetes: Findings from the first investigation with the Omnipod® 5 System. Diabetes Res Clin Pract 2022;190:109998.

Novel Therapies for the Treatment of Cardiovascular Disease

Abdul Aziz A. Asbeutah, MD*, Zachary D. Goldberger, MD, MS

KEYWORDS

- Heart failure • Cardiology • SGLT2 inhibitors • Sacubitril-valsartan • Ivabradine

KEY POINTS

- In the last decade, several new cardiovascular therapies have become pillars in the treatment of heart failure and hypertension.
- Angiotensin-Neprilysin and Sodium-Glucose Co-transporter 2 inhibitors reduce cardiovascular mortality and heart failure hospitalization in patients with heart failure.
- Novel therapies for treating resistant hypertension are being developed.
- Practicing physicians should become familiar with novel cardiovascular therapies, their indications, and common side effects.

INTRODUCTION

Cardiovascular disease (CVD) is the most common cause of death in the United States.[1] Over the last decade, randomized clinical trials of several pharmacologic agents have demonstrated a reduction in cardiovascular mortality and other secondary outcomes. Angiotensin-Neprilysin Inhibitors (ARNI's) and Sodium-Glucose Co-transporter 2 inhibitors (SGLT2i) have now become pillars in the treatment of heart failure. Ivabradine, a selective funny channel inhibitor, is a novel negative chronotropic agent used as an add-on therapy in heart failure.[2] Practitioners must be familiar with the indications and side effects of newer therapies as they are now frequently prescribed. Two new hypertension therapies are also in investigational stages. Subcutaneous injections of zilebesiran inhibits the hepatic production of angiotensinogen; aprocitentan is a dual endothelin antagonist. Finally, mavacamten, a novel cardiac myosin inhibitor, has emerged as a pharmacologic treatment for hypertrophic obstructive cardiomyopathy (HOCM).

Department of Medicine, Division of Cardiovascular Medicine, University of Wisconsin-Madison Hospitals and Clinics, Madison, WI, USA
* Corresponding author. 600 Highland Avenue, Madison, WI 53792-3248.
E-mail address: asbeutah@wisc.edu

HEART FAILURE THERAPIES

Cardiovascular disease is the leading cause of death in the United States with over greater than 920,000 related deaths in 2020.[1] With an aging population, coupled with an increase in risk factors, the prevalence of CVD, especially coronary artery disease and heart failure, will continue to increase. According to prediction models, greater than 8 million people in the United States will be living with heart failure in 2030.[3] Prior studies have shown that heart failure exhibits a major health burden with respect to hospitalizations, overall survival, and premature life years lost, like many forms of cancer.[4,5]

Several therapeutics have emerged over the last 10 years and have led to a marked decline in heart failure morbidity and mortality. The introduction of SGLT2i, ARNI's, and the continued use of prior approved heart failure therapies has led to a reduction in cardiovascular mortality, heart failure hospitalizations, and improved quality of life.[1,2,4,6–8] However impactful, these new medications are expensive, posing limitations to widespread use in eligible patients.[9]

Sodium-Glucose Co-transporter 2 Inhibitors

Sodium Glucose co-transporter 2 inhibitor therapies have revolutionized the treatment of diabetes, chronic kidney disease, and heart failure. Sodium Glucose co-transporter 2 inhibitor therapy has led to a reduction in hemoglobin A1C levels, progression of chronic kidney disease, and reduced heart failure hospitalizations and cardiovascular mortality.[6,7,10–13] Initially developed for the treatment of diabetes, they have now become an American Heart Association (AHA)/American College of Cardiology(ACC)/Heart Failure Society of America (HFSA) class 1 indication for patients with heart failure with reduced ejection fraction (HFrEF), with an ejection fraction lesser than or equal to 40% and a Class 2a indication among patients with heart failure with mildly reduced ejection fraction (HFmrEF), an ejection fraction (EF) of 41% to 49%, and heart failure with preserved ejection fraction (HFpEF), defined as an EF greater than 50%.[2] Importantly, SGLT2i therapies are approved for the treatment of heart failure irrespective of diabetes, based on data mainly derived from the Dapagliflozin and Prevention of Adverse Outcomes in Heart Failure (DAPA-HF) and Empagliflozin Outcome Trial in patients with chronic HFrEF (EMPEROR-Reduced) trials.[6,7]

Mechanism of action

Sodium Glucose co-transporter 2 inhibitor therapies induce glycosuria by inhibiting the reabsorption of sodium and glucose in the proximal convoluted tubule.[14] Several mechanisms have been described on how SGLT2 inhibition leads to cardiac protection including blood pressure lowering, natriuresis, weight reduction, preventing cardiac remodeling, and decreasing oxidative stress.[15] It is important to recognize there will be an expected "dip" in the estimated glomerular filtration rate (eGFR) shortly after starting SGLT2i therapy.[16]

Heart Failure with Reduced Ejection Fraction

Empagliflozin was the first SGLT2i approved for patients with HFrEF regardless of diabetes based on results from the EMPEROR-Reduced trial.[6] Empagliflozin was studied in a double-blind placebo-controlled trial among patients with a left ventricular EF less than 40% and New York Heart Association (NYHA) class II-IV symptoms at 10 mg daily in addition to other guideline-directed medical therapy (GDMT) for HFrEF compared to placebo. There was a significant reduction in the primary composite outcome of index cardiovascular death or hospitalization for heart failure. It is important to note that the primary outcome was mainly driven by hospitalizations for heart failure and cardiovascular death was not significantly different between treatment groups.[6]

Dapagliflozin was studied in a placebo-controlled randomized trial among patients with a left ventricular EF of lesser than or equal to 40%, NYHA class II-IV symptoms at a dose of 10 mg daily in addition to maximally tolerated guideline medical therapy for HFrEF.[7] There was a significant reduction in the primary composite outcome of cardiovascular death or hospitalization for heart failure. Importantly, dapagliflozin was associated with a decrease in cardiovascular mortality when analyzed independently. Of note, this was the first trial to show decreased cardiovascular mortality of SGLT2i's in patients with HFrEF, regardless of diabetes status.[7]

Heart Failure with Mildly Reduced and Preserved Ejection Fraction

With the proven cardiovascular benefits of SGLT2i therapies in HFrEF, several trials have subsequently studied the effect of SGLT2i therapy in patients with heart failure HFmrEF and HFpEF.[10,11] Among patients with an EF greater than 40% and NYHA class II-IV symptoms on GDMT, empagliflozin was initiated in a randomized fashion at a dose of 10 mg per day with the hypothesis that clinical benefits seen among HFrEF patients would be similar.[10] There was a significant reduction in the primary composite outcome event of death from cardiovascular causes or hospitalization for heart failure among patients randomized to empagliflozin. The primary outcome was mainly driven by heart failure hospitalizations and there was no significant reduction in cardiovascular mortality when assessed individually. In sub-group analyses, the primary outcome was significant up to and including an EF less than 60%, there was no significant clinical benefit among patients with an EF greater than 60%.[10]

In the landmark DELIVER trial, patients with an EF greater than 40% and NYHA class II-IV symptoms on GDMT were randomized to dapagliflozin 10 mg daily versus placebo. At a median of 2.3 years, the primary outcome of worsening heart failure or cardiovascular death was significantly reduced in the dapagliflozin group, however, again mainly driven by heart failure hospitalizations or urgent heart failure related visits without a significant reduction in cardiovascular mortality.[11] The primary outcome was significantly reduced among patients with a left ventricular EF greater than or equal to 50%, but not among patients with HFmrEF.[11]

Based on these landmark trials, the AHA/ACC/HFSA Guideline for the Management of Heart Failure awards SGLT2i therapy a class 1 indication for patients with HFrEF and a class 2a indication among patients with HFmrEF and HFpEF.[2,6,7,10,11] **Fig. 1** summarizes the use of SGLT2i therapy in heart failure.

Side effects

Sodium Glucose co-transporter 2 inhibitor therapies induce glycosuria by inhibiting the re-absorption of sodium and glucose in the proximal convoluted tubule.[14] As such, it is prudent to inform patients about proper genital hygiene before prescribing an SGLT2i as they have been associated with infections ranging from simple urinary tract infections, and more rarely to major genital infections such as Fournier's gangrene.[17] Another rare side effect of SGLT2i is euglycemic diabetic ketoacidosis. Other side effects may include volume depletion leading to hypotension and orthostatic hypotension. It is also important not to prescribe SGLT2i therapies to patients with type 1 diabetes mellitus or end-stage renal disease due to an increased risk of euglycemic diabetic ketoacidosis. In the peri-operative setting, SGLT2i therapies should be held 3 to 4 days before planned elective surgery to minimize the risk of ketoacidosis and urinary tract infections.[18]

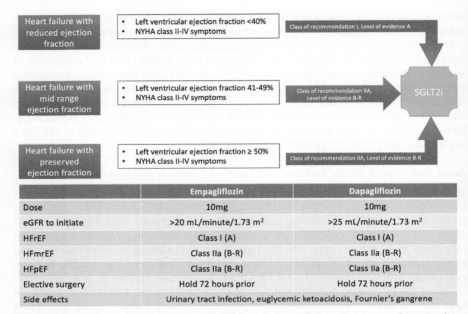

Fig. 1. Sodium-Glucose Co-transporter 2 inhibitors in heart failure. Summary of SGLT2i therapy in heart failure with class of recommendation and level of evidence. eGFR: estimated Glomerular Filtration rate, HFmrEF: Heart failure with mid-range ejection fraction, HFpEF: Heart Failure with preserved ejection fraction, HFrEF: Heart failure with reduced ejection fraction, NYHA: New York Heart Association, SGLT2i: Sodium-Glucose Co-transporter 2 inhibitor.

Angiotensin-Neprilysin Inhibitors

Indications and mechanism of action

Sacubitril-valsartan is a novel combination drug that combines a neprilysin inhibitor, sacubitril, and valsartan, an angiotensin receptor blocker. Neprilysin is an endopeptidase that degrades natriuretic peptides such as atrial natriuretic peptide (ANP), brain natriuretic peptide (BNP), and bradykinin.[19] By inhibiting the breakdown of ANP, sacubitril promotes natriuresis, leading to systemic vasodilation and blood pressure reduction.[19] The AHA/ACC/HFSA Guideline for the Management of Heart Failure awards sacubitril-valsartan a class 1 indication for patients with HFrEF and a class 2b indication among patients with HFmrEF and HFpEF with any ejection fraction in women and up to 60% among men.[2]

Trials

There have been 2 landmark trials that studied the impact of sacubitril-valsartan on cardiovascular outcomes across a spectrum of left ventricular ejection fractions (LVEF).[8,20] The Prospective Comparison of Angiotensin Receptor–Neprilysin Inhibitor (ARNI) with Angiotensin-Converting–Enzyme Inhibitor (ACEi) to Determine Impact on Global Mortality and Morbidity in Heart Failure (PARADIGM-HF) trial was a double-blind, randomized controlled trial that included patients with an LVEF lesser than or equal to 35%, with NYHA class II-IV symptoms. Patients were randomized to sacubitril-valsartan to a total dose of 200 mg twice daily versus enalapril 10 mg twice daily, in addition to GDMT. The primary outcome was a composite of death from cardiovascular causes or hospitalization for heart failure. The trial was stopped early after a median follow-up of 27 months due to substantially significant benefits in the sacubitril-valsartan group (P < .001). There was also a significant reduction in total mortality, cardiovascular mortality, and heart failure hospitalizations, all statistically significant. There was a significant 17.7% reduction in cardiovascular mortality or first hospitalization for heart failure compared to enalapril. This was a pivotal trial with overwhelming evidence in support of sacubitril-valsartan as a pillar in HFrEF management.[8]

Sacubitril-valsartan was also studied among patients with reduced LVEF in the setting of acute myocardial infarction (MI), in which 90% of patients had successful coronary reperfusion.[21] Patients with MI in the last 7 days complicated by reduced LVEF ($\leq$40%) or pulmonary edema were randomized to sacubitril-valsartan or ramipril in addition to GDMT. The primary outcome was death from cardiovascular causes or incident heart failure. Over 22 months, there was no observed significant difference in cardiovascular mortality or heart failure hospitalization in either group. In this trial, there was no superiority for sacubitril-valsartan in reducing heart failure hospitalizations or cardiovascular mortality in comparison to ramipril.[21] This trial shows that in the acute setting of ischemic cardiomyopathy with successful reperfusion, sacubitril-valsartan was non-superior to traditional ACE inhibitor therapy, which is important from a cost-perspective since most patients will be burdened by multiple new costly medications after hospitalization with an MI.

With the substantial benefit in cardiovascular outcomes among patients with HFrEF, sacubitril-valsartan compared to valsartan was studied in a population of patients with a LVEF of greater than or equal to 40%, and NYHA class II-IV symptoms, structural heart disease, and elevated natriuretic peptides.[20] The primary outcome was a composite of total hospitalizations for heart failure and death from cardiovascular causes. There was no significant difference in death from cardiovascular causes in the sacubitril–valsartan group compared to the valsartan group. There were numerically fewer, but not statistically significant hospitalizations for heart failure in the sacubitril-valsartan group. However, in a subgroup analysis, there was a significant reduction in the primary outcome among patients with a median left ventricular EF lesser than or equal to 57% and among women prescribed sacubitril-valsartan. Based on this subgroup analysis, sacubitril-valsartan has been given, and class 2b indication for patients with HFmrEF and HFpEF in women with an EF greater than or equal to 40% and in men with an LVEF less than 60%.[2,20]

How to initiate sacubitril-valsartan in an outpatient setting and side effects

Sacubitril-valsartan is dosed twice daily and comes in 3 standard doses, 24 mg/26 mg, 49 mg/51 mg, and 97 mg/103 mg. The usual starting dose is 24 mg/26 mg twice a day and it is up-titrated to a target dose of 200 mg twice a day according to tolerability and blood pressure response.[22] During the initiation phase of sacubitril-valsartan, BNP levels may increase to above pre-initiation levels mainly due to neprilysin inhibition leading to reduced breakdown of BNP. Pro-NT-BNP levels may be of better predictive value and cause less clinical confusion when measured in the initial 2 months of initiation of sacubitril-valsartan.[23] Of note, in the PARADIGM-HF trial, 18% and 6% of patients had doubled and tripled their circulating BNP level in the first 8 to 10 weeks of sacubitril-valsartan initiation, respectively.[23] **Fig. 2** summarizes the use of sacubitril-valsartan in patients with heart failure.

The combined use of ACE inhibitors and sacubitril-valsartan is not recommended, mainly due to the increased risk of life-threatening angioedema. It is important to note that initiation of sacubitril-valsartan among patients on an ACE inhibitor requires a 36-hours washout period to minimize the risk of angioedema.[24] Among patients

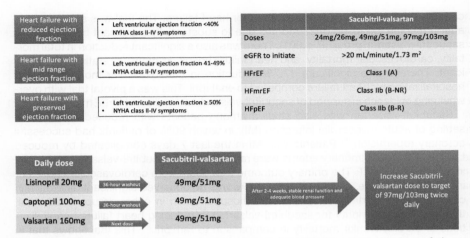

Fig. 2. Sacubitril-valsartan indications and recommended initiation strategy in heart failure. Summary of sacubitril-valsartan therapy in heart failure with class of recommendation and level of evidence. eGFR: estimated Glomerular Filtration rate, HFmrEF: Heart failure with mid-range ejection fraction, HFpEF: Heart Failure with preserved ejection fraction, HFrEF: Heart failure with reduced ejection fraction, NYHA: New York Heart Association.

already prescribed an angiotensin receptor blocker (ARB), sacubitril-valsartan can be started instead of the ARB at the time of the next dose. Even though sacubitril-valsartan does not cause ACE inhibition, there is still a risk of angioedema mainly due to the neprilysin inhibition leading to decreased degradation of bradykinin. The most common reported side effect reported in the PARADIGM-HF trial was symptomatic hypotension in around 14% of patients randomized to sacubitril-valsartan in comparison to 9.2% among patients prescribed enalapril.[8] Interestingly, there were significantly fewer hyperkalemic events (potassium >6.0 mmol/L) in the sacubitril-valsartan group compared to the enalapril group, this is postulated to be due to the natriuretic effect of sacubitril.[8]

Ivabradine

Ivabradine is a novel heart rate-reducing medication that selectively inhibits the funny channel (I_f) in the sinoatrial (SA) node, prolonging the spontaneous depolarization of the SA node leading to reduced heart rates. Ivabradine is selective to the SA node and does not affect systemic blood pressure or myocardial contractility.[25] Ivabradine has been tested in several cardiac conditions including inappropriate sinus tachycardia, HFrEF, and stable coronary artery disease.[26–28]

Ivabradine is currently indicated for patients with LVEF lesser than or equal to 35%, heart rate greater than or equal to70 beats per minute (bpm) on a maximally tolerated beta-blocker dose, and in sinus rhythm. In the Systolic Heart failure treatment with the I_f inhibitor ivabradine Trial (SHIFT), ivabradine was associated with reduced heart failure hospitalizations and deaths due to heart failure. However, there was no significant reduction in all-cause mortality compared to placebo.[26] In the AHA/ACC/HFSA Guideline for the Management of Heart Failure, ivabradine has been designated a 2a classification for patients with HFrEF, NYHA class II-III symptoms, in normal sinus rhythm with a heart rate greater than or equal to 70bpm on maximally tolerate beta-blocker.[2] It is important to note that in the SHIFT trial, only 25% of patients were on optimal beta-blocker dose, hence, it is important to up-titrate the beta-blocker to the maximum tolerated dose before considering ivabradine. This is prudent since beta-blockers with proven cardiovascular mortality benefits have superior outcomes compared to ivabradine. Notable side effects in the SHIFT trial were bradycardia (5%) and visual brightness "phosphenes" (3%), in the first few months after initiation. **Fig. 3** illustrates the use of ivabradine in HFrEF.[26]

Ivabradine was also studied among patients with chronic stable coronary artery disease on GDMT without heart failure and a heart rate greater than 70 bpm and titrated to a goal heart rate of 55 bpm to 60 bpm to test the hypothesis that reduction in heart rates would lead to a reduction in cardiovascular mortality or nonfatal MI. At 3 months, patients assigned to ivabradine had a significantly lower mean heart rate; however, there was no associated significant reduction in their primary endpoint and possibly a signal of increased risk of cardiovascular events among patients with Canadian Cardiovascular Society Class II or higher anginal symptoms.[27]

Hypertension

Zilebesiran

The renin-angiotensin-aldosterone system plays a major role in blood pressure regulation. Zilebesiran, an injectable small interfering RNA therapeutic agent has been

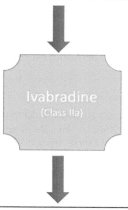

Fig. 3. Ivabradine use in heart failure with reduced ejection fraction. Summary of ivabradine use in heart failure with class of recommendation. BPM: beats per minute.

developed to reduce hepatic angiotensinogen messenger RNA production.[29–31] Currently, there has been only 1 phase 1 randomized controlled trial of zilebesiran and ambulatory blood pressure monitoring. The 4-part trial compared varying doses of zilebesiran to placebo, zilebesiran under varying salt dietary conditions, and irbesartan. The primary outcome of the study was the frequency of adverse events. Overall, single doses of zilebesiran greater than or equal to200 mg were associated with a dose-dependent reduction in blood pressure at 8 weeks, sustained for up to 24 weeks. Additionally, high salt intake attenuated the effect of zilebesiran; however, the blood pressure lowering effects were enhanced in the arm also receiving irbesartan. The study only included 107 patients, however, with promising results. There was no significant increase in adverse events in the zilebesiran arm compared to placebo, the most common being an injection site reaction. There were no reports of hypotension, hyperkalemia, or worsening of renal function resulting in medical intervention. The results of the phase 2 randomized trial (KARDIA-1) are expected to be published in early 2024.[32]

Aprocitentan

Aprocitentan, a novel dual endothelin antagonist, has been developed for the treatment of resistant hypertension.[33] Endothelin has been postulated to play a role in vasoconstriction and pathogenesis in hypertension and several prior trials have been conducted for the treatment of resistant hypertension.[34–37] A phase 3 multicenter, randomized placebo-controlled trial compared aprocitentan added to standard anti-hypertensive therapy compared to standard anti-hypertensive therapy in patients with a sitting systolic blood pressure greater than or equal to 140 despite being treated with 3 anti-hypertensive agents including a diuretic.[38] The trial consisted of 3 sequential phases of varying doses of aprocitentan. The primary endpoint was changes in office systolic blood pressure from baseline to week 4 and from withdrawal baseline to week 40, respectively. A total of 730 patients were randomized and a total of 577 patients completed the trial. The mean change in systolic blood pressure at 4 weeks was −15.3 mm Hg for aprocitentan at 12.5 mg, −15.2 mm Hg for aprocitentan at 25 mg, and −11.5 mm Hg for placebo. After 4 weeks of withdrawal, office systolic blood pressure significantly increased with placebo versus aprocitentan by a mean difference of 5.8 mm Hg. Mild fluid retention was the most reported side effect, with increasing incidence linearly with aprocitentan dosing. During the trial, a total of 11 patients died, none of which were directly attributed to aprocitentan.[38] Aprocitentan has still not been approved by the Food and Drug Administration for the treatment of resistant hypertension.

Mavacamten

Hypertrophic cardiomyopathy is an autosomal dominant condition that affects around 1:500 individuals in the United States.[39] HOCM is an entity in which there is dynamic obstruction of the left ventricular outflow tract (LVOT) that could lead to chest pain, syncope, arrhythmias, and sudden cardiac death. Treatment of HOCM has traditionally been aimed at reducing the LVOT gradient by utilizing beta-blockers, calcium channel blockers, and disopyramide. Mavacamten, a novel cardiac myosin inhibitor, has now emerged as an approved pharmacologic treatment for HOCM. Mavacamten is a selective beta-cardiac myosin ATPase inhibitor, it acts by decreasing the phosphate release from beta-cardiac myosin and also decreases the number of available actin binding heads, hence, decreasing cardiac contractility.[40,41]

Several trials have been conducted to assess the efficacy of mavacamten among patients with HOCM.[42–44] The mavacamten for treatment of symptomatic obstructive hypertrophic cardiomyopathy (EXPLORER-HCM) trial randomized patients with HOCM with a left ventricular wall thickness greater than 15 mm and an LVOT gradient greater than 50 mm Hg to mavacamten or placebo and aimed to examine the change in functional status, peak oxygen consumption, and changes in quality of life. All patients had an LVEF of at least 55% and all were at least 18 year old. At 30 weeks, patients randomized to mavacamten had significant improvements in NYHA functional class, improved peak oxygen consumption, improved post-exercise LVOT gradient, and improvements in their Kansas City cardiomyopathy questionnaire scores.[43] In the EXPOLRER-HCM trial, 11 serious adverse events occurred in the group randomized to mavacamten, while 20 adverse events occurred in the placebo group. Four patients in the mavacamten group developed a form of stress cardiomyopathy and 2 patients developed new-onset atrial fibrillation.[42] The VALOR-HCM trial was a randomized control trial of 108 patients with HOCM, randomized to either mavacamten or placebo. The study aimed to assess the safety and efficacy of mavacamten in addition to background therapy for HOCM. Patients who were randomized to mavacamten were started at 5 mg daily and titrated up according to tolerability, LVEF, and LVOT gradient. At the end of the trial, patients who received placebo were crossed over to receive 5 mg of mavacamten daily. The primary endpoint, proceeding with septal reduction therapy at week 16, for mavacamten versus placebo, was 17.9% versus 76.8% ($P<.0001$).[44]

Mavacamten should not be used among patients with an LVEF less than 55%. Additionally, routine echocardiographic surveillance is required throughout treatment to assess the LVOT and LVEF. At any time during therapy, if the LVEF drops below 50%, the drug should be discontinued.[45] Currently, mavacamten is used in patients with HOCM who have NYHA class II-III symptoms despite adequate background therapy. The European Society of Cardiology guidelines for the treatment of cardiomyopathies state that mavacamten could be considered as an add-on therapy among patients with HOCM who remain symptomatic despite optimal background therapy.[46]

SUMMARY

In summary, the last decade has seen several ground-breaking advancements in cardiovascular medicine. Several medications have revolutionized heart failure management and led to improvements in cardiovascular mortality and overall morbidity. Mavacamten, a cardiac myosin inhibitor, has been approved for the treatment of HOCM and has led to improvements in the LVOT gradient and quality of life. Promising therapies such as zilebesiran and oral aprocitentan are on the horizon for treating resistant hypertension. With these advancements in cardiovascular medicine, practitioners must be aware of the indications and complications of these therapies.

CLINICS CARE POINTS

- Novel medications for the treatment of CVD have emerged in the last 10 years and helped increase survival and reduce morbidity.
- It is important to educate patients about the importance of medications in heart failure and titrate doses of guideline medical therapy to maximal tolerated doses to derive maximal benefit
- Recognizing the need for early initiation of therapy and recognizing the side effects of GDMT is important for general medical providers.

- Newer therapies including subcutaneous injectable zilebesiran and oral aprocitentan are emerging promising therapies for resistant hypertension.
- Mavacamten, a novel cardiac myosin inhibitor, is now an approved pharmacologic treatment for HOCM.

DISCLOSURE

The authors have nothing to disclose.

REFERENCES

1. Tsao CW, Aday AW, Almarzooq ZI, et al. Heart Disease and Stroke Statistics-2023 Update: A Report From the American Heart Association. Circulation 2023; 147:e93–621.
2. Heidenreich P, Bozkurt B, Aguilar D, et al. 2022 AHA/ACC/HFSA Guideline for the Management of Heart Failure: A Report of the American College of Cardiology/American Heart Association Joint Committee on Clinical Practice Guidelines. J Am Coll Cardiol 2022;79:e263–421.
3. Heidenreich PA, Albert NM, Allen LA, et al. Forecasting the impact of heart failure in the United States: a policy statement from the American Heart Association. Circ Heart Fail 2013;6:606–19.
4. Merlo M, Pivetta A, Pinamonti B, et al. Long-term prognostic impact of therapeutic strategies in patients with idiopathic dilated cardiomyopathy: changing mortality over the last 30 years. Eur J Heart Fail 2014;16:317–24.
5. Stewart S, Ekman I, Ekman T, et al. Population impact of heart failure and the most common forms of cancer: a study of 1 162 309 hospital cases in Sweden (1988 to 2004). Circ Cardiovasc Qual Outcomes 2010;3:573–80.
6. Packer M, Anker SD, Butler J, et al. Effect of Empagliflozin on the Clinical Stability of Patients With Heart Failure and a Reduced Ejection Fraction: The EMPEROR-Reduced Trial. Circulation 2021;143:326–36.
7. McMurray JJV, Solomon SD, Inzucchi SE, et al. Dapagliflozin in Patients with Heart Failure and Reduced Ejection Fraction. N Engl J Med 2019;381:1995–2008.
8. McMurray JJ, Packer M, Desai AS, et al. Angiotensin-neprilysin inhibition versus enalapril in heart failure. N Engl J Med 2014;371:993–1004.
9. Sandhu AT, Heidenreich PA. The Affordability of Guideline-Directed Medical Therapy: Cost Sharing is a Critical Barrier to Therapy Adoption. Circulation 2021;143: 1073–5.
10. Anker SD, Butler J, Filippatos G, et al. Empagliflozin in Heart Failure with a Preserved Ejection Fraction. N Engl J Med 2021;385:1451–61.
11. Solomon SD, McMurray JJV, Claggett B, et al. Dapagliflozin in Heart Failure with Mildly Reduced or Preserved Ejection Fraction. N Engl J Med 2022;387:1089–98.
12. Zinman B, Wanner C, Lachin JM, et al. Empagliflozin, Cardiovascular Outcomes, and Mortality in Type 2 Diabetes. N Engl J Med 2015;373:2117–28.
13. Heerspink HJL, Stefánsson BV, Correa-Rotter R, et al. Dapagliflozin in Patients with Chronic Kidney Disease. N Engl J Med 2020;383:1436–46.
14. Kalra S. Sodium-glucose co-transporter-2 (SGLT2) inhibitors: A review of their basic and Clinical Pharmacology. Diabetes Therapy 2014;5:355–66.
15. Lopaschuk GD, Verma S. Mechanisms of cardiovascular benefits of sodium glucose co-transporter 2 (SGLT2) inhibitors. JACC (J Am Coll Cardiol): Basic to Translational Science 2020;5:632–44.

16. Adamson C, Docherty KF, Heerspink HJL, et al. Initial decline (DIP) in estimated glomerular filtration rate after initiation of dapagliflozin in patients with heart failure and reduced ejection fraction: Insights from DAPA-HF. Circulation 2022;146: 438–49.

17. Kasbawala K, Stamatiades GA, Majumdar SK. Fournier's Gangrene and Diabetic Ketoacidosis Associated with Sodium-Glucose Co-Transporter 2 (SGLT2) Inhibitors: Life-Threatening Complications. Am J Case Rep 2020;21:e921536.

18. Preiser J-C, Provenzano B, Mongkolpun W, et al. Perioperative management of oral glucose-lowering drugs in the patient with type 2 diabetes. Anesthesiology 2020;133:430–8.

19. Iborra-Egea O, Gálvez-Montón C, Roura S, et al. Mechanisms of action of sacubitril/valsartan on cardiac remodeling: a systems biology approach. NPJ Syst Biol Appl 2017;3:12.

20. Solomon SD, McMurray JJV, Anand IS, et al. Angiotensin-Neprilysin Inhibition in Heart Failure with Preserved Ejection Fraction. N Engl J Med 2019;381:1609–20.

21. Pfeffer MA, Claggett B, Lewis EF, et al. Angiotensin Receptor-Neprilysin Inhibition in Acute Myocardial Infarction. N Engl J Med 2021;385:1845–55.

22. Du AX, Westerhout CM, McAlister FA, et al. Titration and Tolerability of Sacubitril/Valsartan for Patients With Heart Failure in Clinical Practice. J Cardiovasc Pharmacol 2019;73:149–54.

23. Myhre PL, Vaduganathan M, Claggett B, et al. B-Type Natriuretic Peptide During Treatment With Sacubitril/Valsartan: The PARADIGM-HF Trial. J Am Coll Cardiol 2019;73:1264–72.

24. Eworuke E, Welch EC, Haug N, et al. Comparative Risk of Angioedema With Sacubitril-Valsartan vs Renin-Angiotensin-Aldosterone Inhibitors. J Am Coll Cardiol 2023;81:321–31.

25. Tse S, Mazzola N. Ivabradine (Corlanor) for Heart Failure: The First Selective and Specific I f Inhibitor. PT 2015;40:810–4.

26. Swedberg K, Komajda M, Böhm M, et al. Ivabradine and outcomes in chronic heart failure (SHIFT): a randomised placebo-controlled study. Lancet 2010;376: 875–85.

27. Fox K, Ford I, Steg PG, et al. Ivabradine in stable coronary artery disease without clinical heart failure. N Engl J Med 2014;371:1091–9.

28. Benezet-Mazuecos J, Rubio JM, Farré J, et al. Long-term outcomes of ivabradine in inappropriate sinus tachycardia patients: appropriate efficacy or inappropriate patients. Pacing Clin Electrophysiol 2013;36:830–6.

29. Kahlon T, Carlisle S, Otero Mostacero D, et al. Angiotensinogen: more than its downstream products: evidence from population studies and novel therapeutics. JACC Heart Fail 2022;10:699–713.

30. Mullick AE, Yeh ST, Graham MJ, et al. Blood pressure lowering and safety improvements with liver angiotensinogen inhibition in models of hypertension and kidney injury. Hypertension 2017;70:566–76.

31. Uijl E, Mirabito Colafella KM, Sun Y, et al. Strong and sustained antihypertensive effect of small interfering RNA targeting liver angiotensinogen. Hypertension 2019;73:1249–57.

32. Desai AS, Webb DJ, Taubel J, et al. Zilebesiran, an RNA Interference Therapeutic Agent for Hypertension. N Engl J Med 2023;389:228–38.

33. Clozel M. Aprocitentan and the endothelin system in resistant hypertension. Can J Physiol Pharmacol 2022;100:573–83.

34. Dhaun N, Goddard J, Kohan DE, et al. Role of endothelin-1 in clinical hypertension: 20 years on. Hypertension 2008;52:452–9.

35. Weber MA, Black H, Bakris G, et al. A selective endothelin-receptor antagonist to reduce blood pressure in patients with treatment-resistant hypertension: a randomised, double-blind, placebo-controlled trial. Lancet 2009;374:1423–31.

36. Nakov R, Pfarr E, Eberle S. HEAT Investigators. Darusentan: an effective endothelinA receptor antagonist for treatment of hypertension. Am J Hypertens 2002;15: 583–9.

37. Krum H, Viskoper RJ, Lacourciere Y, et al. The effect of an endothelin-receptor antagonist, bosentan, on blood pressure in patients with essential hypertension. Bosentan Hypertension Investigators. N Engl J Med 1998;338:784–90.

38. Schlaich MP, Bellet M, Weber MA, et al. Dual endothelin antagonist aprocitentan for resistant hypertension (PRECISION): a multicentre, blinded, randomised, parallel-group, phase 3 trial. Lancet 2022;400:1927–37.

39. Butzner M, Leslie DL, Cuffee Y, et al. Stable Rates of Obstructive Hypertrophic Cardiomyopathy in a Contemporary Era. Front Cardiovasc Med 2022;8:765876.

40. Dong T, Alencherry B, Ospina S, et al. Review of Mavacamten for Obstructive Hypertrophic Cardiomyopathy and Future Directions. Drug Des Devel Ther 2023;17:1097–106.

41. Kawas RF, Anderson RL, Ingle SRB, et al. A small-molecule modulator of cardiac myosin acts on multiple stages of the myosin chemomechanical cycle. J Biol Chem 2017;292:16571–7.

42. Olivotto I, Oreziak A, Barriales-Villa R, et al. Mavacamten for treatment of symptomatic obstructive hypertrophic cardiomyopathy (EXPLORER-HCM): a randomised, double-blind, placebo-controlled, phase 3 trial. Lancet 2020;396:759–69.

43. Heitner SB, Jacoby D, Lester SJ, et al. Mavacamten Treatment for Obstructive Hypertrophic Cardiomyopathy: A Clinical Trial. Ann Intern Med 2019;170:741–8.

44. Desai MY, Owens A, Wolski K, et al. Mavacamten in Patients With Hypertrophic Cardiomyopathy Referred for Septal Reduction: Week 56 Results From the VALOR-HCM Randomized Clinical Trial. JAMA Cardiol 2023;8:968–77.

45. Ho CY, Olivotto I, Jacoby D, et al. Study Design and Rationale of EXPLORER-HCM: Evaluation of Mavacamten in Adults With Symptomatic Obstructive Hypertrophic Cardiomyopathy. Circ Heart Fail 2020;13:e006853.

46. Arbelo E, Protonotarios A, Gimeno JR, et al. 2023 ESC Guidelines for the management of cardiomyopathies. Eur Heart J 2023;44:3503–626.

Infectious Disease Updates for Primary Care

Denise J. McCulloch, MD, MPH[a,b],
Paul S. Pottinger, MD, FACP, FIDSA[b,*]

KEYWORDS

- RSV • Influenza • COVID-19 • Vulvovaginal candidiasis • DoxyPEP

KEY POINTS

- Respiratory syncytial virus threatens infants and older adults, but new vaccines and a monoclonal antibody provide protection.
- Seasonal influenza remains a public health menace, but immunizations and antivirals may reduce risk of severe disease.
- COVID-19 still afflicts thousands of Americans every day—immunizations for all, and antivirals for those at highest risk, can help save lives.
- In men who have sex with men and transwomen, doxycycline taken after condomless sex may dramatically reduce the risk of syphilis and chlamydia.
- Women suffering from drug-resistant vulvovaginal candidiasis now have a safe, effective treatment option.

INFECTIOUS DISEASE UPDATES FOR PRIMARY CARE

The last year has brought exciting developments in the prevention and treatment of infectious diseases for primary care: new vaccines to prevent respiratory syncytial virus (RSV), influenza, and COVID-19; a new treatment of drug-resistant vaginal yeast infections; and—despite the increasing incidence of bacterial sexually transmitted diseases (STDs)—we also have exciting news about repurposing an old antibiotic for prevention.

RESPIRATORY VIRUS UPDATES
Introduction

Primary care providers are the front line in caring for patients with acute respiratory infections—and are also ideally positioned to help prevent them. Internists are more likely to assess vaccination status and to recommend and stock vaccines than

---

[a] Vaccine and Infectious Disease Division, Fred Hutchinson Cancer Center, 1100 Fairview Avenue North, E5-110, Seattle, WA 98109-1023, USA; [b] Department of Medicine, Division of Allergy & Infectious Diseases, University of Washington School of Medicine, Seattle, WA, USA
* Corresponding author. 1959 NE Pacific Street, Box 356130, Seattle, WA 98195.
E-mail address: abx@uw.edu
Twitter: @McCullochMD (D.J.M.); @PaulPottingerMD (P.S.P.)

Med Clin N Am 108 (2024) 965–979
https://doi.org/10.1016/j.mcna.2024.02.003
0025-7125/24/© 2024 Elsevier Inc. All rights reserved.

subspecialists.[1] Internists provide around half of all vaccination services among Medicare patients.[2] Outpatient visits for influenzalike illness account for tens of millions of outpatient visits annually.[3,4] Although the burden of illness from respiratory viruses is significant, new developments in the field provide novel measures to prevent and treat these infections.

Respiratory syncytial virus

RSV is a familiar nemesis to pediatricians, as it is the leading cause of hospitalization among US infants.[5] But it has only recently gained attention for its role in causing morbidity and mortality among adults, particularly elderly individuals and those with cardiac or pulmonary comorbidities.[6,7] Multiple studies have demonstrated a similar burden of illness from RSV and influenza,[8–10] but until recently there were no vaccines for RSV. Fortunately, new tools to protect patients from RSV have been developed (**Fig. 1**).

Prevention of respiratory syncytial virus in older adults

In 2023, the Food and Drug Administration (FDA) approved two new protein-based vaccines for RSV for adults older than 60 years. Both were shown in large phase 3 trials to be well tolerated and efficacious in preventing symptomatic RSV lower respiratory tract disease (**Table 1**).[11] A messenger RNA (mRNA) RSV vaccine is also in development, with preliminary phase 2 to 3 trial results demonstrating this vaccine to be safe and similarly efficacious (see **Table 1**).[12]

Regarding adverse events related to RSV vaccination, two categories of severe adverse events are noted for both the Pfizer and GSK vaccine products, although the absolute number of events in each of these categories was extremely small. First, both trials observed an increased number of participants with atrial fibrillation in the vaccine group, including some individuals with new-onset atrial fibrillation, although the numbers were too small to make definitive conclusions about the relationship between atrial fibrillation and the RSV vaccine. Second, trials for both vaccines observed three cases of inflammatory neurologic events, including Guillain-Barré syndrome and acute disseminated encephalomyelitis (ADEM), in individuals who received the vaccine (see **Table 1**). Both atrial fibrillation and inflammatory neurologic events will be monitored in postmarketing surveillance for both products. Until more is known about the frequency and causality of these rare adverse events, patients should be informed that these complications were seen in the vaccine trials, but at very low rates (<0.02%), and that the risk of these adverse events must be weighed against the patient's risk of severe RSV disease. Thus, rather than make a blanket recommendation for RSV vaccination among all individuals in a certain age group or risk category, the Advisory Committee on Immunization Practices (ACIP) recommended that the

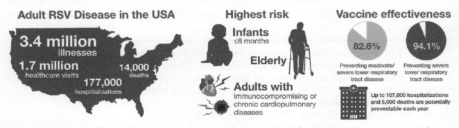

Fig. 1. Overview of RSV in America. (*From* Falsey AR, Walsh EE. Respiratory syncytial virus Prefusion F vaccine. Cell. 2023 Jul 20;186(15):3137–3137.e1. https://doi.org/10.1016/j.cell.2023.05.048. PMID: 37478816.)

Table 1
Vaccines for respiratory syncytial virus in older adults

	Arexvy (GSK)	Abrysvo (Pfizer)	mRNA-1345 (Moderna)
FDA approved at time of writing	Yes	Yes	No
Vaccine type	Adjuvanted protein–based vaccine	Unadjuvanted bivalent protein–based vaccine	mRNA vaccine
Age	Adults ≥ 60	Adults ≥ 60	Adults ≥ 60
Dosing	Single dose	Single dose	Single dose
Vaccine efficacy[a]	82.6%	85.7%	83.7%
Serious adverse events	No difference between vaccine and placebo	No difference between vaccine and placebo	No difference between vaccine and placebo
Unsolicited adverse events	Increased incidence of atrial fibrillation in vaccine group	Increased incidence of atrial fibrillation in vaccine group	—
Inflammatory neurologic events	2–3[b] events among 17,992 participants	3 events among 18,622 participants	None among 17,793 vaccinated participants

[a] Vaccine efficacy defined as efficacy against symptomatic, lab-confirmed lower respiratory disease with ≥ 2 or ≥ 3 signs/symptoms.
[b] Three events were initially reported; one was subsequently reclassified as being due to hypoglycemia and dementia rather than ADEM.[11]

decision to immunize a patient against RSV be made via a process of shared clinical decision-making, taking into account the patient's preferences and risk for severe illness.[11]

Respiratory syncytial virus prevention in infants

Before 2023, the only pharmacologic tool for RSV prevention in infants was palivizumab, a monoclonal antibody requiring monthly intramuscular injections throughout the RSV season. Because of its high cost and frequent dosing requirements, its use was limited to only the highest-risk infants. In 2023, nirsevimab, a new long-acting monoclonal antibody, was approved for prevention of RSV lower respiratory tract disease in infants as a one-time dose (**Table 2**). Because of the high efficacy, safety, and cost-effectiveness of nirsevimab compared with palivizumab, the ACIP recommends nirsevimab for all infants aged younger than 8 months who are born during or entering their first RSV season.[13]

In addition to nirsevimab, a second new measure was approved in 2023 for prevention of RSV lower respiratory disease in infants: Abrysvo, the same Pfizer RSV vaccine described earlier, given to expecting mothers during pregnancy. A trial of this vaccine in pregnancy demonstrated vaccine efficacy against medically attended severe lower respiratory tract illness in infants of 81.8% in the first 90 days after birth and 69.4% in the first 180 days (see **Table 2**).[14] Vaccine efficacy against medically attended RSV-associated lower respiratory tract illness in the first 90 days was 57.1%. In the trial, the vaccine was administered between 24 and 36 weeks gestation, and people at increased risk of preterm birth were excluded. Although it did not reach statistical significance, in the trial there were more preterm births, preeclampsia, low-birth-weight infants, and neonatal jaundice in the vaccine group compared with placebo. Postmarketing surveillance of preterm birth and hypertensive disorders of pregnancy is

Table 2
Respiratory syncytial virus prevention in infants

	Palivizumab	Nirsevimab	Abrysvo (Pfizer)
Mechanism	Passive immunization—monoclonal antibody	Passive immunization—monoclonal antibody	Immunization of birth parent during pregnancy
Dosing	Monthly during RSV season	Single dose prior to, or at the start of, RSV season	Single dose at 32–36 wk gestation
Administration	Intramuscular	Intramuscular	Intramuscular
Target population	Highest-risk infants	• All infants younger than 8 mo entering their first RSV season • Infants 8–19 mo old at increased risk of severe RSV entering their second RSV season	Pregnant people at 32–36 wk gestation
Efficacy	39%–78% reduction in hospitalization resulting from RSV[15]	79.0% vs medically attended RSV LRTI; 80.6% efficacy vs RSV LRTI hospitalization	81.8% vs severe LRTI in first 90 days 69.4% vs severe LRTI in first 180 days
Adverse effects	No significant difference from placebo	No significant difference from placebo	Potential increased risk of preterm birth and hypertensive disorders of pregnancy

planned, and the FDA approval specifies a dosing interval of 32 to 36 weeks to reduce the risk for preterm birth.

Protecting infants from respiratory syncytial virus—the bottom line

In the past year, the approvals of nirsevimab for infants and maternal immunization with Abrysvo have provided dramatic advances in infant RSV prevention. The two have not been compared head-to-head, but both provide moderate to high efficacy against severe RSV in young infants. The choice to use infant monoclonal vs maternal immunization will likely depend on cost and logistical considerations, which may differ across health systems. In situations where both are available, patients and providers may choose nirsevimab due to its more favorable side-effect profile. But, some birth parents may wish to receive an injection themselves, rather than have their infant require another injection after delivery. In either case, this is a choice of one product or the other: there is no recommendation to administer both products to protect the same child.

Diagnostics

The gold-standard test for RSV is reverse transcription polymerase chain reaction (RT-PCR) of a nasal or nasopharyngeal swab. Other commonly used tests are less sensitive and may lead to underdiagnosis: in adults, the sensitivity of rapid antigen testing compared with RT-PCR is 64%.[16] Ideally, testing of symptomatic patients would include multiplex testing for SARS-CoV-2 and influenza, as respiratory viral infections may be difficult to distinguish from one another based on symptoms alone.[17] Home-based self-testing for RSV has not yet been approved but is in development.[18]

Treatment

Unfortunately, although great advances have been made in RSV prevention, the mainstay of treatment continues to be supportive care. Studies of novel antivirals are ongoing. This makes protection of vulnerable patients through vaccination or monoclonal antibody administration all the more critical.

Challenges and areas of uncertainty

Although the development of new vaccines and monoclonals for RSV represent a tremendous step forward for RSV prevention, several areas of uncertainty remain.

- The durability of the RSV vaccine response is unknown, and whether booster doses will be needed over time has not yet been determined.
- There is scant data regarding simultaneous administration of either RSV vaccine with vaccines for influenza, SARS-CoV-2, and other indications for this age group, such as the recombinant zoster vaccine (Shingrix by GSK) and pneumococcal vaccines. Early data suggested the possibility of slightly decreased influenza immune response when coadministered with RSV,[11] whereas a subsequent study demonstrated that coadministration of influenza and RSV vaccination was safe and noninferior to administration of each vaccine alone.[19]
- Although both RSV vaccines for older adults demonstrated protection against symptomatic, lab-confirmed lower respiratory disease, these studies were not powered to provide data on efficacy against hospitalization, intensive care unit admission, or death—key metrics in understanding the value of these novel immunizations.
- With vaccine fatigue[20,21] and high levels of vaccine-related misinformation over the course of the COVID pandemic,[22] it remains to be seen how widely RSV vaccines will be used and in particular whether they will be used by the patients most vulnerable to severe disease. At the time of writing, only 17% of US adults older than 60 years have received an RSV vaccine.[23]

Influenza

Prevention

Trivalent and quadrivalent vaccines. Annual influenza vaccines are formulated to include the strains most likely to be circulating during the upcoming influenza season. Previously, the seasonal influenza vaccine was trivalent and included two influenza A strains and one influenza B strain; circulation of two influenza B strains prompted the addition of a second influenza B strain, making a quadrivalent vaccine. Trivalent vaccines were phased out in 2021 to 2022 period, with all available influenza vaccines in the United States being quadrivalent since then. However, with the shifting epidemiology of respiratory viruses during the SARS-CoV-2 pandemic, the influenza B/Yamagata strain has not been seen since March 2020. The World Health Organization and FDA have recommended that this strain be removed from future influenza vaccines; the timeline for this change is unclear.[24]

Adjuvanted, high-dose, and recombinant vaccines. Aging is associated with a decline in immune function, with increased vulnerability to infections and decreasing response to vaccinations.[25] Given the need for improved protection against influenza in elderly populations, several effective vaccine strategies have been developed for use in this age group.

The ACIP recommends that adults older than 65 years receive either high-dose inactivated influenza vaccine, recombinant influenza vaccine, or adjuvanted inactivated influenza vaccine. Large trials comparing standard dose with enhanced vaccines for older adults have demonstrated 12% to 30% higher relative efficacy for high-dose and adjuvanted vaccines.[26–29] However, if none of these is available at the time of immunization, a standard dose influenza vaccine can be given instead. Of note: a recent study also demonstrated superiority of the high-dose recombinant vaccine, compared with standard dose, in adults aged 50 to 64 years,[30] raising the possibility that in the future, high-dose vaccines could become recommended for populations younger than 65 years as well, if additional studies support this finding.

Egg allergies. Most influenza vaccines are produced in chicken eggs. Thus, until recently, individuals with severe egg allergy (symptoms other than urticaria) were recommended to be vaccinated in a medical setting "supervised by a health care provider who is able to recognize and manage severe allergic reactions." Thankfully, this is no longer the case: current ACIP guidance indicates that no additional safety precautions are needed for influenza vaccination based on an egg allergy alone, regardless of severity.[31] This recommendation is based on a significant body of evidence demonstrating that administration of live and inactivated influenza vaccines is safe in recipients with egg allergy, including those with anaphylaxis.[32]

Diagnostics
Outpatient diagnosis of influenza infection. The most recent Centers for Disease Control and Prevention guidelines for influenza recommend choosing molecular testing (PCR, nucleic acid amplification test) over rapid antigen tests whenever possible, due to low sensitivity of antigen testing.[33]

Home-based self-testing. Home-based self-swabbing for respiratory virus testing became commonplace during the SARS-CoV-2 pandemic. Until recently, testing was available only for SARS-CoV-2. However, a home-based molecular test has now been FDA approved for SARS-CoV-2 and influenza, and home-based self-testing for RSV is in development.[18] Uptake of novel tests for multiple viruses will likely depend on cost, insurance coverage, availability, and provider awareness.

Treatment
Oseltamivir remains the standard of care for treatment of influenza in most cases (**Table 3**). In 2018 baloxavir was approved in for treatment of influenza A and B infections and is another option for outpatient therapy with comparable efficacy.[34] Baloxavir is a first-in-class influenza antiviral with an enticing feature: treatment consists of just a single dose. Although there is a greater body of literature supporting the use of oseltamivir, baloxavir could be considered in certain clinical situations, such as when a single-dose regimen is needed or the patient has a history of intolerance to oseltamivir (see **Table 3**). There is also some evidence for superiority of baloxavir compared with oseltamivir for influenza B infection,[35] suggesting that preferential use in these cases may be helpful.

Influenza challenges and uncertainties
- Because of concerns for the prognosis of patients experiencing severe influenza infection and for possibility of antivirals driving drug resistance, the question has been raised whether using combination therapy would improve outcomes and/or mitigate this risk.[38] A randomized trial was conducted to answer this question but found that the combination of baloxavir plus a neuraminidase inhibitor did not improve outcomes compared with a neuraminidase inhibitor alone.[39] As a result,

Table 3
Outpatient treatment and postexposure prophylaxis for influenza

	Oseltamivir	Baloxavir
Key treatment populations	• Pregnant people • Hospitalized patients • Immunocompromised patients	• Concerns about ability to adhere to 5-day course of oseltamivir • History of adverse reaction to oseltamivir • Consider for influenza B infection—some evidence for greater efficacy than oseltamivir[35]
Dosing schedule—treatment	5-day course	Single dose
Price (approximate) for a course of treatment	$50–100 for 5-day course (generic)	$160–210 for a single dose
Most common adverse effects	Nausea, vomiting, headache	Diarrhea
Contraindications	—	Should not be used in highly immunocompromised patients due to development of resistance
Postexposure prophylaxis	• Begin within 48 hours of influenza exposure • 7-day course of once-daily dosing after last known influenza exposure	• Begin within 48 hours of influenza exposure • Single dose

Of note, although the 2011 CDC guidance suggested using double-dose oseltamivir (150 mg BID) in severely ill patients, studies have not shown benefit,[36,37] and the 2018 CDC guidelines for treatment of influenza indicate that higher doses of oseltamivir should not be routinely used.[33].

combination therapy with oseltamivir and baloxavir is not currently recommended for the routine treatment of influenza.
- Another area of uncertainty is around coadministration of vaccines for influenza, SARS-CoV-2, and RSV. Present ACIP guidance is that influenza and SARS-CoV-2 vaccines can be given at the same time, ideally in different limbs; the ACIP also indicates that the coadministration of the RSV vaccine with other vaccines is acceptable, while acknowledging that data are limited and evolving.[31]

SARS-CoV-2

Prevention
Updated 2023 to 2034 COVID-19 vaccines replaced the original and bivalent COVID vaccines. The 2023 to 2024 updated vaccine targets the XBB lineage of the Omicron variant and is more closely matched to currently circulating strains than prior versions of the vaccine. Vaccine schedules have been updated and simplified, so that receipt of a single dose of an updated COVID-19 mRNA vaccine, or two doses of a Novavax COVID-19 vaccine, is now considered fully vaccinated. In the past 2 years, however, uptake of updated vaccines has been poor, with approximately 20% of US adults receiving the 2022 to 2023 bivalent booster.[40] As of 12/1/2023, only 16% of US adults had received the 2023 to 2024 updated COVID vaccine.[41]

Diagnostics
Since the end of the official public health emergency, COVID-19 testing has become less available, with access to molecular testing (PCR) being particularly limited. Rapid antigen

tests are now widely available and have shown to be reliable for detecting the Omicron variant.[42,43] However, newer data suggest that early antigen testing may be less sensitive than it was earlier in the pandemic in populations with high rates of prior COVID-19, high rates of vaccination, or both.[44] Specifically, viral loads were found to peak at day 4 to 5 after symptom onset, with peak antigen test sensitivity on day 4. Therefore, it should be emphasized that the sensitivity of antigen testing early in the course of illness is low and that SARS-CoV-2 should not be considered "ruled out" in patients with compatible symptoms and negative antigen testing soon after symptom onset.

Treatment

A full review of the treatment of COVID-19 is beyond the scope of this article. In general: as of early 2024, because of the virulence attenuation of commonly circulating strains of SARS-CoV-2, primary care providers can thoughtfully recommend antiviral treatment of patients who are at risk of infection complications, especially those who are older than 60 years, those who are immunosuppressed, and those with chronic cardiopulmonary conditions. These patients comprise most of the 1000 to 1500 Americans who currently die of COVID-19 each week. Younger, otherwise healthy patients will almost always recover from a self-limited illness and may reasonably choose not to take antivirals. Thorough guidelines can be found on the NIH Covid Treatment Guidelines Web site https://www.covid19treatmentguidelines.nih.gov/, which includes information on outpatient evaluation, triage, and follow-up. Following is a brief summary of outpatient antivirals for patients who do not require supplemental oxygen.

Ritonavir-boosted nirmatrelvir (Paxlovid). Ritonavir-boosted nirmatrelvir is the preferred therapy for nonhospitalized patients with COVID-19 and is currently given as a 5-day course.[45] In high-risk patients treated within 3 days of symptom onset, nirmatrelvir/ritonavir (n/r) demonstrated a relative risk reduction in COVID-19–related hospitalization or death by 89%.[46] However, it is a strong CYP3A inhibitor and has significant interactions with several other drugs, which may preclude its use in some individuals. Some of these drug interactions can produce life-threatening side effects; therefore, drug interactions should be checked in all patients before treatment initiation. The University of Liverpool provides a useful tool for checking for drug interactions: https://www.covid19-druginteractions.org/checker.

However, many drug interactions can be mitigated by briefly holding or reducing doses of concomitant medications. For instance, statins, which are commonly prescribed medications in older patients with cardiovascular risk factors—a group of patients at higher risk for complications of COVID-19—interact with nirmatrelvir/ritonavir, but adverse effects from this drug interaction can be avoided as outlined in **Table 4**.

Remdesivir. For patients who cannot receive nirmatrelvir/ritonavir due to drug interactions or other reasons, the next best therapy is a 3-day course of remdesivir.[45] A randomized, double-blind, placebo controlled trial of nonhospitalized patients with COVID-19 and at least one risk factor for disease progression demonstrated that a 3-day course of intravenous remdesivir resulted in an 87% lower risk of hospitalization or death, compared with placebo.[47]

Molnupiravir. If patients cannot take nirmatrelvir/ritonavir, and remdesivir not feasible or otherwise contraindicated, high-risk patients can be prescribed molnupiravir.[45] Among nonhospitalized, high-risk, unvaccinated adults, molnupiravir reduced the risk of hospitalization or death from 9.7% to 6.8%.[48] However, a subsequent study among vaccinated high-risk adults did not show a reduction in hospitalization or death with molnupiravir.[49]

Table 4
Drug interactions between statins and nirmatrelvir/ritonavir and strategies for mitigation

Statin	Effect	Situations Where It is Safe to Stop Statin (Such as Primary Prevention)	Situations Where It is Unsafe to Stop Statin (eg, Recent MI, Secondary Prevention)
Atorvastatin	Increased atorvastatin levels due to inhibition of CYP3A4 by n/r	Stop atorvastatin during n/r; restart 3 days after the last dose	Reduce atorvastatin dose to 10 mg daily during n/r; resume normal dose 3 days after completing n/r
Rosuvastatin	Increased rosuvastatin levels due to ritonavir inhibition of drug transporters	Stop rosuvastatin during n/r (5 days)	Decrease dose to 10 mg/day during coadministration with n/r (5 day)
Simvastatin Lovastatin	Massive increase (100-fold) in simvastatin and lovastatin levels; increased risk of toxicity including rhabdomyolysis	Stop simvastatin or lovastatin at least 12 hours before starting n/r Resume 5 days after completing n/r. Concurrent administration of n/r with simvastatin or lovastatin is **contraindicated.**	Stop simvastatin or lovastatin at least 12 hours before starting n/r Resume 5 days after completing n/r. Concurrent administration of n/r with simvastatin or lovastatin is **contraindicated.**
Pravastatin	No interaction	No change	No change

Adapted from https://www.acc.org/-/media/Clinical/PDF-Files/Approved-PDFs/2022/06/24/19/07/COVID-Drug-Clinical-Bulletin.pdf. *Adapted from* https://www.covid19-druginteractions.org/checker; *Adapted from* https://www.accessdata.fda.gov/drugsatfda_docs/label/2023/217188s000lbl.pdf

Challenges and areas of uncertainty

Rebound. Although there is substantial evidence that people can experience viral and symptomatic rebound during the course of COVID-19, studies of whether this is associated with antiviral use have produced mixed results.[50,51] Although a causal role for antivirals in rebound remains to be elucidated, there is consensus that concerns about rebound should not prevent the use of antivirals in appropriate patients and that high-risk patients benefit from antiviral therapy, particularly when it is initiated early in the course of infection.[45] Whether a second course of Paxlovid for people with rebound symptoms and viremia could be effective is unknown; clinical trials are underway.[52,53]

Treatment duration. Although nirmatrelvir/ritonavir (Paxlovid) is approved as a 5-day treatment course, and this has been shown to be effective in general patient populations, there is concern that this treatment duration is insufficient in immunocompromised patients, who may experience prolonged viral replication.[54,55] A clinical trial in immunocompromised patients to compare 5, 10, and 15 days of nirmatrelvir/ritonavir is ongoing.[53]

Long COVID/postacute sequelae of COVID-19. The effects of COVID-19 may linger for months or longer. These postacute sequelae of COVID-19 (PASC) may involve any combination of body systems, often including debilitating fatigue. A substantial portion of Americans experience a constellation of issues long after their respiratory infection has resolved. In 2022, approximately 8% of respondents to a large survey indicated that they had experienced PASC, with highest burden among Hispanic respondents.[56] PASC can happen to anyone, but risk factors include unvaccinated status, older age, severe infection, and immunosuppression. The best way for patients to reduce risk of PASC is to be immunized with the latest vaccine. We have hoped that prompt antiviral treatment would reduce the risk of PASC, but this was not found in a recent survey of COVID-19 survivors.[57] No medications have FDA approval for the treatment of PASC. This condition may be very debilitating and discouraging for patients and doctors alike. The CDC offers an online resource that includes linkages to observational and clinical trials that all patients should consider joining: https://covid19.nih.gov/covid-19-topics/long-covid.

VAGINAL YEAST INFECTIONS

Vulvovaginal candidiasis (VVC) is a common complaint among women in primary care, especially among those who have recently taken antibiotics. *Candida albicans* is the leading cause, which is fortunate because most *C albicans* remains susceptible to first-line treatment. Patients usually respond promptly to treatment with a single dose of oral fluconazole or a course of topical triazole cream (eg, clotrimazole). When patients fail to improve, two main explanations should be considered:

First, the diagnosis of VVC should be confirmed. Understandably, women may mistake another vaginal discharge syndrome for "yeast." Impostors include bacterial vaginosis and sexually transmitted infections such as trichomoniasis and gonorrhea—none of which will respond to triazoles.

Second, if VVC is confirmed, fluconazole resistance should be ruled out using culture and sensitivity of a vaginal swab or fluid specimen. Often, Candida species such as glabrata will be partially resistant to fluconazole and the topical triazoles—these cases can be stubborn and often require repeated courses of compounded or OTC boric acid suppositories. In 2022, the FDA approved a new treatment option for these patients: ibrexafungerp. This is a novel triterpenoid antifungal that blocks glucan synthesis in most yeast species, including *Candida glabrata*. Prescribers may think of this as an "oral echinocandin." A 1-day course is highly efficacious in most women suffering from drug-resistant VVC, and the drug is well tolerated (with gastrointestinal upset in 10%–15% of patients).[58] Ibrexafungerp should only be used when first-line treatments have failed, not only to preserve their spectrum of activity over time but also because of the high cost of this medication, approximately $500 to $600.

SEXUALLY TRANSMITTED INFECTION PREVENTION USING DOXYCYCLINE

The incidence of sexually transmitted infections (STIs) such as syphilis, chlamydia, and gonorrhea has increased strikingly in recent years.[59] Two recent studies demonstrated a substantial reduction in risk of these bacterial infections among men who have sex with men and transgender women, by simply taking a dose of doxycycline after condomless sex. In the DoxyPEP trial,[60] people with elevated risk of acquiring STIs (some living with HIV, others participating in HIV preexposure prophylaxis) were randomized to swallow 200 mg of doxycycline postexposure prophylaxis within 72 hours following condomless sex or to receive usual care. Both groups underwent STI testing at least every 3 months and were followed-up for a year. The overall incidence of a bacterial STI among doxycycline recipients was 24% versus 48% among those receiving standard of care. Another trial called Doxyvac[61] reached similar conclusions. Based on these findings, the CDC encourages primary care providers to discuss benefits and risks of this strategy with their patients.[62] Some talking points to consider are as follows:

- Doxycycline postexposure prophylaxis (PEP) should be taken within 24 hours of condomless sex if at all possible—there may still be benefit if taken any time within 72 hours. Benefits beyond that time are unlikely.
- Even in the doxycycline PEP arm, there was still an alarmingly high (although lower) rate of STIs. In other words, doxycycline PEP was beneficial but certainly not perfect. Therefore, men who have sex with men and transgender women who try it should continue to be carefully monitored for STI acquisition, including screening at least every 3 months.
- Cisgender women and men who have sex with women were not included in these trials. Unfortunately, a well-designed trial focused on protecting women at high risk from STIs using the same protocol recently failed to detect benefit.[63] If such patients are eager to try this technique, that decision can be individualized in light of specific risk factors and preferences, but they should understand that current evidence is against this practice.
- Either doxycycline monohydrate or hyclate may be used. In either case, patients should avoid consuming calcium-rich foods or vitamins within 2 hours of their dose. As always, this medication should be taken with plenty of water to reduce risk of nausea and esophagitis. Recipients may develop photosensitivity.
- There is a concern that doxycycline PEP may result in the development of drug-resistant microbes such as methicillin-resistant *Staphylococcus aureus* and *Neisseria gonorrhea*. While colleagues at CDC grapple with this public health question, clinicians talking with their patients should balance this theoretic issue with the potential harms (including accelerated drug resistance) associated with the increased overall antibiotic consumption among those who develop bacterial STIs.

DISCLOSURE

Dr P.S. Pottinger has nothing to disclose. Dr D.J. McCulloch has nothing to disclose.

REFERENCES

1. Lutz CS, Kim DK, Black CL, et al. Clinicians' and Pharmacists' Reported Implementation of Vaccination Practices for Adults. Am J Prev Med 2018;55(3):308–18.
2. Wilkinson E, Jetty A, Petterson S, et al. Primary Care's Historic Role in Vaccination and Potential Role in COVID-19 Immunization Programs. Ann Fam Med 2021; 19(4):351–5.
3. Molinari N-AM, Ortega-Sanchez IR, Messonnier ML, et al. The annual impact of seasonal influenza in the US: Measuring disease burden and costs. Vaccine 2007;25(27):5086–96.
4. Matias G, Haguinet F, Lustig RL, et al. Model estimates of the burden of outpatient visits attributable to influenza in the United States. BMC Infect Dis 2016; 16(1):641.
5. Suh M, Movva N, Jiang X, et al. Respiratory Syncytial Virus Is the Leading Cause of United States Infant Hospitalizations, 2009-2019: A Study of the National (Nationwide) Inpatient Sample. J Infect Dis 2022;226(Suppl 2):S154–63.
6. Prasad N, Walker TA, Waite B, et al. Respiratory Syncytial Virus-Associated Hospitalizations Among Adults With Chronic Medical Conditions. Clin Infect Dis 2021; 73(1):e158–63.
7. Tseng HF, Sy LS, Ackerson B, et al. Severe Morbidity and Short- and Mid- to Long-term Mortality in Older Adults Hospitalized with Respiratory Syncytial Virus Infection. J Infect Dis 2020;222(8):1298–310.

8. Ambrosch A, Luber D, Klawonn F, et al. Focusing on severe infections with the respiratory syncytial virus (RSV) in adults: Risk factors, symptomatology and clinical course compared to influenza A/B and the original SARS-CoV-2 strain. J Clin Virol 2023;161:105399. https://doi.org/10.1016/j.jcv.2023.105399.

9. Ackerson B, Tseng HF, Sy LS, et al. Severe Morbidity and Mortality Associated With Respiratory Syncytial Virus Versus Influenza Infection in Hospitalized Older Adults. Clin Infect Dis 2019;69(2):197–203.

10. Falsey AR, Hennessey PA, Formica MA, et al. Respiratory syncytial virus infection in elderly and high-risk adults. N Engl J Med 2005;352(17):1749–59.

11. Melgar M, Britton A, Roper LE, et al. Use of Respiratory Syncytial Virus Vaccines in Older Adults: Recommendations of the Advisory Committee on Immunization Practices - United States, 2023. MMWR Morb Mortal Wkly Rep 2023;72(29): 793–801.

12. Wilson E, Goswami J, Baqui AH, et al. Efficacy and Safety of an mRNA-Based RSV PreF Vaccine in Older Adults. N Engl J Med 2023;389(24):2233–44.

13. Jones JM, Fleming-Dutra KE, Prill MM, et al. Use of Nirsevimab for the Prevention of Respiratory Syncytial Virus Disease Among Infants and Young Children: Recommendations of the Advisory Committee on Immunization Practices - United States, 2023. MMWR Morb Mortal Wkly Rep 2023;72(34):920–5.

14. Kampmann B, Madhi SA, Munjal I, et al. Bivalent prefusion f vaccine in pregnancy to prevent rsv illness in infants. N Engl J Med 2023;388(16):1451–64.

15. Group TI RS. Palivizumab, a Humanized respiratory syncytial virus monoclonal antibody, reduces hospitalization from respiratory syncytial virus infection in high-risk infants. Pediatrics 1998;102(3):531–7.

16. Onwuchekwa C, Moreo LM, Menon S, et al. Underascertainment of Respiratory Syncytial Virus Infection in Adults Due to Diagnostic Testing Limitations: A Systematic Literature Review and Meta-analysis. J Infect Dis 2023;228(2):173–84.

17. McCulloch DJ, Rogers JH, Wang Y, et al. Respiratory syncytial virus and other respiratory virus infections in residents of homeless shelters - King County, Washington, 2019-2021. Influenza Other Respir Viruses 2023;17(6):e13166. https://doi.org/10.1111/irv.13166.

18. Adalja AA. At-home infectious disease testing: An idea whose time has come. Antimicrobial Stewardship & Healthcare Epidemiology 2022;2(1):e170.

19. Athan E, Baber J, Quan K, et al. Safety and immunogenicity of bivalent RSVpreF vaccine coadministered with seasonal inactivated influenza vaccine in older adults. Clin Infect Dis 2023. https://doi.org/10.1093/cid/ciad707.

20. Su Z, Cheshmehzangi A, McDonnell D, et al. Mind the "Vaccine Fatigue". Front Immunol 2022;13:839433.

21. Barouch DH. Covid-19 Vaccines — Immunity, Variants, Boosters. N Engl J Med 2022;387(11):1011–20.

22. Lee SK, Sun J, Jang S, et al. Misinformation of COVID-19 vaccines and vaccine hesitancy. Sci Rep 2022;12(1):13681.

23. Vaccination Trends—Adults. Centers for Disease Control and Prevention. 2023. Available at: https://www.cdc.gov/respiratory-viruses/data-research/dashboard/vaccination-trends-adults.html#:~:text=The%20percent%20of%20adults%20age,%25%20. [Accessed 18 December 2023].

24. Information for the 2023-2024 Flu Season. Centers for Disease Control and Prevention, National Center for Immunization and Respiratory Diseases (NCIRD). 2023. Available at: https://www.cdc.gov/flu/season/faq-flu-season-2023-2024.htm. [Accessed 6 December 2023].

25. Haq K, McElhaney JE. Immunosenescence: Influenza vaccination and the elderly. Curr Opin Immunol. Aug 2014;29:38–42.

26. DiazGranados CA, Dunning AJ, Kimmel M, et al. Efficacy of high-dose versus standard-dose influenza vaccine in older adults. N Engl J Med 2014;371(7): 635–45.

27. Dunkle LM, Izikson R, Patriarca P, et al. Efficacy of Recombinant Influenza Vaccine in Adults 50 Years of Age or Older. N Engl J Med 2017;376(25):2427–36.

28. Izurieta HS, Thadani N, Shay DK. Corrections. Comparative effectiveness of high-dose versus standard-dose influenza vaccines in US residents aged 65 years and older from 2012 to 2013 using Medicare data: a retrospective cohort analysis. Lancet Infect Dis 2015;15(3):263.

29. McElhaney JE, Beran J, Devaster JM, et al. AS03-adjuvanted versus non-adjuvanted inactivated trivalent influenza vaccine against seasonal influenza in elderly people: a phase 3 randomised trial. Lancet Infect Dis 2013;13(6):485–96.

30. Hsiao A, Yee A, Fireman B, et al. Recombinant or Standard-Dose Influenza Vaccine in Adults under 65 Years of Age. N Engl J Med 2023;389(24):2245–55.

31. Grohskopf LABL, Ferdinands JM, Chung JR, et al. Prevention and Control of Seasonal Influenza with Vaccines: Recommendations of the Advisory Committee on Immunization Practices — United States, 2023–24 Influenza Season. MMWR Recomm Rep (Morb Mortal Wkly Rep) 2023;72.

32. Greenhawt M, Turner PJ, Kelso JM. Administration of influenza vaccines to egg allergic recipients: A practice parameter update 2017. Ann Allergy Asthma Immunol 2018;120(1):49–52.

33. Uyeki TM, Bernstein HH, Bradley JS, et al. Clinical Practice Guidelines by the Infectious Diseases Society of America: 2018 Update on Diagnosis, Treatment, Chemoprophylaxis, and Institutional Outbreak Management of Seasonal Influenzaa. Clin Infect Dis 2019;68(6):895–902.

34. Hayden FG, Sugaya N, Hirotsu N, et al. Baloxavir Marboxil for Uncomplicated Influenza in Adults and Adolescents. N Engl J Med 2018;379(10):913–23.

35. Ison MG, Portsmouth S, Yoshida Y, et al. Early treatment with baloxavir marboxil in high-risk adolescent and adult outpatients with uncomplicated influenza (CAPSTONE-2): a randomised, placebo-controlled, phase 3 trial. Lancet Infect Dis 2020;20(10):1204–14.

36. Lee N, Hui DSC, Zuo Z, et al. A Prospective Intervention Study on Higher-Dose Oseltamivir Treatment in Adults Hospitalized With Influenza A and B Infections. Clin Infect Dis 2013;57(11):1511–9.

37. Effect of double dose oseltamivir on clinical and virological outcomes in children and adults admitted to hospital with severe influenza: double blind randomised controlled trial. BMJ 2013;346:f3039.

38. Dunning J, Baillie JK, Cao B, et al, International Severe Acute Respiratory and Emerging Infection Consortium ISARIC. Antiviral combinations for severe influenza. Lancet Infect Dis 2014;14(12):1259–70.

39. Kmeid J, Vanichanan J, Shah DP, et al. Outcomes of Influenza Infections in Hematopoietic Cell Transplant Recipients: Application of an Immunodeficiency Scoring Index. Biol Blood Marrow Transplant 2016;22(3):542–8.

40. COVID-19 vaccinations in the United States. Centers for Disease Control and Prevention; 2023. Available at: https://covid.cdc.gov/covid-data-tracker. [Accessed 6 December 2023].

41. Vaccination Trends—Adults. Centers for Disease Control and Prevention. 2023. https://www.cdc.gov/respiratory-viruses/data-research/dashboard/vaccination-trends-adults.html. [Accessed 6 December 2023].

42. Stanley S, Hamel DJ, Wolf ID, et al. Limit of Detection for Rapid Antigen Testing of the SARS-CoV-2 Omicron and Delta Variants of Concern Using Live-Virus Culture. J Clin Microbiol 2022;60(5):001400.

43. Soni A, Herbert C, Filippaios A, et al. Comparison of Rapid Antigen Tests' Performance Between Delta and Omicron Variants of SARS-CoV-2. Ann Intern Med 2022;175(12):1685–92.

44. Frediani JK, Parsons R, McLendon KB, et al. The New Normal: Delayed Peak SARS-CoV-2 Viral Loads Relative to Symptom Onset and Implications for COVID-19 Testing Programs. Clin Infect Dis 2023. https://doi.org/10.1093/cid/ciad582.

45. Therapeutic management of nonhospitalized adults with COVID-19. National Institutes of Health; 2023. Available at: https://www.covid19treatmentguidelines. nih.gov/management/clinical-management-of-adults/nonhospitalized-adults–therapeutic-management/. [Accessed 22 December 2023].

46. Hammond J, Leister-Tebbe H, Gardner A, et al. Oral Nirmatrelvir for High-Risk, Nonhospitalized Adults with Covid-19. N Engl J Med 2022;386(15):1397–408.

47. Gottlieb RL, Vaca CE, Paredes R, et al. Early Remdesivir to Prevent Progression to Severe Covid-19 in Outpatients. N Engl J Med 2021;386(4):305–15.

48. Jayk Bernal A, Gomes da Silva MM, Musungaie DB, et al. Molnupiravir for Oral Treatment of Covid-19 in Nonhospitalized Patients. N Engl J Med 2021;386(6): 509–20.

49. Butler CC, Hobbs FDR, Gbinigie OA, et al. Molnupiravir plus usual care versus usual care alone as early treatment for adults with COVID-19 at increased risk of adverse outcomes (PANORAMIC): an open-label, platform-adaptive randomised controlled trial. Lancet 2023;401(10373):281–93.

50. Edelstein GE, Boucau J, Uddin R, et al. SARS-CoV-2 Virologic Rebound With Nirmatrelvir–Ritonavir Therapy. Ann Intern Med 2023;176(12):1577–85.

51. Harrington PR, Cong J, Troy SB, et al. Evaluation of SARS-CoV-2 RNA Rebound After Nirmatrelvir/Ritonavir Treatment in Randomized, Double-Blind, Placebo-Controlled Trials - United States and International Sites, 2021-2022. MMWR Morb Mortal Wkly Rep 2023;72(51):1365–70.

52. A study to learn about a repeat 5-day treatment with the study medicines (called nirmatrelvir/ritonavir) in people 12 Years old or older with return of COVID-19 symptoms and SARS-CoV-2 positivity after finishing treatment with nirmatrelvir/ritonavir. National Library of Medicine; 2023. Available at: https://clinicaltrials.gov/study/NCT05567952?cond=COVID&term=paxlovid&locStr=USA&country=United%20States&distance=50&page=2&rank=11. [Accessed 18 December 2023].

53. A Study to Learn About the Study Medicines (Nirmatrelvir Plus Ritonavir) in People Aged 12 Years or Older With COVID-19 and a Compromised Immune System. 2023. Available at: https://clinicaltrials.gov/study/NCT05438602?cond=immunocompromised&intr=nirmatrelvir%2F%20ritonavir&rank=2&tab=table. [Accessed 22 December 2023].

54. Baang JH, Smith C, Mirabelli C, et al. Prolonged Severe Acute Respiratory Syndrome Coronavirus 2 Replication in an Immunocompromised Patient. J Infect Dis 2020;223(1):23–7.

55. Avanzato VA, Matson MJ, Seifert SN, et al. Case Study: Prolonged Infectious SARS-CoV-2 Shedding from an Asymptomatic Immunocompromised Individual with Cancer. Cell 2020;183(7):1901–12.e9.

56. Adjaye-Gbewonyo D, Vahratian A, Perrine CG, Bertolli J. Long COVID in Adults: United States, 2022. NCHS Data Brief. 2023;(480):1-8.

57. Durstenfeld MS, Peluso MJ, Lin F, et al. Association of nirmatrelvir for acute SARS-CoV-2 infection with subsequent Long COVID symptoms in an observational cohort study. J Med Virology 2024. https://doi.org/10.1002/jmv.29333.
58. Jallow S, Govender NP. Ibrexafungerp: A First-in-Class Oral Triterpenoid Glucan Synthase Inhibitor. J Fungi 2021.
59. https://www.cdc.gov/nchhstp/newsroom/fact-sheets/std/std-us-2021.html
60. Luetkemeyer AF, Donnell D, Dombrowski JC, et al. Postexposure Doxycycline to Prevent Bacterial Sexually Transmitted Infections. New England J Medicine 2023 Apr 6;388(14):1296–306.
61. Molina JM, Bercot B, Assoumou A, et al. ANRS 174 Doxyvac: an open-label randomized trial to prevent STIs IN MSM ON PrEP. Conference on Retroviruses and Opportunistic Infections February 2023. Available at: https://www.croiconference.org/abstract/anrs-174-doxyvac-an-open-label-randomized-trial-to-prevent-stis-in-msm-on-prep/.
62. https://www.cdc.gov/std/treatment-guidelines/clinical-primary.htm#CautionsFor DoxyPEP
63. Stewart J, Oware K, Donnell D, et al. Doxycycline postexposure prophylaxis for prevention of stis among cisgender women. Conference on Retroviruses and Opportunistic Infections February 2023. Available at: https://www.croiconference.org/abstract/doxycycline-postexposure-prophylaxis-for-prevention-of-stis-among-cisgender-women/.

Advances in Outpatient Therapies and Treatment of Benign Prostatic Hyperplasia

A Comprehensive Review for Men's Health

Talia A. Helman, MD[a],*, Brendan M. Browne, MD, MS[a]

KEYWORDS

- Prostatic hyperplasia • Lower urinary tract symptoms • Treatment • Therapies

KEY POINTS

- Benign prostatic hyperplasia is a condition that affects a majority of men at some point throughout their lives.
- Prostate growth causes bladder outlet obstruction and leads to bothersome lower urinary tract symptoms.
- Enucleation (either anatomic endoscopic enucleation of prostate or robotic simple prostatectomy) provides lowest retreatment rates and best chance of eliminating catheter-dependence.

INTRODUCTION AND DEFINITION

Benign prostatic hyperplasia (BPH) is a condition that affects a majority of men at some point throughout their life. Prostate growth causes bladder outlet obstruction and leads to bothersome lower urinary tract symptoms (LUTS). BPH/LUTS is one of the most common conditions of aging men with over 70% of men over 70 having symptoms[1] and can negatively impact their quality of life (QoL). Treatments include behavioral modifications, medications, and surgical treatments, with considerable recent advances particularly in the procedural options for BPH, which is the focus of this review.

Pretreatment Assessment

Patient comorbidities, severity of symptoms, and outcome priorities should be assessed prior to embarking on treatment, particularly as some newer treatments

a Division of Urology, Department of Surgery, Emory University, 1365 Clifton Road NorthEast, Building B 1st Floor, Suite 1400, Atlanta, GA 30322, USA
* Corresponding author. Emory University, 1365 Clifton Road NorthEast, Building B 1st Floor, Suite 1400, Atlanta, GA 30322.
E-mail address: thelman@emory.edu

Med Clin N Am 108 (2024) 981–991
https://doi.org/10.1016/j.mcna.2024.03.009
0025-7125/24/© 2024 Elsevier Inc. All rights reserved.

excel in certain outcome domains at the expense of others. It is helpful to quantify baseline symptoms—done with the International Prostate Symptom Score (IPSS), which scores symptom severity (ie, frequency, urgency, etc.) and QoL. Additionally, physicians should evaluate comorbidities that may worsen urinary symptoms, for example, uncontrolled diabetes causing frequency or sleep apnea worsening nocturia.

When considering invasive procedures, treatment should be tailored to the size of the prostate and patient-specific factors. Prostate size often correlates with clinical success and retreatment rates, with larger prostates having higher rates of retreatment for some procedures. Prostate sizing with transrectal or abdominal ultrasound, computed tomography, MRI, or cystoscopy helps select appropriate treatment. For small-to-average prostates most surgical options are viable, however, once the prostate grows greater than 80 g some treatments become less efficacious and should be avoided. Additional factors, such as anticoagulation (AC) status, prior prostate surgery, degree of bladder dysfunction, and patient's desire to maintain normal ejaculatory function can help guide treatment selection.

Pharmacologic Therapy

Medication is a common early treatment for BPH, with the goal of alleviating symptoms, improving bladder emptying, and preventing disease progression. Classes of medication for treatment of BPH/LUTS include

- α-adrenergic antagonists (alpha blockers)
- 5-α reductase inhibitors (5-ARIs)
- Phosphodiesterase-5 (PDE-5) inhibitors
- Anticholinergics
- β3-adrenergic agonists (beta agonists)

Alpha-blockers and 5-ARIs have been used for LUTS for decades, with notable improvements in IPSS, but known adverse effects (AEs) of orthostasis, retrograde ejaculation (RE), ejaculatory dysfunction (EjD), and decreased libido. These AEs are uncommon, and these medications are widely used in treatment of LUTS. Terazosin and doxazosin are non-selective alpha blockers with increased incidence of systemic AE, particularly orthostasis. Newer generation alpha blockers, tamsulosin and silodosin, directly target alpha-1a receptors decreasing orthostasis and reducing risk of falls. Negatively, increased alpha-1 selectivity has higher likelihood of causing RE, alfuzosin has demonstrated reduced risk for those looking to preserve ejaculatory function. Combining alpha-blockers and 5-ARIs (finasteride or dutasteride) is considered safe for enhanced efficacy and reduction of LUTS progression, especially for larger prostates and persistent symptoms on monotherapy.

In the early 2000s, PDE-5 inhibitors were added to the treatment armamentarium for LUTS. Tadalafil (5 mg daily) decreases IPSS by 6 points and offers simultaneous treatment for BPH and erectile dysfunction (ED).[2] PDE-5 inhibitors can also be used safely in combination with alpha-blockers with minimal additional AE, including back pain, headache, nasopharyngitis, and upper respiratory tract infection.[3]

Historically, clinicians have been hesitant to use anticholinergic medications for BPH/LUTS due to fear of acute urinary retention (AUR). However, anticholinergics and newly approved β3 agonists—mirabegron and vibegron—have demonstrated safe and effective for men with predominant overactive symptoms (eg, frequency, urgency)[4] even with enlarged prostates.[5] Post-void residual should be monitored to ensure no chronic retention develops. β3 agonists are particularly useful in older men to avoid the risk of dementia from anticholinergics.[6] Mirabegron (25–50 mg daily) and Vibegron can be cost prohibitive to patients, however, most insurances will cover if a patient has trialed and not tolerated an anticholinergic for overactive bladder or who have a clinical reason to avoid anticholinergics (eg, dementia).

Surgical Treatment

The availability and low morbidity of medication has led to a reduction surgery; however, many men still undergo surgical treatment for BPH. Indications for surgical treatment can be disease or patient factors:

Disease Factors	Patient Factors
• Renal insufficiency from bladder outlet obstruction • Refractory urinary retention • Recurrent urinary tract infections (UTIs) • Bladder stones • Gross hematuria from BPH	• Persistent LUTS despite medication • Medication AEs • Patient preference to avoid long-term medication

Surgical treatment modalities for BPH range from maximally invasive, open simple prostatectomy (OSP) to contemporary robotic approaches, transurethral treatments in the operating room, and minimally invasive surgical techniques (MISTs). Significant advances within the past decade allow treatment to be tailored to specific patient anatomy and personal preferences.

Endoscopic Resection and Vaporization

Transurethral Resection of Prostate (TURP) remains the most frequently utilized procedure due to its effectiveness with a range of prostate sizes and widely available equipment. The procedure works well for moderate-to-severe LUTS, achieving an average IPSS reduction of 17 points at 1 year postop. Return of symptoms can occur with time, as any residual adenoma grows to cause repeat obstruction. Five year surgical retreatment rates for TURP range from 5% to 17%.[7,8] AEs are similar to those of other transurethral surgery with low risk of urinary incontinence (1%), urethral stricture (1%–2%), and postoperative AUR (3%).[8] ED is generally not impacted by TURP, but EjD is common, reported in 45% to 90% across different series.

New electrodes including a rollerball, vaportrode, and most recently plasma button have been developed that allow for Transurethral Vaporization of the Prostate (TUVP), simultaneously destroying adenoma and cauterizing blood vessels, speeding treatment compared to TURP which requires first-pass cut followed by coagulation. Symptom improvement, reoperation rates, and transfusion rates are comparable to TURP.[9] Since these procedures were long the only options, guidelines offer no size criteria for TURP or TUVP and in skilled hands larger prostates (> 80 g) can be effectively treated.

Prostatic Laser Ablation

Surgical lasers for BPH management have further revolutionized treatment. The Nd:YAG laser was the first introduced in the 1990s, but it caused persistent irritative voiding symptoms from deep tissue penetration.[10] After several iterations, the Greenlight (KTP) laser was developed, whose wavelength is preferentially absorbed by hemoglobin, improving hemostasis and decreasing tissue penetration, producing the technique of photovaporization of prostate (PVP). The GOLIATH trial comparing PVP to TURP in prostates greater than 80 g found an equivalent reduction in IPSS scores by 7 points at 6 months posttreatment.[11] Five year retreatment rates for PVP are reported at 8.9%, comparable to TURP.[12]

Recent development of holmium and thulium technology moved these lasers to the forefront of urologic surgery, serving as multiuse platforms for both prostate and kidney stone treatment. With shallower depth of penetration than KTP lasers, holmium and thulium are more accurate with less irritative tissue effect, enabling their use for prostate ablation and enucleation.[13]

Prostate Enucleation

The anatomy of the prostate includes 3 distinct zones: peripheral, central, and transition (**Fig. 1**). The transition zone is responsible for urinary obstruction and is contained by a pseudocapsule, offering an identifiable surgical plane. Enucleation dissects the transition zone circumferentially along the pseudocapsule to maximally open the urine channel. This approach was originally performed via open surgery (ie, "simple prostatectomy"), but now is commonly approached cystoscopically or robotically.

Anatomic Endoscopic Enucleation of Prostate

Anatomic endoscopic enucleation of prostate (AEEP) secured its place for BPH treatment in the form of holmium laser enucleation of prostate (HoLEP) in 1990s.[14] This approach can use any number of energy sources, including holmium, thulium, greenlight laser, or bipolar electrocautery to remove the entire prostate transition zone with a scope.

HoLEP has the longest experience and consistently reports less bleeding, shorter catheter times, and shorter hospital stay than other resection techniques.[15] A meta-analysis of almost 70 randomized controlled trials comparing HoLEP, TURP, and PVP found HoLEP to have superior symptom improvement.[16] Improvement in voiding symptoms is supported by urodynamics studies showing superior voiding pressure and flow rates for HoLEP compared with TURP.[17] Moreover, enucleation is ideal for

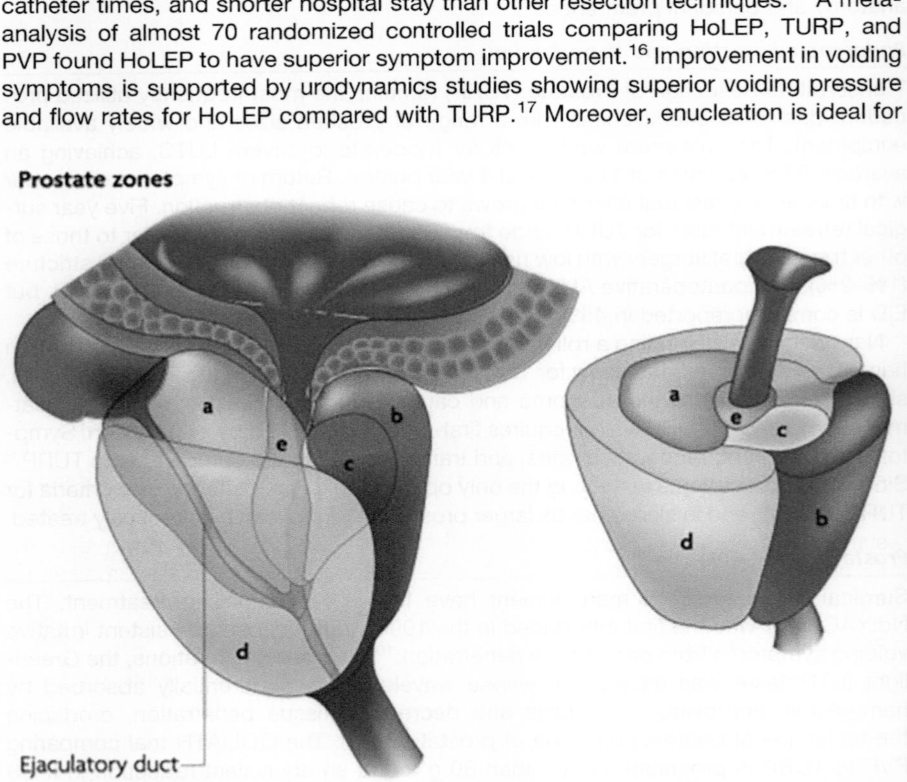

Prostate zones

Ejaculatory duct

Fig. 1. Prostate zones: (a) central zone, (b) fibromuscular zone, (c) transitional zone, (d) peripheral zone, and (e) periurethral gland region. (Reprinted with permission from De Marzo, A.M., et al., Inflammation in prostate carcinogenesis. Nat Rev Cancer, 2007. 7(4): p. 256-69.eMarzo et. al.)

catheter-dependent patients; for men with any degree of bladder contractility preoperatively, 89% to 98% are catheter-free post-HoLEP. Men with entirely acontractile bladders are still 62% catheter free, likely via valsalva voiding.[18]

AEs of HoLEP are comparable to TURP with 0% to 2% transfusion rates and AUR, short-term urinary incontinence is seen in approximately 5% of patients.[7] ED is largely unchanged, but AEEP has high rates of EjD, reporting 70% to 92%.[19] New ejaculation-preserving techniques have been described, decreasing the rate to 5% to 27%,[19] more consistent with other transurethral procedures. HoLEP or ThuLEP can be performed on anticoagulated patients, with meta-analysis of patients on AC undergoing HoLEP showing no increased AE.[20]

AEEP is the most durable of all transurethral outlet procedures. Long-term follow-up showed 0.7% retreatment for BPH/LUTS at 10 years following HoLEP.[21] Enucleation is size independent, showing efficacy with prostate size even greater than 300 g without increasing catheterization time, hospital stay, or complications.[22] Critics of AEEP often site the difficult learning curve, but its utilization is growing, likely driven by superior outcomes.[23] Furthermore, since the COVID pandemic, there is growing adoption of same-day catheter removal and discharge, advancing the frontier for this procedure.

Surgical Prostate Enucleation

The advent of the DaVinci Robotic system (Intuitive Technologies, Sunnyvale, California, USA) transitioned the traditional OSP into the twenty-first century. Robotic simple prostatectomy (RSP) follows the same surgical planes, but now done with pneumoperitoneum that reduces bleeding and transfusion rates.[24] RSP shows similar improvement in urinary parameters as HoLEP and can also easily manage prostates greater than 100 g.[25] The standard RSP is done transabdominal, opening the bladder to access the prostate, the downside being longer catheter duration and hospital stay compared with HoLEP.

The new, single-port robotic system is designed to function in smaller spaces, allowing transvesical simple prostatectomy. Here resection is performed exclusively within the bladder, never entering the peritoneum. Early reports show this approach to be safe and effective, with decreased blood loss, decreased opioid use, and minimal postoperative incontinence (3%) compared with OSP[26] and similar safety outcomes to HoLEP.[27]

Minimally Invasive Surgical Techniques

Surgical intervention for BPH has markedly shifted toward less-invasive techniques that aim to reduce patient discomfort and inconvenience while providing effective symptom relief. MISTs have increased in utilization over the past decade, especially for men with medical comorbidities or men who prefer less-invasive, outpatient procedures, often with only local anesthesia.

Prostatic Urethral Lift

The US Food and Drug Administration (FDA)-approved prostatic urethral lift (PUL), commercially available as UroLift (Teleflex, Pleasanton, CA) in 2013. The placement of transprostatic nonabsorbable implants widens the prostatic lumen without resecting prostatic tissue. In the L.I.F.T. study, PUL was compared against sham (ie, cystoscopy alone) in prostates of 30 to 80 g without a median lobe; PUL was found to be superior to sham in improved IPSS of 11 points at 1 year, but its efficacy lost impact at 5 year follow up (though symptoms were still improved from baseline).[28] When compared against TURP, PUL was inferior for IPSS reduction at 12 and 24 month follow-up.[29] PUL demonstrates higher 5 year retreatment rates than other modalities with 10% to 20% requiring additional surgery.[12,30]

PUL has minimal impact on ED or EjD,[28] which can be attractive to patients. While observational studies have demonstrated efficacy in larger prostates and/or treatment of median lobes,[31] current guidelines recommend PUL only in patients with prostate volume of 30 to 80 g without an obstructing median lobe. PUL is relatively well tolerated and safe, with main AEs being mild dysuria, hematuria, and urinary urgency. Unfortunately, UroLift clips can interfere with prostate MRI,[32] which may not be ideal for patients at high risk for prostate cancer or those on active surveillance.

Water Vapor Thermal Therapy

Water vapor thermal therapy (WVTT), commercially available as Rezum (Boston Scientific, Marlborough, MA), delivers steam directly into the prostate adenoma, inducing coagulative necrosis to reduce prostate size. This platform was approved by the FDA in 2015 for prostates of 30 to 80 g with or without a median lobe. Using transurethral lidocaine lubricant and pudendal nerve block, this procedure is commonly done without general anesthesia (GA), frequently in a clinic or ambulatory cystoscopy setting. The steam initially induces prostate swelling and therefore a Foley catheter is needed for a few days following treatment.

In a study of WVTT versus sham surgery for prostates of 30 80 g, 5-year follow-up showed sustained symptom relief for WVTT, with IPSS more than 11 points below pretreatment (50% reduction from baseline compared to 20% for sham, $P < .0001$).[33] WVTT offers the ability to treat patients in the office and those with a median lobe, an advantage over PUL. Procedural AEs were minimal, including dysuria, hematuria, frequency, urgency, and hematospermia which resolved within 3 weeks. Surgical retreatment is also low, at 4.4% after 5 years,[33] which makes WVTT one of the more cost-effective MISTs.

Temporarily Implanted Prostatic Devices

Temporarily implanted prostatic device (TIPD), commercially available as iTind (Olympus, Hadera, Israel), is a small, nitinol metal frame temporarily implanted into the prostatic urethra. This outward force leads to compressive necrosis and tissue loss. iTind is placed under conscious sedation and left in place for 5 to 7 days to achieve desired effect, then removed in the office with a retrieval string and catheter.

This device is new and has only early clinical data, but current guidelines support its use for prostates between 25 and 75 g, without a median lobe.[5] When compared with sham, TIPD had a greater percentage of patients with 7 or greater point IPSS improvement (72.6% vs 50%, $P = .048$), but the entire cohort IPSS reduction for TIPD was not statistically different than sham (-9 vs -6.6, $P = .063$).[34] Device-related AEs include irritative urinary symptoms, with most resolving after removal of device. The reported serious AEs included AUR, UTI, and sepsis, occurring in greater than 5% of patients. There was no reported impact on sexual function. Four year follow-up showed sustained improvement in IPSS and QoL, but 11% underwent additional surgical treatment for LUTS.[35]

Prostate Artery Embolization

Prostate artery embolization (PAE) is a new option for minimally invasive treatment of BPH. Performed by experienced interventional radiologists (IRs), embolization causes ischemic necrosis and decreased prostate size to relieve urinary obstruction. First reported in 2000 for the treatment of refractory hematuria,[36] this procedure has evolved to treat AUR in poor surgical candidates, and is now more frequently used in healthy patients who wish to avoid transurethral procedures or GA.

PAE is predominantly done under intravenous sedation as an outpatient procedure using fluoroscopic guidance to identify and treat the prostatic artery branch of the internal iliac. Following embolization of the prostatic artery, patients are typically discharged on the same day with a urinary catheter for a few days while edema subsides. Variable anatomy, atherosclerosis, and vascular tortuosity make this procedure technically challenging, and PAE is not offered by all IR centers.

Following embolization, prostate volume can decrease to 25% to 40% with similar IPSS (−16.22) and QoL (−3) improvements as TURP after 1 year.[37] Retreatment was more likely in PAE (relative risk [RR] 3.30), with some reports showing up to 19% surgical retreatment within 1 year.[38] PAE does have a lower risk of major AEs (RR 0.75) including hematuria, AUR, and pelvic pain, as well as reduced risk of EjD (RR 0.51), while ED was the same between the two groups.[38] For catheter-dependent patients, PAE was able to achieve a 70% catheter-free rate.[39]

PAE has unique risks compared to other treatments. Specifically, risk of nontarget embolization (NTE) and postembolization syndrome (PES). NTE is rare, but can obstruct collateral arterial branches leading to ischemia of the bladder, rectum, penis, or other pelvic structures. Meanwhile, PES can cause significant pelvic pain, fever, body aches, nausea, and vomiting. These symptoms are generally able to be managed medically and subside within a few weeks posttreatment.

Overall, this therapy is very well tolerated and is a good addition to the treatment armamentarium for BPH, particularly in poor surgical candidates and patients with hematuria.

Aquablation

Aquablation (PROCEPT BioRobotics, Redwood City, CA) is another new BPH treatment with significant promise. This platform uses a robotic-guided high-pressure water jet to perform heat-free ablation of the prostatic adenoma. The patient's prostate anatomy is mapped in real time with transrectal ultrasound, marking the urethral sphincter, bladder neck, and prostate capsule to ablate tissue within those boundaries. Aquablation received FDA approval in 2018 based on the WATER trial, which treated prostates up to 80 g, and the subsequent WATER II trial supported the clinical efficacy in prostates up to 150 g. This treatment requires GA and usually includes overnight hospital observation.

The WATER trial found better IPSS reduction for Aquablation compared to TURP (−14.1 vs −10.8, $P = .02$) at 5 year follow-up,[40] supported by WATER II in larger prostates with a 15.8 point improvement after 5 years.[41] Durability was also better than TURP, with 5 year retreatment rates 1.6% for prostates more than 80 g[40] and 3.7% for prostates 80 to 150[41] and a 14% lower chance of medical retreatment compared to TURP. Notably, Aquablation demonstrated superior preservation of ejaculatory function, with lower rates of RE than TURP (6% vs 23.1%, $P = .0015$).[40] ED was not impacted by either treatment.

Early in the Aquablation experience, the "cautery-free" approach had considerable postoperative hemorrhage, with transfusion rates ranging up to 10%. However, adjustments to the technique, using focal bladder neck cautery decreased transfusion rates to less than 1% without increasing EjD.[42]

Aquablation has shown encouraging clinical results. The technology standardizes treatment using ultrasound guidance that facilitates more complete transitional zone tissue ablation (though not quite enucleation). Similarly, use of real-time ultrasound reduces the risk of capsular perforation, damage to the urethral sphincter or bladder neck. To its detriment, Aquablation is not currently widely accessible as it requires a dedicated single-function robotic platform. Nevertheless, this technology clearly demonstrates the opportunity for future robotic BPH treatment.

Optilume Benign Prostate Hyperplasia

The newest addition to the BPH MIST offerings is Optilume BPH (Laborie, Portsmouth, NH). FDA approved in July 2023, Optilume BPH is a transurethral catheter coated with paclitaxel for in-office dilation of the prostatic urethra in glands greater than 80 g. The balloon fractures the prostatic anterior commissure, opening a wider channel, and paclitaxel prevents refusion of the lobes, maintaining patency. The PINNACLE trial reported an 11.5 point IPSS improvement at 1 year, significantly better than sham (4.8 points improvement).[43] No difference in sexual function was seen; however, patients must abstain from sex or use condoms for 30 days to avoid exposure of paclitaxel to their partner. More data are needed to determine where this fits in the spectrum of BPH options.

Several other outpatient MISTs are coming down the pipeline, but still lacking meaningful clinical data.

SUMMARY

Treatment of BPH has made remarkable strides in the past decade with new surgical treatments and pharmacologic options to address patient-specific symptoms while minimizing side effects, especially sexual function. As the population of men who suffer from BPH continue to age, MISTs offer many advantages especially for older patients with significant morbidity precluding them from more invasive procedures. Patients should be counseled, while the degree of symptom improvement and durability of the procedure are variable based on patient characteristics, these techniques are less likely to relieve symptoms with the same impact or duration as a more invasive surgery. The aim of any surgical intervention is to capture men resistant or intolerant to medication before impending bladder dysfunction becomes irreversible.

Given the large prevalence of this disease and patient's interest in maximizing symptom relief while minimizing interruption of their day-to-day life, we expect that new BPH treatments will continue to be explored.

CLINICS CARE POINTS

- Patient preferences should be taken into account when selecting treatment for LUTS, including patient anatomy, severity of disease, as well as patient's interest in avoiding general anesthesia (GA) or maintaining ejaculatory function versus avoiding need for future retreatment.

- Medical therapy is effective for reducing LUTS and can help avoid surgery for BPH. Alpha blockers and 5-ARIs are a cornerstone of treatment, but β3-agonists can be safely used for men with overactive-predominant LUTS.

- Enucleation (either anatomic endoscopic enucleation of prostate or robotic simple prostatectomy) provides lowest retreatment rates and best chance of eliminating catheter-dependence.

- Multiple new minimally invasive surgical treatments (MISTs) are available with promising results for relieving LUTS with outpatient treatment, but some carry a higher retreatment rate than treatments in the operating room (OR).

- For patients highly interested in preserving antegrade ejaculation, MISTs, Aquablation, or prostate artery embolization (PAE) offer the lowest rates of ejaculatory dysfunction (EjD).

DISCLOSURE

T. Helman has no disclosures. B. Browne: Cook Medical educational consultant, aGUaRx scientific advisory board.

REFERENCES

1. Platz EA, Smit E, Curhan GC, et al. Prevalence of and racial/ethnic variation in lower urinary tract symptoms and noncancer prostate surgery in U.S. men. Urology (Ridgewood, N.J.) 2002;59(6):877–83.
2. Goldfischer E, Kowalczyk JJ, Clark WR, et al. Hemodynamic effects of once-daily tadalafil in men with signs and symptoms of benign prostatic hyperplasia on concomitant $\alpha 1$ -adrenergic antagonist therapy: results of a multicenter randomized, double-blind, placebo-controlled trial. Urology (Ridgewood, N.J.) 2012; 79(4):875–82.
3. Fawzi A, Kamel M, Salem E, et al. Sildenafil citrate in combination with tamsulosin versus tamsulosin monotherapy for management of male lower urinary tract symptoms due to benign prostatic hyperplasia: A randomised, double-blind, placebo-controlled trial. Arab Journal of Urology 2017;15(1):53–9.
4. Matsukawa Y, Takai S, Majima T, et al. Comparison in the efficacy of fesoterodine or mirabegron add-on therapy to silodosin for patients with benign prostatic hyperplasia complicated by overactive bladder: A randomized, prospective trial using urodynamic studies. Neurourol Urodyn 2019;38(3):941–9.
5. Sandhu JS, Bixler BR, Dahm P, et al. Management of lower urinary tract symptoms attributed to benign prostatic hyperplasia (BPH): AUA guideline amendment 2023. J Urol 2024;211(1):11–9.
6. Zheng YB, Shi L, Zhu XM, et al. Anticholinergic drugs and the risk of dementia: A systematic review and meta-analysis. Neurosci Biobehav Rev 2021;127:296–306.
7. Wymer KM, Narang G, Slade A, et al. Evaluation of the cost-effectiveness of surgical treatment options for benign prostatic hyperplasia. Urology 2023;171: 96–102.
8. Ottaiano N, Shelton T, Sanekommu G, et al. Surgical complications in the management of benign prostatic hyperplasia treatment. Curr Urol Rep 2022;23(5): 83–92.
9. Yip SK, Chan NH, Chiu P, et al. A randomized controlled trial comparing the efficacy of hybrid bipolar transurethral vaporization and resection of the prostate with bipolar transurethral resection of the prostate. J Endourol 2011;25(12): 1889–94.
10. Kabalin JN, Bite G, Doll S. Neodymium: YAG laser coagulation prostatectomy: 3 years of experience with 227 patients. J Urol 1996;155(1):181–5.
11. Bachmann A, Tubaro A, Barber N, et al. 180-W XPS greenlight laser vaporisation versus transurethral resection of the prostate for the treatment of benign prostatic obstruction: 6-month safety and efficacy results of a european multicentre randomised trial—The GOLIATH Study. Eur Urol 2014;65(5):931–42.
12. Kaplan S, Kaufman RP Jr, Mueller T, et al. Retreatment rates and postprocedural complications are higher than expected after BPH surgeries: a US healthcare claims and utilization study. Prostate Cancer Prostatic Dis 2023. https://doi.org/ 10.1038/s41391-023-00741-8.
13. Kronenberg P, Cerrato C, Juliebø-Jones P, et al. Advances in lasers for the minimally invasive treatment of upper and lower urinary tract conditions: a systematic review. World J Urol 2023;41(12):3817–27.

14. Fraundorfer MR, Gilling PJ. Holmium:YAG laser enucleation of the prostate combined with mechanical morcellation: preliminary results. Eur Urol 1998;33(1): 69–72.
15. Aho T, Armitage J, Kastner C. Anatomical endoscopic enucleation of the prostate: The next gold standard? Yes. Andrologia 2020;52(8):e13643.
16. Cornu JN, Ahyai S, Bachmann A, et al. A Systematic Review and Meta-analysis of Functional Outcomes and Complications Following Transurethral Procedures for Lower Urinary Tract Symptoms Resulting from Benign Prostatic Obstruction: An Update. Eur Urol 2015;67(6):1066–96.
17. Tan AH, Gilling PJ, Kennett KM, et al. A randomized trial comparing holmium laser enucleation of the prostate with transurethral resection of the prostate for the treatment of bladder outlet obstruction secondary to benign prostatic hyperplasia in large glands (40 to 200 grams). J Urol 2003;170(4 Pt 1):1270–4.
18. Lomas DJ, Krambeck AE. Long-term efficacy of holmium laser enucleation of the prostate in patients with detrusor underactivity or acontractility. Urology 2016;97: 208–11.
19. Guldibi F, Altunhan A, Aydın A, et al. What is the effect of laser anatomical endoscopic enucleation of the prostate on the ejaculatory functions? a systematic review. World J Urol 2023;41(12):3493–501.
20. Rivera M, Krambeck A, Lingeman J. Holmium Laser Enucleation of the Prostate in Patients Requiring Anticoagulation. Curr Urol Rep 2017;18(10):77.
21. Elmansy HM, Kotb A, Elhilali MM. Holmium laser enucleation of the prostate: long-term durability of clinical outcomes and complication rates during 10 years of followup. J Urol 2011;186(5):1972–6.
22. Humphreys MR, Miller NL, Handa SE, et al. Holmium laser enucleation of the prostate—outcomes independent of prostate size? J Urol 2008;180(6):2431–5.
23. Weinstein IC, Wu X, Arenas-Gallo C, et al. Adoption and outcomes of holmium laser enucleation of the prostate in the united states. Urology 2023;179:106–11.
24. Lee MS, Assmus MA, Ganesh M, et al. An outcomes comparison between holmium laser enucleation of the prostate, open simple prostatectomy, and robotic simple prostatectomy for large gland benign prostatic hypertrophy. Urology 2023; 173:180–6.
25. Wen Z, Deng XZ, Wang L, et al. Efficacy and safety of transurethral thulium laser enucleation versus robot-assisted prostatectomy for large-volume benign prostatic hyperplasia: a systematic review and meta-analysis. J Robot Surg 2023; 17(6):2633–46.
26. Abou Zeinab M, Kaviani A, Ferguson E, et al. Single-port transvesical versus open simple prostatectomy: a perioperative comparative study. Prostate Cancer Prostatic Dis 2023;26(3):538–42.
27. Palacios DA, Kaouk J, Abou Zeinab M, et al. Holmium laser enucleation of the prostate vs transvesical single-port robotic simple prostatectomy for large prostatic glands. Urology 2023;181:98–104.
28. Roehrborn CG, Barkin J, Gange SN, et al. Five year results of the prospective randomized controlled prostatic urethral L.I.F.T. study. Can J Urol 2017;24(3):8802.
29. Gratzke C, Barber N, Speakman MJ, et al. Prostatic urethral lift vs transurethral resection of the prostate: 2-year results of the BPH6 prospective, multicentre, randomized study. BJU Int 2017;119(5):767.
30. Dutta R, Matz EL, Deebel NA, et al. Persistent need for ongoing medical or surgical therapy despite UroLift: Data from an academic center. Can Urol Assoc J 2023;17(12):E408–11.

31. Rukstalis D, Grier D, Stroup SP, et al. Prostatic urethral lift (PUL) for obstructive median lobes: 12 month results of the MedLift Study. Prostate Cancer Prostatic Dis 2019;22(3):411–9.

32. Benidir T, Austhof E, Ward RD, et al. Impact of prostate urethral lift device on prostate magnetic resonance image quality. J Urol 2023;209(4):752–61.

33. McVary KT, Gittelman MC, Goldberg KA, et al. Final 5-year outcomes of the multi-center randomized sham-controlled trial of a water vapor thermal therapy for treatment of moderate to severe lower urinary tract symptoms secondary to benign prostatic hyperplasia. J Urol 2021;206(3):715–24.

34. Chughtai B, Elterman D, Shore N, et al. The itind temporarily implanted nitinol device for the treatment of lower urinary tract symptoms secondary to benign prostatic hyperplasia: a multicenter, randomized, controlled trial. Urology (Ridge-wood, N.J.) 2021;153:270–6.

35. Amparore D, De Cillis S, Schulman C, et al. Temporary implantable nitinol device for benign prostatic hyperplasia-related lower urinary tract symptoms: over 48-month results. Minerva Urology and Nephrology 2023;75(6):743.

36. DeMeritt JS, Elmasri FF, Esposito MP, et al. Relief of benign prostatic hyperplasia-related bladder outlet obstruction after transarterial polyvinyl alcohol prostate embolization. J Vasc Interv Radiol 2000;11(6):767–70.

37. Malling B, Røder MA, Brasso K, et al. Prostate artery embolisation for benign prostatic hyperplasia: a systematic review and meta-analysis. Eur Radiol 2019;29(1):287–98.

38. Jung JH, McCutcheon KA, Borofsky M, et al. Prostatic arterial embolization for the treatment of lower urinary tract symptoms in men with benign prostatic hyperplasia. Cochrane Database Syst Rev 2020;12(12):CD012867.

39. Kenny AG, Pellerin O, Amouyal G, et al. Prostate Artery Embolization in Patients With Acute Urinary Retention. Am J Med 2019;132(11):e786–90.

40. Oumedjbeur K, Corsi NJ, Bouhadana D, et al. Aquablation versus TURP: 5-year outcomes of the WATER randomized clinical trial for prostate volumes 50-80 mL. Can J Urol 2023;30(5):11650–8.

41. Bhojani N, Bidair M, Kramolowsky E, et al. Aquablation Therapy in Large Prostates (80-150 mL) for Lower Urinary Tract Symptoms Due to Benign Prostatic Hyperplasia: Final WATER II 5-Year Clinical Trial Results. J Urol 2023;210(1):143–53.

42. Elterman DS, Foller S, Ubrig B, et al. Focal bladder neck cautery associated with low rate of post-Aquablation bleeding. Can J Urol 2021;28(2):10610–3.

43. Kaplan SA, Moss J, Freedman S, et al. The PINNACLE Study: A Double-blind, Randomized, Sham-controlled Study Evaluating the Optilume BPH Catheter System for the Treatment of Lower Urinary Tract Symptoms Secondary to Benign Prostatic Hyperplasia. J Urol 2023;210(3):500–9.

Moving?

Make sure your subscription moves with you!

To notify us of your new address, find your **Clinics Account Number** (located on your mailing label above your name), and contact customer service at:

Email: journalscustomerservice-usa@elsevier.com

800-654-2452 (subscribers in the U.S. & Canada)
314-447-8871 (subscribers outside of the U.S. & Canada)

Fax number: 314-447-8029

Elsevier Health Sciences Division
Subscription Customer Service
3251 Riverport Lane
Maryland Heights, MO 63043

Printed and bound by CPI Group (UK) Ltd, Croydon, CR0 4YY

08/05/2025

01864752-0001